OCULAR

SYNDROMES

OCULAR SYNDROMES

WALTER J. GEERAETS, M.D.

Professor of Ophthalmology, Department of Ophthalmology

Associate Professor, Department of Biophysics

Medical College of Virginia
(Health Sciences Division)
Virginia Commonwealth University
Richmond, Virginia

SECOND EDITION

LEA & FEBIGER · *Philadelphia, 1969*

To my teacher

Professor Dr. H. Burkle De La Camp

Preface

Encouraged by many readers of 'Ocular Syndromes' and by their stimulating remarks, several additions have been made in this second edition.

The number of syndromes covered has been expanded from the original 138 to 197 and includes those more recently described in the literature. Also the information given on each syndrome has been extended. References for further reading have been added and the original publication of the author(s) whose name(s) the syndrome bears is given. The 'Cross Reference of Syndromes based on Ocular Manifestations' also includes now the most outstanding systemic findings. Syndromes presenting similar features have been grouped and tabulated for easier comparison. Finally, a glossary has been added for the readers not familiar with ophthalmological terminology.

Some diseases, not truly belonging under the heading and definition of the term 'syndrome' have been included, since they are found occasionally referred to as such in the literature. This, however, will probably add rather than detract from the versatility of the book.

It is hoped that this second edition will serve the purpose of making these syndromes more easily recognizable in the constant strife for a more accurate diagnosis.

Richmond, Virginia   WALTER J. GEERAETS

Preface to the First Edition

This tabulated and cross indexed presentation of syndromes associated with ocular manifestations in alphabetical order and of pocket size offers a quick reference for daily clinical use. It should make the recognition of the many signs and symptoms which form a syndrome easier and as such it should also help in student and resident teaching.

Terse and succinct wording has been used by necessity to ensure this goal but no claim is made of complete and detailed coverage of this topic for which references are given.

Richmond, Virginia   WALTER J. GEERAETS

Contents

NOTICE

Names of syndromes carrying the presyllable "von" or "van" are listed under V in the tabulated part of this book. In the "cross indices" they are listed under the authors' names, disregarding the presyllable, thus insuring adequate coverage (i.e., von Hippel-Lindau is quoted in the tabulated part under "V", but in the cross indices under "H").

Quick Cross Reference
of Syndromes and
Their Synonyms

(in alphabetical order)

Abducens-facial hemiplegia alternans (*see* Millard-Gubler syndrome)

A-β-Lipoproteinemia (*see* Bassen-Kornzweig syndrome)

Acrocephalosyndactylism syndrome (*see* Apert syndrome)

Acrodynia (*see* Feer syndrome)

Acustic neuroma (*see* Cushing (2) syndrome)

Acute infectious neuritis (*see* Guillain-Barré syndrome)

Acute polyradiculitis (*see* Guillain-Barré syndrome)

Addison's disease—Moniliasis—idiopathic hypoparathyroidism (keratoconjunctivitis, cataracts, blepharitis—moniliasis, tetany, skin pigmentation, weakness)

Adherence syndrome (*see* Johnson syndrome)

Adherent lateral rectus syndrome (*see* Johnson syndrome)

Adie (myotonia,—absence of ankle or knee jerk)

Adrenocortical neuroblastoma with orbital metastasis (*see* Hutchinson syndrome)

Adrenocortical syndrome (*see* Cushing (1) syndrome)

Albright (unilateral proptosis, optic nerve involvement,—osteitis fibrosa, skin pigmentations, endorcine dysfunction)

Alport (lens changes, fundus albi punctatus—hemorrhagic nephritis, deafness)

Alternating oculomotor paralysis (*see* Weber syndrome)

Amalric-Dialinas (*see* Dialinas-Amalric syndrome)

Amaurosis fugas syndrome (blindness, retinal arteriolar spasm,—hypertension)

Angelucci (conjunctivitis,—tachycardia, excitability, labile vasomotor system)

Angiokeratoma corporis diffusum syndrome (*see* Fabry-Anderson syndrome)

Angiomatosis retinae (*see:* von Hippel-Lindau syndrome)

Angel tumor syndrome (*see* Cushing (2) syndrome)

Anomalous leukocytic inclusions with constitutional stigamta (*see* Chediak-Higashi syndrome)

Anton (blindness, denial of blindness,—confabulation, allochiria)

Anterior-segment traumatic syndrome (*see* Frenkel syndrome)

Aortic arch syndrome (*see* Takayasu syndrome)

Apert (cranial deformities, loss of vision, ophthalmoplegia,—syndactyly)

Aphasia-agnosia-apraxia syndrome (*see* Arnold Pick syndrome)

Aplasia axialis extracorticalis congenita (*see* Pelizaeus-Merzbacher syndrome)

Arachnodactyly (*see* Marfan syndrome)

Argyll Robertson (loss of pupillary reflex,—involvement of the CNS)

Arnold-Chiari (visual field defect, nystagmus,—pyramidal tract signs, vertebral malformations)

Arnold Pick (apperceptive blindness,—progressive dementia, cerebral atrophy)

Ascher (lack of tone of orbital fascia, blepharochalasis, protrusion of lacrimal gland—goiter, reduplication upper lip)

Ataxia-telangiectasia syndrome (*see* Louis-Bar syndrome)

Avelli (*see* Cestan-Chenais syndrome)

Axenfeld-Schürenberg (congenital cyclic oculomotor paralysis)

Axenfeld (glaucoma, posterior embryotoxon, ring-shaped corneal opacity)

Baader's dermatostomatitis (*see* Stevens-Johnson syndrome)

Babinski-Nageotte (Horner syndrome, nystagmus,—cerebellar hemiataxia, hemiparesis)

Balint (optic ataxia, disturbance of visual fixation,—loss of body coordination)

Bardet-Biedl (*see* Laurence-Moon-Bardet-Biedl syndrome)

Barnard-Scholz (*see* Ophthalmoplegic-retinal degeneration)

Barré-Liéou (corneal hypesthesia, reduced vision—headache, dizziness, ear noises, neck pain)

Basal-frontal syndrome (*see* Foster Kennedy syndrome)

Bassen-Kornzweig (retinitis pigmentosa-steatorrhea, acanthocytosis, neuropathy)

Batten-Mayou (retinal pigment disturbance, optic atrophy,—amaurotic idiocy, convulsions)

Behcet (iritis, keratitis, uveitis,—ulcerations of mucous membranes, skin lesions)

Behr (heredofamilial optic atrophy,—abortive hereditary ataxia, mental deficiency)

Benedikt (oculomotor paralysis,—contralateral hemichorea)

Bernard-Horner (*see* Horner syndrome)

Besnier-Boeck-Schaumann (*see* Schaumann syndrome)

Bielschowsky-Lutz-Cogan (paralysis int. rectus muscle, contralateral nystagmus on lateral gaze)

Bing (ptosis, paralysis extraocular muscles, glaucoma, chorioretinitis)

Blepharochalasis with struma and double lip (*see* Ascher syndrome)

Bloch-Sulzberger (retinal pseudoglioma, optic nerve involvement, nystagmus,—bullous skin eruptions and pigmentations)

Boeck's sarcoid (*see* Schaumann syndrome)

Bogorad (unilateral lacrimation,—excessive salivation)

Bonnet-Dechaume-Blanc (arteriovenous retinal angiomas,—angiomas of mesencephalon and thalamus)

Bonnevie-Ullrich (congenital cataracts—pterygeal folds of neck, hyperelastic skin, edema neck and extremities, hypertrichosis)

Bourneville (retinal tumor,—adenoma sebaceum, epilepsy, mental deficiency)

Brailsford-Morquio (*see* Morquio-Brailsford syndrome)

Carotid artery-cavernous sinus fistula syndrome (exophthalmos, secondary glaucoma, papilledema, retinopathy,—unilateral headache, subjective buzzing intracranial noise)

Cartilagenous-arthritic-ophthalmic-deafness syndrome (uveitis,—deafness, rheumatic arthritis, joint dislocations)

Cat-scratch-oculoglandular (Parinaud oculoglandular)

Cavernous sinus syndrome (*see* Foix syndrome)

Central nervous system deficiency syndrome (visual loss, bitemporal optic atrophy,—deafness, tinnitus, unsteady gait, tingling in legs)

Cephalo-oculo-cutaneous telangiectasis (*see* Louis-Bar syndrome)

Cerebellar peduncle syndrome (*see* Weber syndrome)

Cerebellomedullary malformation (*see* Arnold-Chiari syndrome)

Cerebellopontine angle syndrome (*see* Cushing (2) syndrome)

Cerebroretinal arteriovenous aneurysm syndrome (*see* Bonnet-Dechaume-Blanc syndrome)

Cerebroretinal degeneration (*see* Batten-Mayou syndrome)

Cervical sympathetic paralysis syndrome (*see* Horner syndrome)

Cestan (1) (*see* Cestan-Chenais syndrome)

Cestan (2) (*see* Raymond syndrome)

Cestan-Chenais (Horner syndrome, nystagmus,—flaccid paralysis of soft palate and vocal cord, contralateral hemiplegia, ataxia)

Charcot-Marie-Tooth (nystagmus, optic atrophy,—progressive muscular atrophy)

Charcot-Wilbrand (visual agnosia, loss of ability to revisualize images)

Charlin (inflammation anterior segment of the eye, orbital pain,—rhinorrhea)

Chauffard-Still (*see* Felty syndrome)

4

Chediak-Higashi (decreased iris pigmentation, corneal edema, elevated disc—hepatosplenomegaly, recurrent infections)

Chiasmal syndrome (*see* Cushing (3) syndrome)

Chondroectodermal dysplasia (*see* Ellis-van Crefeld syndrome)

Chondro-osteo-dystrophy (*see* Hurler syndrome)

Chronic renal tubular insufficiency syndrome (*see* pseudohypoparathyroidism syndrome)

Claude (III and IV nerve paralysis,—contralateral hemianesthesia and hemiataxia)

Claude Bernard-Horner syndrome (*see* Horner syndrome)

Cockayne (retinal pigmentary degeneration, optic atrophy,—dwarfism, deafness, mental retardation)

Cogan (interstitial keratitis,—vestibuloauditory symptoms)

Cole-Rauschkolb-Toomey (*see* Zinsser-Engman-Cole syndrome)

Cone dysfunction (macular degeneration, field defects, decreased visual acuity)

Congenital brevicollis (*see* Klippel-Feil syndrome)

Congenital encephalo-Ophthalmic dysplasia (*see* Krause syndrome)

Congenital epiblepharon-inferior oblique insufficiency syndrome (narrow interpupillary distance, epicanthus, inferior oblique insufficiency, keratitis,—chubby cheeks)

Congenital facial diplopia (*see* Moebius syndrome)

Congenital familial dysautonomia (*see* Riley-Day syndrome)

Congenital muscular hypertrophy-cerebral (*see* de Lange syndrome)

Congenital oculofacial paralysis (*see* Moebius syndrome)

Congenital paralysis of 6th and 7th nerves (*see* Moebius syndrome)

Congenital poikiloderma with juvenile cataract (*see* Rothmund syndrome)

Congenital rubella syndrome (*see* Rubella syndrome)

Congenital spinocerebellar ataxia-cataract-oligophrenia syndrome (*see* Marinesco-Sjögren syndrome)

Conjunctivo-urethro-synovial (*see* Reiter syndrome)

Cranial arteritis (*see* Temporal-arteritis syndrome)

Craniofacial dysostosis (*see* Crouzon syndrome)

Crocodile tear (*see* Bogorad syndrome)

Crouzon (exophthalmos, strabismus, papilledema,—prognathism, maxilla atrophy, deformity anterior fontanel)

Cushing (1) (ocular muscle palsies, visual field changes, optic atrophy—obesity, hirsutism, skin pigmentation, osteo porosis)

Cushing (2) (paralysis V-VIII, decreased corneal sensitivity,—tinnitus, deafness, defect in labyrinthine function)

Cushing (3) (progressive bitemporal hemianopsia, optic atrophy)

Cutis hyperelastica (*see* Ehlers-Danlos syndrome)

Dacryosialoadenopathy (*see* Mikulicz-Radecki syndrome)

Dandy-Walker (ptosis, paralysis VI nerve, papilledema,—hydrocephalus)

Deaf-mutism-retinal degeneration syndrome (*see* Dialinas-Amalric syndrome)

Degos (atrophic skin of eye lids, diplopia, choroidal changes—skin lesions, gastro-intestinal involvement)

de Lange (antimongoloid slant palpebral fissures, myopia anisocoria, pale discs—mental retardation, multiple skeletal abnormalities)

Dejean (exophthalmia, diplopia,—superior maxillary pain, numbness V 1 & 2)

Déjerine-Klumpke (Horner syndrome,—paralysis and atrophy of small muscles of upper extremities)

Déjerine-Roussy (hemianopsia,—transient hemiplegia, hemiataxia, choreoathetotic movements)

Denial-visual hallucination syndrome (*see* Anton syndrome)
Dermatostomatitis (*see* Stevens-Johnson syndrome)
Dermatostomatoophthalmic syndrome (*see* Behcet syndrome)
Devic (optic neuritis,—ascending myelitis)
Dialinas-Amalric (retinal pigmentary anomalies—deaf-mutism)
Diffuse angiokeratosis (*see* Fabry-Anderson syndrome)
Dissociation of lateral gaze syndrome (*see* Raymond syndrome)
Dolichostenomelia (Marfan syndrome)
Dorsolateral medullary syndrome (*see* Wallenberg syndrome)
Double Whammy syndrome (voluntary propulsion of eyes)
Down (hypertelorism, slanted eyelid fissures, myopia, iris spots, lens opacities—mental retardation, skeletal and heart anomalies)
D—Trisomy Syndrome (*see* Trisomy D syndrome)
Duane (primary global retraction, narrowing palpebral fissure)
Dyscephalic-mandibulo-oculo-facial syndrome (*see* Hallermann-Streiff syndrome)
Dysgenesis mesodermalis corneae et irides (*see* Riegers syndrome)
Dysgenesis mesostromalis (*see* Riegers syndrome)
Dyskeratosis congenita with pigmentation (*see* Zinsser-Engman-Cole syndrome)
Dysostosis cranio-facialis (*see* Crouzon syndrome)
Dysostosis multiplex (*see* Hurler syndrome)
Dystrophia adiposogenitalis (*see* Fröhlich syndrome)
Dystrophia mesodermalis congenita (*see* Marfan syndrome)
Dwarfism with retinal atrophy and deafness (*see* Cockayne syndrome)

E—Syndrome (*see* Trisomy—18 syndrome)
Eaton-Lambert (ocular myoclonus, decreased vision, corneal haze—weakness, fatigue, peripheral paresthesia)
Ehlers-Danlos (Hyperelasticity of palpebral skin, ptosis, epicanthus, hypotony extraocular muscles, increased intraocular pressure, thin sclera and cornea, keratoconus, subluxated lens, retinopathy—cutaneous hyperelasticity, atrophic skin, excessive articular laxity)
Ekman (*see* van der Hoeve syndrome)
Elastorrhexis (*see* Groenblad-Strandberg syndrome)
Ellis—van Crefeld (congenital cataract, strabismus—talipes, polydactyly(sceletal anomalies, heart defects, mental deficiency)
Embryonic fixation syndrome (*see* Waardenburg syndrome)
Empty-sella (decerased vision, optic atrophy, visual field defects—acromegalic features)
Encephalitis hemorrhagica superioris (*see* Wernicke syndrome)
Encephalitis periaxialis diffusa (*see* Schilder syndrome)
Encephalofacial angiomatosis (*see* Sturge-Weber syndrome)
Encephalo-ophthalmic syndrome (*see* Krause syndrome)
Epidermolysis bullosa (*see* Goldscheider syndrome)
Epiloia syndrome (*see* Bourneville syndrome)
Erb-Goldflam (ptosis, strabismus—general muscle weakness)
Erythema multiforme exudativum (*see* Stevens-Johnson syndrome)
Espildora-Luque (ophthalmic artery emboly—contralateral temporary hemiplegia)
Essential lipoid histiocytosis (*see* Niemann-Pick syndrome)
Eyelid-malar-mandible syndrome (*see* Franceschetti syndrome)

Fabry-Anderson (conjunctival varicosis, corneal opacities, swelling of eye lids—angiokeratosis of skin, disturbed sweat secretion, pain in limbs)
Familial amaurotic idiocy (*see* Tay-Sachs syndrome)

Familial hemolytic icterus (*see* Gänsseln syndrome)
Familial myoclonia syndrome (*see* Unverrichts syndrome)
Familial-osteodystrophy (*see* Morquio-Brailsford syndrome)
Feer (conjunctival injection, pronounced photophobia,—muscle hypotony, irritability, profuse sweating, skin exfoliation palms and soles)
Felty (scleromalacia—rheumatic arthrities, splenomegaly, oral lesions, leukopenia)
Fibrodysplasia elastica generalisata (*see* Ehlers-Danlos syndrome)
Fiessinger-leroy (*see* Reiter syndrome)
Fisher (external and internal ophthalmoplegia,—ataxia, loss of deep reflexes)
Foix (paralysis III, IV, VI and ophthalmic branch V, proptosis, lid and conjunctival edema,—external jugular vein less distended on affected side, postauricular edema)
Foster Kennedy (homolateral optic atrophy, contralateral papilledema,—anosmia (frontal lobe tumor)
Foville (paralysis VI, nystagmus,—peripheral facial palsy, contralateral hemiplegia)
Foville's peduncular syndrome (*see* Foville syndrome)
Frankl Hochwart (choked disc, concentric field constriction, limited upward gaze,—hypopituitarism, ataxia, bilateral deafness)
Franceschetti (lid coloboma, oblique lid fissure with lateral downward slope,—fish-like face, high palate, abnormal dentation)
Frenkel (retinal pigment disturbance, traumatic involvement of anterior eye segment)
Fröhlich (impaired scotopic vision, optic atrophy, bitemporal hemianopsia,—adiposity, genital hypoplasia, a.o.)
Fuchs (1) (unilateral heterochromia irides, cyclitis, secondary cataract)
Fuchs (2) (severe conjunctivitis,—mucosa ulcers, swelling of face, fever, cyanosis)
Fuch's sign (*see* Pseudo Graefe syndrome)
Fuller Albright (*see* Albright syndrome)
Funds albipunctatus with hemeralopia and xerosis (*see* Uyemura syndrome)

Gänsslen (microphthalmia, epicanthus, increased PD-splenomegaly, hemolytic crises, polydactyly, a.o.)
Gargoylism (*see* Hurler syndrome)
Gaucher (macular infiltration, pinguecula of brown-yellowish color, strabismus—hypertonia, opisthotonus, dysphagia, cachexia (infantile form); hepatosplenomegaly, lymphadenopathy, skin pigmentations (chronic form))
Geniculate neuralgia (*see* Hunt syndrome)
Genital dwarfism (*see* Turner syndrome)
Giant cell arteritis (*see* Temporal arteritis syndrome)
Glaucomatocyclitic crisis (*see* Posner-Schlossman syndrome)
Glosso-pharyngo-labial syndrome (*see* Bing syndrome)
Glucocerebroside storage disease (*see* Gaucher syndrome)
Goldenhar (epibulbar dermoids, colobomata—sceletal deformities, preauricular fistulas)
Goldscheider (conjunctival shrinkage, keratitis—skin lesions, growth and mental retardation)
Gonadal dysgenesis (*see* Turner syndrome)
Gorlin-Chaudhry-Moss (lid defect, nystagmus, astigmatism—craniofacial dysostosis)
Gorlin-Goltz (cataract, glaucoma, prominent supraorbital ridges—multiple basal cell nevi, rib anomalies, cysts in jaws, medulloblastoma)
Gougerot-Sjögren (*see* Sjögren syndrome)
Gowers-Paton-Kennedy (*see* Foster Kennedy syndrome)

Gradenigro (ipsilateral paralysis VI, homolateral spasm internal rectus, photophobia, lacrimation—inner ear infection, mastoidities)

Graefe, von (*see* Moebius syndrome)

Greig (wide spacing of orbits, enophthalmos, epicanthus, paralysis VI, astigmatism —mental deficiency, skull deformation)

Groenblad-Strandberg (angioid streaks, macular degeneration—pseudoxanthoma elasticum)

Guillain-Barré (possible external ophthalmoplegia, facial nerve paralysis with exposure keratitis,—polyneuritis, absent tendon reflexes)

Gynecomastia-aspermatogenesis syndrome (*see* Klinefelter syndrome)

Hallermann-Streiff (microphthalmia, nystagmus, strabismus, cataract—malformation of skull, facial skeleton, joints, dental defects)

Hallgren (retinitis pigmentosa, optic atrophy, cataract, nightblindness, blindness, nystagmus—deafness, ataxia, mental deficiency)

Hand-Schüller-Christian (exophthalmos, xanthomatous tumors, blepharitis, retinal Hemorrhages exudates,—skin xanthomatosis, diabetes insipidus, skull defects)

Harada (*see* Vogt-Koyanagi-Harada syndrome)

Hare (*see* Pancoast syndrome)

Heefordt (bilateral granulomatous uveitis,—swelling parotid gland, lymphadenopathy)

Heidenhain (cortical blindness,—presenile dementia, ataxia, rigidity)

Hematologic—metabolic bone disorder (*see* Gänsslen syndrome)

Hemifacial Microsomia (microphthalmos, colobomata—facial sceletal deformities, hemifacial muscle hypoplasia)

Hemorrhagic polioencephalitis superior (*see* Wernicke syndrome)

Hennebert (nystagmus,—vertigo)

Heparitinuria (*see* Sanfillipo-Good syndrome)

Hepatolenticular degeneration (*see* Wilson syndrome)

Hereditary benign intraepithelial dyskeratosis (*see* von Sallmann-Paton-Witkop syndrome)

Hereditary familial congenital hemorrhagic nephritis (*see* Alport syndrome)

Hereditary retinitis pigmentosa—deafness syndrome (*see* Usher syndrome)

Heredopathia atactica polyneuritiformis syndrome (*see* Refsum syndrome)

Herpes zoster auricularis (*see* Hunt syndrome)

Herrenschwand, von (enophthalmos, ptosis, miosis, heterochromia,—decreased sweating ipsilateral side of face)

Herrick (retinopathy, vitreous hemorrhages, scleral icterus, telangiectasis of conjunctival vessels—severe anemia, joint pain, hepatosplenomegaly, cardiomegaly)

Heterochromic cyclitis syndrome (*see* Fuchs (1) syndrome)

Hippel-Lindau, von (secondary glaucoma, retinal angiomatosis, vitreous hemorrhages—cerebral angiomatosis, epilepsy, psychic disturbances)

Histamine cephalalgia (*see* Raeders syndrome)

Hoeve, van der—Halbertsma—Waardenburg (*see* Waardenburg syndrome)

Hoeve, van der (blue sclerae, keratoconus—brittle bones, deafness, ligaments hyperflexible)

Holmes-Adie (*see* Adie syndrome)

Homocystinuria (dislocated lens—mental retardation, sparseness of hair)

Horner (enophthalmos, ptosis, miosis—anhidrosis, facial hemiatrophy)

Horton's headache (see Raeder syndrome)

Hunt (absent corneal reflex, decreased lacrimation—ear involvement, facial palsy, decreased salivation)

Hunter (MPS II) (retinal pigmentary degeneration—mild gargoylike features, hepatosplenomegaly)

Hurler (MPS I) (milky corneae, thick lids, internal strabismus—retarded normal development, dorso lumbar kyphosis, head deformities, a.o.)
Hutchinson (exophtalmos, lid hematoma, extraocular muscle palsy, optic nerve path.—anemia, abdominal tumor)
Hyperchondroplasia (see Marfan syndrome)
Hyperostosis frontalis interna syndrome (*see* Morgagni syndrome)
Hypertelorism (*see* Greig syndrome)
Hypertensive diencephalic (*see* Page syndrome)
Hypophyseal-sphenoidal syndrome (*see* Foix syndrome)
Hypothalamique-carrefour (visual loss—hypertension, hemianesthesia, apraxia)

Idiopathic fibroedema (*see* Melkersson-Rosenthal syndrome)
Incontinentia pigmenti (*see* Bloch-Sulzberger syndrome)
Infantile acrodynia (*see* Feer syndrome)
Inferior nucleus ruber syndrome (*see* Claude syndrome)
Internuclear ophthalmoplegia (*see* Bielschowsky-Lutz-Cogan syndrome)
Interoculo-irido-dermato-auditive dysplasia (*see* Waardenburg syndrome)
Intracranial exostosis (*see* Morgagni syndrome)
Inverse jaw-winking syndrome (*see* Marcus Gunn syndrome)
Inverted Marfan syndrome (*see* Marchesani syndrome)
Iridoplegia interna (*see* Adie syndrome)

Jacod (ophthalmoplegia, optic atrophy,—trigeminal neuralgia, cervical lymphadenopathy)
Jadassohn-Lewandowski (corneal dystrophy—keratosis and hyperhidrosis of palms and soles, pachyonychia, bullous skin lesions)
Jahnke (*see* Sturge-Weber syndrome)
Jaw winking syndrome (*see* Marcus Gunn syndrome)
Johnson (pseudoparalysis of lateral or superior rectus muscles)
Juvenile amaurotic family idiocy (*see* Batten-Mayou syndrome)

Kearns-Sayre (*see* Ophthalmoplegia-retinal degeneration syndrome)
Keratosulfatoria (*see* Morquio-Brailsford syndrome)
Klinefelter (reduced incident of color blindness in male-small testes, sterility, gynecomastia, mild mental retardation)
Klippel-Feil (squint—platybasia, brevicollis)
Kloepfer (blindness,—blistering in sunlight, stagnation in growth, imbecility)
Klüver-Bucy (psychic blindness—changes in emotional behavior, deficiency of memory)
Klumpke (*see* Déjerine-Klumpke syndrome)
Koerber-Salus-Elschnig (lid retraction,—nystagmus, ocular muscle paresesheadaches, ataxia, positive Babinski)
Krause (microphthalmos, blindness, glaucoma, cataract, retinal dysplasia—hydrocephalus or mirocephaly, mental retardation, heterotopia)

Landry's paralysis (*see* Guillain-Barré syndrome)
Lannois-Gradenigro (*see* Gradenigro syndrome)
Lateral bulbar syndrome (*see* Wallenberg syndrome)
Laurence-Moon-Bardet-Biedl (nystagmus, strabisums, visual loss, scotoma, fundus pathology,—obesity, hypogenitalism, polydactyly, mental deficinecy)
Lawford (*see* Sturge-Weber syndrome)
Leber (bilateral optic atrophy,—vertigo, headaches)

9

Lenoble-Aubineau (nystagmus,—head and limb tremor, myoclonia)
Lipoid granuloma (*see* Hand-Schüller-Christian syndrome)
Lobstein (*see* van der Hoeve syndrome)
Louis-Bar (pseudoophthalmoplegia, conjunctival telangiectasia—cerebellar ataxia, telangiectasis of skin, scanning speech)
Lowe (nystagmus, glaucoma, anterior segment anomalies,—mental retardation, acidosis, osteomalacia)
Lower radicular syndrome (*see* Déjerine-Klumpke syndrome)
Luetic-otitic-nystagmus syndrome (*see* Hennebert syndrome)

Macroglobulinemia syndrome (*see* Waldenström syndrome)
Malignant atrophic papulosis (*see* Degos syndrome)
Mandibulo-facial dysostosis (*see* Franceschetti syndrome)
Mandibulofacial syndrome (*see* Franceschetti syndrome)
Marchesani (myopia, glaucoma, ectopia lentis,—brachydactyly, reduced growth)
Markus (*see* Adie's syndrome)
Marcus Gunn (ptosis, but elevation with movement of the mandible)
Marfan (myopia, ectopia lentis, coloboma,—arachnodactyly, congenital heart defects, relaxed ligaments)
Marinesco-Sjögren (Aniridia, cataracts,—cerebellar ataxia, oligophrenia)
Matorell (*see* Takayasu syndrome)
Mayou-Batten (see Batten-Mayou syndrome)
McCune-Albright (*see* Albright syndrome)
Medullary tegmental paralysis (*see* Babinski -Nageotte syndrome)
Melanophoric nevus syndrome (*see* Naegeli syndrome)
Melkersson-Rosenthal (ectropion lower lid, exposure keratitis—chron. face edema, facial palsy, furrowed tongue)
Ménière (nystagmus,—vertigo, tinnitus, progressive deafness)
Meningocutaneous syndrome (*see* Sturge-Weber syndrome)
Metabolic craniopathy (*see* Morgagni syndrome)
Meyer-Schwickerath-Weyers(microphthalmia, iris anomalies, glaucoma—syndactyly, polydactyly, developmental anomalies of nose and oral cavity)
Micrognathia-glossoptosis syndrome (*see* Pierre Robin syndrome)
Microphthalmos syndrome (*see* Meyer-Schwickerath-Weyers syndrome)
Miescher's cheilitis garnulomatosis (*see* Melkersson-Rosenthal syndrome)
Mikulicz (*see* Mikulicz-Radecki syndrome)
Mikulicz-Radecki (enlargement of lacrimal glands,—enlargement of salivary glands)
Mikulicz-Sjögren (*see* Mikulicz- Radecki syndrome)
Millard-Gubler (diplopia, paralysis V_1,—hemiplegia of arm and leg)
Mille (*see* Sturge-Weber syndrome)
Moebius (ptosis, proptosis, weakness of adductor muscles—facial diplegia, deafness, digital defects)
Mongolism (*see* Down syndrome)
Mongoloid idiocy (*see* Down syndrome)
Morgagni (optic atrophy, hyperostosis frontalis interna)
Morquio-Brailsford (MPS IV) (hazy cornea—sceletal deformities, dwarfism)
MPS I (*see* Hurler syndrome)
MPS II (*see* Hunter syndrome)
MPS III (*see* Sanfillipo-Good syndrome)
MPS IV (*see* Morquio-Brailsford syndrome)
MPS V (*see* Scheie syndrome)
Mucocutaneous ocular syndrome (*see* Fuchs (2) syndrome)

Mucosal-respiratory syndrome (*see* Stevens-Johnson syndrome)
Multiple basal cell nevi syndrome (*see* Gorlin-Goltz syndrome)
Myasthenia gravis (*see* Erb-Goldflam syndrome)
Myasthenic syndrome (*see* Eaton-Lambert syndrome)
Myoclonic syndrome (*see* Eaton-Lambert syndrome)
Myotonic pupil (*see* Adie syndrome)

Naegeli (nystagmus, papillitis, retinal pseudoglioma,—keratosis, pigmentary skin changes)
Naffziger (ptosis, small pupil,—reduced hand grip)
Nasal nerve syndrome (*see* Charlin syndrome)
Nasociliaris nerve syndrome (*see* Charlin syndrome)
Negri-Jacod (*see* Jacod syndrome)
Neurinomatosis (*see* von Recklinghausen syndrome)
Neurofibromatosis (*see* von Recklinghausen syndrome)
Neuromyelitis optica (*see* Devic syndrome)
Neuroretinoangiomatosis syndrome (*see* Bonnet-Dechaume-Blanc syndrome)
Niemann-Pick (reduced vision, retinopathy—mental retardation, hepatosplenomegally, seizures, skin pigmentation)
Nonsyphilitic interstitial keratitis (*see* Cogan syndrome)
Noonan (hypertelorism, ptosis, slanting palpebral fissure—pulmonary stenosis, webbed neck, short stature, cubitus valgus, micrognathia, mental retardation)
Nothnagel oculomotor paresis,—cerebellar ataxia)
Nystagmus-myoclonia syndrome (*see* Lenoble-Aubineau syndrome)
Nystagmus retractorius syndrome (*see* Koerber-Salus-Elschnig syndrome)

Ocular contusion syndrome (*see* Frenkel syndrome)
Ocular hypertelorism syndrome (*see* Greig syndrome)
Ocular myoclonus syndrome (*see* Eaton-Lambert syndrome)
Oculoauriculovertebral dysplasia (*see* Goldenhar syndrome)
Oculobuccogenital syndrome (*see* Behcet syndrome)
Oculocerebellar-tegmental (paralysis of associated ocular movements,—hemiplegia)
Oculodentodigital dysplasia (*see* Meyer-Schwickerath-Weyers syndrome)
Oculomandibulodyscephaly (*see* Hallerman-Streiff syndrome)
Oculo-oro-genital syndrome (Keratoconjunctivities, optic atrophy,—stomatitis, scrotal dermatitis, pharyngeal erythema)
Oligophrenia-ichthyosis-spastic diplegia syndrome (*see* Sjögren-Larsson syndrome)
Ophthalmic-sylvian syndrome (*see* Espildora-Luque syndrome)
Ophthalmoencephalomyelopathy (*see* Devic syndrome)
Ophthalmoplegia-ataxia-areflexia syndrome (*see* Fisher syndrome)
Ophthalmoplegia-cerebellar ataxia syndrome (*see* Nothnagel syndrome)
Ophthalmoplegic-migraine syndrome (supra-orbital pain, oculomotor paralysis,—migraine headaches possible)
Ophthalmoplegic-retinal degeneration syndrome (retinitis pigmentosa, ocular myopathy—possible sceletal muscle involvement)
Optical myelitis (*see* Devic syndrome)
Optic atrophy-ataxia syndrome (*see* Behr syndrome)
Optic neuromyelitis (*see* Devic syndrome)
Orbital apex-sphenoidal syndrome (*see* Rollet syndrome)
Orbital floor syndrome (*see* Déjean syndrome)
Osteitis fibrosa disseminata (*see* Albright syndrome)
Osteodystrophia fibrosa (*see* Albright syndrome)
Osteogenesis imperfecta (*see* Hoeve, van der, syndrome)

Otitic hydrocephalus syndrome (*see* Symond syndrome)
Otomandibular dysostosis (*see* Hemifacial Microsomia)
Oxycephaly (*see* Crouzon syndrome)

Pachyonychia congenita (*see* Jadassohn-Lewandowski syndrome)
Page (lacrimation,—hypertension, hot flashes, tachycardia)
Pancoast (enophthalmos, ptosis, miosis,—shoulder pain, paresthesia arm and hand)
Painful ophthalmoplegia (*see* Tolosa-Hunt syndrome)
Paralysis agitans (*see* Parkinson syndrome)
Paratrigeminal paralysis (*see* Raeder syndrome)
Parinaud (papilledema, displaced pupils, diplopia, a.o.—vertigo)
Parinaud's oculoglandular syndrome (conjunctivitis,—preauricular and cervical adenopathy, fever)
Parkinson (blepharospasm, nystagmus, convergence paresis, pupillary disorders,—loss of facial expression, "cog wheel" rigidity, tremor)
Parry-Romberg (*see* Romberg syndrome)
Patau (*see* Trisomy-D1 syndrome)
Pelizaeus-Merzbacher (nystagmus, visual impairment, retinopathy, optpic nerve involvement retarded development, ataxia, abnormal reflexes)
Petrosphenoidal space syndrome (*see* Jacod syndrome)
Pfaundler-Hurler (*see* Hurler syndrome)
Pick (2) (*see* Arnold Pick syndrome)
Pierre Robin (myopia, congenital glaucoma, retinal disinsertion,—micrognathia, cleft palate)
Pigmentary retinal lipoid neuronal heredodegeneration (see Batten-Mayou syndrome)
Pigmented choroidal vessels (*see* Siegrist syndrome)
Pineal-neurologic-ophthalmic syndrome (*see* Frankl Hochwart syndrome)
Pink Disease (*see* Feer syndrome)
Pituitary basophilism (*see* Cushing (1)syndrome)
Platybasia syndrome (*see* Arnold-Chiari syndrome)
Polyarthritis Enterica (*see* Reiter syndrome)
Pontine syndrome (*see* Raymond syndrome)
Pontocerebellar-angle tumor syndrome (*see* Cushing (2) syndrome)
Posner-Schlossman (glaucomatouscyclitic crisis—allergy)
Posterior cervical sympathetic syndrome (*see* Barré-Liéou syndrome)
Posterior embryotoxon (*see* Axenfeld syndrome)
Posterior thalamic syndrome (*see* Déjerine-Roussy syndrome)
Presenile dementia-cortical degeneration syndrome (*see* Heidenhain syndrome)
Primary splenic neutropenia with arthritis (*see* Felty syndrome)
Progeria of adults (*see* Werner syndrome)
Progressive facial hemiatrophy (*see* Romberg syndrome)
Progressive hemifacial atrophy (*see* Romberg syndrome)
Progressive neuritic muscular atrophy (*see* Charcot-Marie-Tooth syndrome)
Progressive peroneal muscular atrophy (*see* Charcot-Marie-Tooth syndrome)
Pseudo-Graefe (anomalies in lid movement with ocular gaze)
Pseudohypoparathyroidism syndrome (strabismus,—obesity, short stature, tetany, mental retardation)
Pseudoparalytic syndrome (*see* Erb- Goldflam syndrome)
Pseudotonic pupillotonia (*see* Adie syndrome)
Pseudoxanthoma elasticum (*see* Groenblad-Strandberg syndrome)
Psychic paralysis of visual fixation syndrome (*see* Balint syndrome)
Pterygolymphangiectasia (*see* Bonnevie-Ullrich syndrome)

Pulseless disease (*see* Takayasu syndrome)

Raeder (ocular pain, enophthalmos, ptosis, hypotonia, miosis,—facial pain)
Ramsay Hunt (*see* Hunt syndrome)
Raymond (abducens palsy,—hemiplegia, anesthesia)
Recklinghausen, von (proptosis, ptosis, muscle palsies, hydrophthalmos,— nodular swellings, café-au-lâit spots, spontaneous fractures, fibromata)
Refsum (nightblindness, retinal degeneration—ataxia, ichthyosis, deafness, polyneurities)
Reiter (conjunctivitis,—urethritis, arthritis)
Retinitis pigmentosa-deafness-ataxia syndrome (*see* Hallgren syndrome)
Retinitis pigmentosa-polydactyly-adiposogenital syndrom (*see* Laurence-Moon-Bardet-Biedl syndrome)
Retinocerebral angiomatosis (*see* von Hippel-Lindau syndrome)
Retinohypophysary syndrome (impaired central vision, field defects, optic neuritis, —glycosuria vertigo, psychic disturbances)
Retraction syndrome (*see* Duane syndrome)
Retrolenticular syndrome (*see* Déjerine-Roussy syndrome)
Reversed coarctation syndrome (*see* Takayasu syndrome)
Rheumatoid arthritis with hypersplenism (*see* Felty syndrome)
Riegers (congenital glaucoma, iris hypoplasia, microcornea—dental anomalies, wide' face)
Riley-Day (corneal anesthesia, keratitis, lack of tear production—excessive salivation, failure to thrive, skin blotching)
Robin (*see* Pierre Robin syndrome)
Rochon-Duvigneaud (ophthalmoplegia, decreased corneal sensitivity, papilledema—decreased sensitivity V_1)
Rollet (exophthalmos, ptosis, ophthalmoplegia, optic atrophy, corneal anesthesia,—vasomotor disturbances, hyperesthesias)
Romberg (enophthalmos, ptosis, iris involvement, keratitis—atrophy half side of face, seizures, trigeminal neuralgia)
Rothmund (bilateral cataracts,—skin pigmentation, telangiectasis)
Rothmund-Thomson (*see* Rothmund syndrome)
Rubella syndrome (glaucoma, keratitis, cataract, optic atrophy—hearing loss, pneumonia, diarrhea, low birth weight)
Rubinstein-Taybi (antimongoloid slant of lid fissure, strabismus—motor and mental retardation, obnormalities face and extremities)
Rubro spinal cerebellar peduncle syndrome (*see* Claude syndrome)

Sabin-Feldman (chororetinitis—convulsions, microcephaly)
Saenger (*see* Adie syndrome)
Sallmann, von-Paton-Witkop (perilimbal conjunctival lesions—oral lesions)
Sanfillipo-Good (MPS III) (retinal pigmentary changes—mental deficiency, seizures, mild gargoyl features)
Sarcoidosis (*see* Schaumann syndrome)
Scalenus anticus syndrome (*see* Naffziger syndrome)
Schaumann (granulomatous uveitis, vitreous floaters, retinopathy,— hilar nodes, lymphadenopathy)
Scheie (MPS V) (progressive corneal clouding, scotomata—broad facies, limitation of motion)
Schilder (nystagmus, extraocular palsy,—spastic paralysis, mental deficiency, tremor)
Schirmer (*see* Sturge-Weber syndrome)

Schüller-Christian-Hand (*see* Hand-Schüller-Christian syndrome)
Seabright-Bantam (*see* Pseudohypoparathyroidism)
Secreto-inhibitor syndrome (*see* Sjögren syndrome)
Serous meningitis syndrome (*see* Symonds syndrome)
Shaking palsy (*see* Parkinson syndrome)
Sickle cell disease (*see* Herrick syndrome)
Siegrist (exophtalmos, fundus pigment anomalies,—hypertension, albuminuria)
Sjögren (deficient lacrimal secretion, keratoconjunctivitis sicca,—polyarthritis, dryness of mucous membranes)
Sjögren-Larsson (atypical retinitis pigmentosa, reduced vision, hypertelorism—oligophrenia, ichthyosis, tremor, speech defect.)
Spheno- cavernous (proptosis, external ophthalmoplegia,—paresis 5th nerve)
Spielmeyer-Vogt (*see* Batten-Mayou syndrome)
Spinal miosis (*see* Argyll Robertson syndrome)
Spurway (*see* van der Hoeve syndrome)
Stevens-Johnson (keratoconjunctivitis, chemois,—skin and mucous membrane eruptions and ulcerations)
Still-Chauffard (*see* Uveitis-rheumatoid arthritis syndrome)
Stillings's syndrome (*see* Duane syndrome)
Sturge-Weber (unilateral hydrophthalmos, retinal glioma, choroidal angiomata,—skin vascular nevi, symptoms of CNS involvement)
Superior hemorrhagic polioencephalopathic syndrome (*see* Wernicke syndrome)
Superior orbital fissure syndrome (*see* Rochon-Duvigneaud syndrome)
Superior pulmonary sulcus (*see* Pancoast syndrome)
Suprarenal syndrome (*see* Cushing (1) syndrome)
Swift-Feer (see Feer syndrome)
Sylvian-aqueduct syndrome (*see* Koerber-Salus-Elschnig syndrome)
Symonds (papilledema, retinal hemorrhages, 6th nerve palsy, diplopia, optic atrophy,—drowsiness, otitis media, meningeal involvement, headaches)
Syndroma muco-cutaneo-oculare (*see* Stevens-Johnson syndrome)
Synostosis cervical vertebrae (*see* Klippel-Feil syndrome)
Systemic elastodystrophy (*see* Groenblad-Strandberg syndrome)
Systemic mucopolisaccharidosis (1) see Hurler; (2) see Hunter; (3) see Sanfillipo-Good; (4) see Morquio-Brailsford; (5) see Scheie syndromes)

Takayasu (iris atrophy, cataracts, vascular retinopathy, transient visual loss—absent pulse, orthostatic syncope, facial atrophy)
Tapetal-like reflex syndrome (ring scotoma, yellow spots in posterior pole of the fundus)
Tay-Sachs (cherry red macular apot, optic atrophy—mental retardation, convulsions)
Tegmental syndrome (*see* Benedict syndrome)
Telangiectasia-pigmentation-cataract syndrome (*see* Rothmund syndrome)
Temporal arteritis (diplopia, optic atrophy, retinal detachment—hyperalgesia of the scalp, pain temporal region)
Temporal lobectomy behavior syndrome (*see* Klüver-Bucy syndrome)
Temporal syndrome (*see* Gradenigro syndrome)
Terry (*see* Groenblad-Strandberg syndrome)
Thalamic syndrome (*see* Déjerine-Roussy syndrome)
Thalamic hyperesthetic anesthesia syndrome (*see* Déjerine-Roussy syndrome)
Tolosa-Hunt (ptosis, visual impairment, ocular muscle involvement)
Tonic pupil (*see* Adie syndrome)
Treacher Collins (*see* Franceschetti syndrome)

Trisomy 13–15 (D-Trisomy) anophthalmia, microphthalmia, hyperteolrism, shallow orbits, iris coloboma, cataracts, optic nerve coloboma—hemangioma, polydactyly, cerebral defects, harelip, finger and hand changes)

Trisomy 18 (unilateral ptosis, corneal opacities—mental retardation, face anomalies, failure of flexion of fingers)

Trisomy 21 (*see* Down syndrome)

Trisomy 22 (high myopia—schizophrenia, micrognathia, large nostrils, flat occiput, overextension of elbows)

Tuberous sclerosis (*see* Bourneville syndrome)

Turk-Stilling (*see* Duane syndrome)

Turner (exophthalmos, ptosis, epicanthal folds, oval corneae—webbed neck, deafness, diminished growth)

Uilrich-Bonnevie (*see* Bonnevie-Ullrich syndrome)

Unilateral facial agenesis (*see* Hemifacial Microsomia)

Unverrichts (amaurosis-epilepsy, myoclonus, dementia)

Usher (retinitis pigmentosa, concentric field contraction—deaf mutism)

Uveitis-rheumatoid arthritis syndrome (uveitis, bandshaped keratopathy, choroidal inflammation—rheumatoid arthritis)

Uveitis-vitiligo-alopecia-poliosis (*see* Vogt-Koyanagi-Harada syndrome)

Uveomeningitis syndrome (*see* Vogt-Koyanagi-Harada syndrome)

Uveoparotid fever (*see* Heerfordt syndrome)

Uveoparotitic paralysis (*see* Heerfordt syndrome)

Uyemura (white spots of fundus, conj. xerosis, nightblindness)

van der Hoeve-Halbertsma-Waardenburg (*see* Waardenburg syndrome)

vascular encephalotrigeminal syndrome (*see* Sturge Weber syndrome)

vermis (nystagmus, papilledema—vomiting, enlarged head, incoordination)

vogt-Koyanagi-Harada (uveitis, secondary cataracts, serous retinal detachment, exudative choroiditis—alopecia, poliosis, hearing defect)

volunlary propulsion of the eye (*see* Double Whammy syndrome)

von Herrenschwand (enophthalmos, ptosis, miosis, heterochromia—decreased sweating ipsilateral side of face)

von Hippel-Lindau (retinal angiomatosis, vitreous hemorrhages, sec. glaucoma—cerebral angiomatosis, epilepsy, psychic disturbances)

von Mikulicz-Radecki (*see* Mikulicz-Radecki syndrome)

von Recklinghausen (proptosis, ptosis, muscle palsies, hydrophthalmos—nodular swelling café-au-lâit spots, spontaneous fractures, fibromata)

von Sallmann-Paton-Witkop (perilimbal conjunctival lesions—oral lesions)

Waardenburg (increased PD, lateral displacement of medial canthi, blepharophimosis, iris heterochromia,—deafness, broad nasal root, albinotic hair strain)

Waldenström (chorioretinal hemorrhages and exudates,—adenopathy, vasospasm of extremities, dyspnea)

Wallenberg (nystagmus, diplopia, Horner's trias,—nausea, difficulty in speaking and swallowing)

Weber (3rd nerve palsy, fixed pupil, ptosis,—Hemiplegia, paralysis face and tongue)

Weber-Cockayne (*see* Goldscheider syndrome)

Weil-Marchesani syndrome (*see* Marchesani syndrome)

Werner (no eye lashes, cataracts,—thin limbs, leanness, small mouth, stretched atrophic skin)

Wernicke (ophthalmoplegia, ptosis,—peripheral neuritis, ataxia, mental disturbances)

Wilson (corneal ring,—liver cirrhosis, muscular rigidity, ascites in late stages)
Wyburn-Mason (*see* Bonnet-Dechaume-Blance syndrome)

Xanthomatous granuloma syndrome (*see* Hand-Schuller-Christian syndrome)
Xanthomatous granuloma syndrome (*see* Hand-Schüller-Christian syndrome)

Zinsser-Engman-Cole (conjunctival keratinization—congenital dyskeratosis, oral lesions, aplastic anemia)

Tabulated Brief Description of Syndromes Involving the Eye and Its Adnexa

(in alphabetical order)

SYNDROME: Addison
SYNONYMS: Addison's disease-moniliasis-idiopathic hypoparathyroidism
GEN. INFORMATION:
The syndrome has been reported with familial occurrence in some cases though the pattern of a possible inheritance is not quite clear. Association with mycoses other than moniliasis is not rare (Del Negro *et al.*: Ann. Int. Med., 1961). Onset usually during end of Ist and beginning of 2nd decade of life. Hypoparathyroidism and hypoadrenal-corticism become evident usually between age 8 to 12 years of life. Laboratory findings: Decreased serum calcium level and increased serum phosphorus. (Injection of parathyroid hormone increases the serum calcium and results in increased urinary excretion of phosphorus.) Low serum sodium and high serum potassium levels. Adrenal insufficiency evident by lack of increased urinary excretion of 17-hydroxy-corticosterone and 17-ketosteroid upon injection of ACTH. Pathology: Atrophy of adrenal cortex. Prognosis for life is poor with death in adrenal crisis.

OCULAR FINDINGS:

Orbit	Eyebrows sparse
Lids	Ptosis, blepharitis, blepharospasm
Motility	
Lacr. App.	
Vision	
Vis. Fields	
Intraoc. Ten.	
Ant. Segm. and Sclera	Keratoconjunctivitis with extreme photophobia, corneal ulcers, vascularization and opacities, episcleritis, keratitic moniliasis
Ocul. Media	Cataracts
Retina and Choroid	Retinal hemorrhages (isolated finding-Leonard, 1946)
Optic Nerve	Papilledema casued by increased cerebrospinal fluid pressure

OTHER CLINICAL FINDINGS:
1. Moniliasis (usually the first appearing finding of this syndrome and most frequently present by age 5 to 6 years. Its association with the hormonal deficiency is not understood as of now)
2. Tetany
3. Progressive weakness
4. Anorexia
5. Progressive skin pigmentation
6. Dry skin and brittle finger and toenails
7. Sparse pubic and axillary hair or total alopecia
8. Intracranial calcifications
9. Epileptiform seizures
10. Poor dentition

BIBLIOGRAPHY:
1. Addison, T.: On the constitutional and local effects of disease of the suprarenal capsules, London, S. Highley, 1855, ibid: Lond. Med. gaz. *43:*517, 1849.
2. Lyle, D. J.: The ocular syndrome of cataract and papilledema in the manifest from of parathyroid deficiency, Am. J. Ophth. *31:*580, 1948.
3. Forbes, G. B.: Clinical features of idiopathic hypoparathyroidism in children, Ann. New York Acad. Sc. *64:*432, 1956.
4. Gass, J. D.: The syndrome of keratojunctivitis, superficial moniliasis, idiopathic hypoparathyroidism and Addison's disease, Am. J. Ophth. *54:*660, 1962.

SYNDROME: Adie

SYNONYMS: Holmes-Adie syndrome, Markus syndrome, Saenger syndrome, tonic pupil, iridoplegia interna, myotonic pupil, pseudotonic pupillotoma

GEN. INFORMATION:

Etiology unknown. More frequent in females. Some genetic factors involved. Manifest in 2nd and 3rd decade. Ocular findings in approximately 80% of the cases. Abnormal sensitivity to a 2.5% solution of methacholin instilled into the conjunctival sac. The tonic pupil constricts while normal pupils are unaffected (Adler and Scheie: Tr. Am. Ophth. Soc. *38:* 183, 1940). Wasserman reaction negative. Progressive selective paseudomotor denervation may produce this syndrome (Petajan *et al.*) Scheie (Arch. Ophth., 1940) has suggested that the site of the lesion is in the post ganglionic fibers after they have left the ciliary ganglion, whereas de Haas (Arch. Ophth., 1959) considers the disturbance to be due to a lesion within the hypothalamic vegetative centers.

OCULAR FINDINGS:

Orbit	
Lids	
Motility	
Lacr. App.	
Vision	
Vis. Fields	
Intraoc. Ten.	
Ant. Segm. and Sclera	Slightly enlarged pupils, delayed or diminished direct and consensual reaction to light, (pupillotonia or bradycoria). Usually unilateral. Consensual reflex is abolished on the affected side but normal on the other. Apparently abolished photomotor reflex. Slow and prolonged reaction on convergence and full reaction to mydriatics and miotics
Ocul. Media	
Retina and Choroid	
Optic Nerve	

OTHER CLINICAL FINDINGS:

1. Loss of tendon reflexes particularly ankle and knee jerk (partial or total).
2. Anhidrosis ⎰ Not in classical syndrome. Described in association
3. Generalized weakness ⎱ with it (Ref. 2 and 4), though with variations in several aspects.

BIBLIOGRAPHY:

1. Adie, W.: Complete and incomplete forms of the benign disorder characterized by tonic pupils and absent tendon reflexes, Brit. J. Ophth., *16:*449, 1932.
2. Ross, A.T.: Progressive selective sudomotor-denervation, Neurology, *8:* 811, 1958.
3. Francois, J.: *Heredity in Ophthalmology,* St. Louis, C.V. Mosby Co., 1961, p. 353
4. Petajan, J. H.; Danforth, R. C.; D'Allesio, D. and Lucas, G. J.: Progressive sudomotor denervation and Adie's syndrome, Neurology *15:* 172, 1965.
5. Adler, F. H.: *physiology of the Eye.* 4th Ed. St. Louis, C. V. Mosby Co., 1965, P. 221.
6. Loewenfeld, I. E. and Thompson, H. S.: The tonic pupil: A re-evaluation, Am. J. Ophth. *63:* 46, 1967

SYNDROME: Albright

SYNONYMS: Fuller Albright syndrome, McCune-Albright syndrome, osteitis fibrosa disseminata, osteodystrophia fibrosa, polyostotic fibrous dysplasia.

GEN. INFORMATION:
Etiology unknown, hereditary for bone lesions (?). The disease is rare. Manifest in childhood and young adults. Serum calcium and phosphorus often normal, but Ca may be elevated (about 20% of patients) and serum phosphorus is diminished in about 40% of patients. Serum phosphatase often elevated. Normal 17-ketosteroid values (d.d adrenocortical tumor). X-ray finding: Cystic bone deformation. Pathology: Replacement of bone by fibrous tissue with dense collagenous or fibrillar stroma, Multiple small cystic spaces. Irregular trabeculae. Foci of multinucleated giant cells.

OCULAR FINDINGS:

Orbit	Unilateral proptosis
Lids	
Motility	
Lacr. App.	
Vison	
Vis. Fields	Defects possible, depending on location of bone lesions
Intraoc. Ten.	
Ant. Segm. and Sclera	
Ocul. Media	
Retina and Choroid	
Optic Nerve	Papilledema, optic atrophy

OTHER CLINICAL FINDINGS:
1. Osteitis fibrosa cystica (unilateral) medullary structures replaced by fibrous dysplasia. Pelvic bones and lower extremities most frequently involved (Spontaneous fractures)*
2. Brown pigmented areas of skin (same side as bone lesions) size:from small freckle-like dots to large flat patches. Location:thighs, sacrum, upper spine and neck, scalp. Melanin deposits in inner layer of epidermis in areas of pigment spots*
3. Endocrine dysfunction (precocious puberty in females) early menarche, adolescent external genitalia, breast enlargement.* Precocity in males only occasionally

*Typical for this syndrome

BIBLIOGRAPHY:
1. Albright, F.; Butler, A. M.; Hampton, A. O. and Smith, P.: Syndrome characterized by osteitis fibrosa disseminata, areas of pigmentation and endocrine dysfunction, with precocious puberty in females, New Engl. J. Med. 216: 727, 1937.
2. Albright, F., Scoville, W. B. and Sulkovitch, H. W.: Syndrome characterized by osteitis fibrosa disseminata, areas of pigmentation and gonadal dysfunction, Encocrinol. 22: 411, 1938.
3. Neller, J. L.: Osteitis fibrosa cystica (Albright). Am. J. Dis. Child. 61:690, 1941.
4. Albright, F.: Polysotoic fibrous dysplasia: A defense of the entity, J. Clin. Endocrinol. 7:307, 1947

3

SYNDROME: Alport
SYNONYMS: Hereditary familial congenital hemorrhagic nephritis
GEN. INFORMATION:

Hereditary familial congenital disease. Autosomal dominant inheritance has been suggested possibly modified by a sex linked suppressor gene.* Early death in males, normal life span in females. Lab. findings: Proteinuria, erythrocyturia, leukocyturia, cylindruria of alternating intensity, reduced concentration power of kidneys, hyperaminoaciduria of alanin, glycin, serin and taurin. It has been proposed that similar pathologic changes which have been described for the optic nerve may also affect the stato-acustic nerve.*

OCULAR FINDINGS:

Orbit	
Lids	
Motility	
Lacr. App.	
Vision	Reduced vision
Vis. Fields	
Intraoc. Ten.	
Ant. Segm. and Sclera	
Ocul. Media	Anterior lenticonus (bilateral progressive), subcapsular cataracts. Thinning of lens capsule, decreased number of lens epithelial cells, bulging lens substance. (Lens changes in males only), juvenile arcus of the cornea*
Retina and Choroid	Fundus albi punctatus, retinopathy similar to juvenile macular degeneration (Pichelmaier-Adenauer, 1967)
Optic Nerve	Hyalin bodies of optic nerve head,* pseudoneuritis*

OTHER CLINICAL FINDINGS:
1. Hemorrhagic nephritis
2. Progressive nerve deafness (begin usually after 10 years of age)
3. Increase of α_2 fraction of serumproteins
4. Vestibulary disturbances

*(Friedburg, 1968)

BIBLIOGRAPHY:
1. Alport, A. C.: Hereditary familial congenital hemorrhagic nephritis, Brit. Med. J. *1*:504, 1927.
2. Brownell, R. D.; and Wolter, J. R.: Anterior lenticonus in familial hemorrhagic nephritis, Arch. Ophth. *71*:481, 1964.
3. Sarre, H.: Rother, K.; Schmitt, Ch.; Unger, H. H..; Beickert, P.; and Baitsch, H.: Neue Befunde zur hereditären Nephritis (Alport-Syndrom), Arch. Klin. Med. *212*:1, 1966.
4. Friedburg, D.: Pseudoneuritis und Drusenpapille beim Alport-Syndrom, Kl. Mbl. Augenhk. *152*:379, 1968.

SYNDROME: Amaurosis fugax
SYNONYMS:
GEN. INFORMATION:

Tabagism, and malignant hypertension have been said to be the most frequent causes for this syndrome, since it often occurs in association with heavy smoking or this form of hypertension. However, the sensation of momentary loss of vision may indicate a vascular insufficiency of the vertebral-basilar arterial system and may precede a cerebral vascular accident and it is not infrequently seen in vascular insufficiency problems of the carotic arterial system. Thorpe also mentioned its occurrence in expanding lesions of the frontal and temporal lobes. Amaurosis fugax after angiography has also been described (Lombardi).

OCULAR FINDINGS:

Orbit	
Lids	
Motility	
Lacr. App.	Partial blindness in short attacks to permanent complete blindness. Initially the periods of visual loss last only for several seconds. With increasing severity of the condition the frequency of attacks may increase as well and each episode may become longer, eventually resulting in permanent visual loss
Vision	
Vis. Field	
Intraoc. Ten.	
Ant. Segm. and Sclera	
Ocul. Media	
Retina and Choroid	Retinal arteriolar spasm, signs of arteriolar sclerosis
Optic Nerve	

OTHER CLINICAL FINDINGS:

1. Malignant hypertension
2. Atherosclerosis
3. Expanding lesions of the frontal or temporal lobe (Lombardi)
4. Vascular insufficiency

BIBLIOGRAPHY:

1. Moore, R. F.: *Medical Ophthalmology,* London, J. & A. Churchill, Ltd., 1922.
2. Haney, W. P. and Preston, R. E.: Ocular complications of carotid arteriography in carotid occlusive disease, Arch. Ophth. 67:127, 1963.
3. Guerry, D. III, and Wiesinger, H.: Ocular complications in carotid angiography, Am. J. Ophth. 55:241, 1963.
4. Thorpe, R. M.: Ocular signs in cerebral disease, (in Gay, J. A. and Burde, R. M. (eds.): Clinical concepts in neuro-ophthalmology, Internal. Ophth. Clinics. 7: 707. 1967.
5. Lombardi, G.: *Radiology in Neuro-Ophthalmology,* Baltimore, The Williams & Wilkins Co., 1967.

SYNDROME: Angelucci
SYNONYMS: Critical allergic conjunctivitis syndrome
GEN. INFORMATION:
Etiology unknown (lymphatic condition). Pruriginous cutaneous and mucous reactions which appear and cease rather suddenly. The condition may be local, occurring always at the same site, or it may alternate and be associated with other allergic manifestations.

OCULAR FINDINGS:

Orbit	
Lids	
Motility	
Lacr. App.	
Vision	
Vis. Fields	
Intraoc. Ten.	
Ant. Segm. and Sclera	Chemosis, conjunctivitis (papillary type). Generally watery discharge but may become mucopurulent. Conjunctival smears negative for bacteria, eosinophilic cells usually present. Severe itching, burning and photophobia
Ocul. Media	Perilimbal corneal infiltration (occasional finding)
Retina and Choroid	
Optic Nerve	

OTHER CLINICAL FINDINGS:
1. Tachycardia
2. Vasomotor lability
3. Excitability
4. Allergies (asthma, urticaria, edema, etc.)
5. Dystrophic conditions and endocrine disorders are frequently associated findings

BIBLIOGRAPHY:
1. Angelucci, A: Di una sindrome sconoscita negli infermi di cattarro primaverile, Arch. di ottal., Palermo, *4:*270, 1897-98.
2. Lagrange, H.: The pathogenic problem of so-called critical allergic conjunctivis; specific sensitization, non-specific sensitization, instability of organic colloids, Brit. J. Ophth., 19:241, 1935.
3. Pasteur Vallery-Radot; Blamoutier, P. and Stehelin, J.; Conjonctivites anaphylactiques et crises conjonctivales chez les asthmatiques, Presse Méd. *33,* 1909.
4. Theodore, F. H.: The significance of conjunctival eosinophilia in the diagnosis of allergic conjunctivitis. Eye, Ear, Nose & Throat Monthly, *30:*653, 1951.
5. Theodore, F. H. and Schlossman, A.: *Ocular Allergy,* Baltimore, The Williams & Wilkins Co., 1958.

SYNDROME: Anton
SYNONYMS: Denial-visual hallucination syndrome
GEN. INFORMATION:
Etiology unknown (isolation of diencephalon from occipital lobe would be necessary to result in the features of the syndrome). Lesions of the calcarine -thalamic connections or bilateral destruction of the occipital regions have been claimed by others to cause denial of blindness. Also large tumors of the pituitary may give rise to psychotic symptoms (White and Cobb) including denial of blindness, hallucinations and uncinate fits. These symptoms occur, however, only with large tumors in this region, involving adjacent portions of the brain and having therefore a poor prognosis. The disease is very rare and littel understood.

OCULAR FINDINGS:

Orbit	
Lids	
Motility	
Lacr. App.	
Vision	Blindness of cerebral origin, either due to occipito or parieto-temporal lesions, are often accompanied by denial of blindness (Patients may deny persistantly of having any loss of visual perception. The objects the patient describes and claims to see are regarded as visual hallucinations -(Raney and Nielson)
Vis. Fields	Hemianopsia
Intraoc. Ten.	
Ant. Segm. and Sclera	
Ocul. Media	
Retina and Choroid	
Optic Nerve	

OTHER CLINICAL FINDINGS:
1. Confabulation
2. Denial of blindness
3. Allocheiria—(Reference of a sensation is made to the opposite side to which the stimulus is applied)

BIBLIOGRAPHY:
1. Anton, G.: Ueber die Selbstwahrnehmung der Herderkrankung des Gehirns durch den Kranken bei Rindentaubheit, Arch. Psychiat. Nervenkr., *32*:86, 1899.
2. Raney, A. and Nielsen, J.: Denial of blindness (Anton's symptom), Bull. Los Angeles Neurol. Soc., *7*:150, 1942.
3. Redlich, F. C. and Dorsey, J. F.: Denial of blindness by patients with cerebral disease, Arch. Neurol. Psychiat., *53*:407, 1945.
4. White, J. C. and Cobb, S.: Psychological changes associated with giant Pituitary neoplasms, Arch. Neurol. Psychiat., *74:* 383, 1955
5. Lutt, C. J.: Denial of blindness and Argyll Robertson pupils without syphilis, Bull. Los Angeles Neurol. Soc. *12*:189, 1947.
6. Tyler, H. R.: Cerebral disorders of vision, in Smith, J. L. (ed.) *Neuro-Ophthalmology,* Vol. IV, St. Louis, C. V. Mosby Co., 1968.

SYNDROME: Apert
SYNONYMS: Acrocephalosyndactylism syndrome
GEN. INFORMATION:

Inherited. Most often recessive, sometimes dominant (François). Defect in germ plasm (?). Manifestations congenital. X-ray examinations reveals high vertex of the skull, absence of suture lines and convolutional markings. The syndrome may be associated with other malformations, *i.e.* other skeletal dysplasias, dysraphic stygmata, hemolytic jaundice (Baumatter, 1932). Acrocephaly may also be observed in Bonnevie-Ullrich syndrome, in lipidoses, gargoylism, Bardet-Biedl syndrome, etc. Optic atrophy in Apert's syndrome is either due to compression of the nerve by narrowed optic foramina or to traction on the nerve by the downward displacement of the brain.

OCULAR FINDINGS:

Orbit	Shallow, exophthalmos, wide separation of eyes (hypertelorism)
Lids	Ptosis, inner canthus higher than outer canthus (slant appearance)
Motility	Strabismus, nystagmus, external squint, ophthalmoplegia
Lacr. App.	
Vision	Usually good up to age 6 or 7, diminishing thereafter. Hyperopia
Vis. Fields	Upper field defect frequently (pressure and stretching on lower part of optic disc)
Intraoc. Ten.	
Ant. Segm. and Sclera	Iris coloboma (occasionally)
Ocul. Media	Exposure keratitis, cataracts, ectopia lentis. Megalocornea and keratoconus (single observations)
Retina and Choroid	Medullated nerve fibers, retinal detachment, choroidal coloboma (occasionally)
Optic Nerve	Papilledema with following optic atrophy

OTHER CLINICAL FINDINGS:

1. Oxycephaly ("towerskull")
2. Syndactyly (symmetrically)
3. Synostoses and synarthroses of shoulder and elbows frequently
4. Brevicollis might be associated

5. Agenesia of spinal bones and limbs
6. Headaches
7. Convulsions
8. Loss of smell and hearing
9. Mentality usually normal

BIBLIOGRAPHY:

1. Apert. E.: Acrocephalosyndactylia, Bull. Soc. med. hop. Paris, *23:*1310, 1906.
2. Greig, D. M.: Oxycephaly, Edinburgh M. J., *33:*189, 280, 357, 1926.
3. Mann, J.: A theory of the embryology of oxycephaly, Tr. Ophth. Soc. U. K., *55:*279, 1935.
4. François, J.: *Heredity in Opthhalmology,* St. Louis, C. V. Mosby Co., 1961. p. 608.
5. Seelenfreund, M. and Gartner, S.:Acrocephalosyndactyly (Apert's syndrome), Arch. Ophth. *78:*8, 1967.

SYNDROME: Argyll Robertson
SYNONYMS: Spinal miosis
GEN INFORMATION:
Cause almost always syphilis (rare: epidemic encephalitis, disseminated sclerosis, diabetes, brain tumor, syringomyelia, syringobulbia, chronic alcoholism, injury). Numerous theories exist with regard to the localization of the lesion. The most common ones are: (1) Pretectal area (midbrain tegmentum just ventral to posterior commissure) histologic findings and experimental work did not substantiate this theory; (2) Ciliary ganglion, however, the presence of response to accommodation, miosis and lack of histologic findings are against this localization; (3) Abnormal cholinergic activity. Though this theory accounts for a number of aspects, the poor response to atropine is not explainable by it; (4) Iris nerve fibers. Lesions in axons of ciliary ganglion neurons with degeneration of nerve fibers in the iris has been demonstrated. A number of additional factors would, however, be necessary to substantiate this theory; (5) Combined afferent and efferent central lesion at present regarded the most likely one since on theoretical grounds it will account for all symptoms of the A. R. pupil (Ref. 4).

OCULAR FINDINGS:

Orbit	
Lids	Lid reflex occasionally absent
Motility	
Lacr. App.	
Vision	Vision not significantly impaired
Vis. Fields	
Intraoc. Ten.	
Ant. Segm. and Sclera	No direct and consensual pupil reaction to light but well for accommodation (except in terminal stages when pupil is fixed to all stimuli); Pupil contraction with eserine, but poor dilatation with atropine. Miosis (generally). Irregular pupil. Iris atrophy (occasionally). Occurs unilateral and bilateral. The complete form is preceded by a series of gradual changes of pupillary function. Anisocoria or discoria frequent
Ocul. Media	
Retina and Choroid	
Optic Nerve	

OTHER CLINICAL FINDINGS:
1. Syphilis of CNS (presence of pupillary abnormalities points to it, even if standard serologic tests negative. Immobilization test is then done since false positives rare.) Ref. 3, 4
2. General paresis   3. Tabes dorsalis

BIBLIOGRAPHY:
1. Argyll Robertson, D.: Four cases of spinal miosis: with remarks on the action of light on the pupil, Edinburgh M. J. *15:*487, 1869.
2. Lowenstein, O.: Argyll Robertson pupillary syndrome mechanism and localization, A. J. O., *42:*105, 1956.
3. Smith, J. L.: Seronegative ocular and neurosyphilis, A. J. O. *59:*753, 1965.
4. Kerr, F. W.: The pupil-functional anatomy and clinical correlation.-in: Smith, J. L.: *Neuro-Ophthalmology,* Vol. IV, S. Louis, C. V. Mosby Co., 1968.

SYNDROME: Arnold-Chiari
SYNONYMS: Platybasis syndrome, cerebellomedullary malformation syndrome
GEN. INFORMATION:
Malformation of the hindbrain. Developmental deformity of the occipital bone and upper cervical spine. Recognized in children or adults. The clinical picture may be indistinguishable from that of the Dandy-Walker syndrome in infants. Important differential diagnosis: MS, syringomyelia, progressive bulbar paralysis, amyotrophic lateral sclerosis. X-ray examination shows platybasia and narrowing of the foramen magnum. Air encephalogram may demonstrate herniated cerebellar tonsils. Narrowed foramen magnum with herniation of the brain stem and cerebellum. Adhesive arachnoiditis around herniated tissue. Elongation of lower cranial and upper cervical nerves. Spinal fluid block. Hydromyelia, upper portion of spinal canal. Differentiation from intramedullary tumors may be difficult unless downward displacement of the fourth ventricle and foramen of Magendie can be demonstrated (Liliequist, 1960).

OCULAR FINDINGS:

Orbit	
Lids	
Motility	Horizontal, vertical and rotary forms of nystagmus may exist.* Vertical nystagmus in both, up-and down-gaze is most common. Particular the latter is of diagnostic value. Diplopia (Cogan and Barrows)
Lacr. App.	
Vision	
Vis. Fields	Bitemporal hemianopsia (might have been due to chiasmal injury at time of ventriculostomy (Post)
Intraoc. Ten.	
Ant. Segm. and Sclera	
Ocul. Media	
Retina and Choroid	
Optic Nerve	Papilledema *Characteristic for this syndrome

OTHER CLINCIAL FINDINGS:
1. Spina bifida
2. Meningomyelocele
3. Hydrocephalus*
4. Cranial nerve dysfunctions
5. Headaches
6. Cerebellar ataxia*
7. Bilateral pyramidal tract signs*
8. Motor and sensory disorders

BIBLIOGRAPHY:
1. Arnold, J.: Myelocyste, Transposition von Gewebskeimen und Sympodie, Beitr. z. path Anat. u. z. allgem. Path., Jena, *16*:1, 1894.
2. Chiari, H.: Ueber Veränderungen des Kleinhirns infolge von Hydrocephalie des Grosshirns, Dtsch. med. Wschr., Leipzig, *17*:1172, 1981.
3. Cogan, D. S. and Barrows, L. J.: Platybasia and the Arnold-Chiari malformation, Arch. Ophth., *52*:13, 1954.
4. Gardner, W. J.; et al. The varying expressions of embryonal atresia of the fourth ventricle in adults, J. Neurosurg. *14*:591, 1957.
5. Mahaley, M. S., Jr.: Ocular motility with foramen magnum syndromes, in: Smith, J. L.: *Neuro-Ophthalmology,* Vol, IV, St. Louis C. V. Mosby Co., 1968.

SYNDROME: Arnold Pick

SYNONYMS: Aphasia-agnosia-apraxia syndrome, Pick syndrome (2)

GEN. INFORMATION:

Blindness is caused by widerspread cortical atrophy. Pathologically, the atrophied lobe shows shrunken gyri with widened sulci. The atrophy involves not only the gray but also the white cortical matter. Females are more frequently affected. It may occur in several members of a family. Manifest between 40 and 70 years. Onset with loss of interest and initiative and impairment of attention and concentration. Electroencephalography and pneumoencephalography reveal cerebral atrophy.

OCULAR FINDINGS:

Orbit	
Lids	
Motility	
Lacr. App.	
Vision	Apperceptive blindness, inability to fix reflex upon objects within his gaze
Vis. Fields	Visual agnosia and visual field defects in this syndrome are due to circumscribed atrophy in the occipital lobe
Intraoc. Ten.	
Ant. Segm. and Sclera	
Ocul. Media	
Retina and Choroid	
Optic Nerve	Optic neuritis (isolated finding-(Urechias) does not belong to the typical findings) (Best)

OTHER CLINICAL FINDINGS:

1. Presenile or progressive dementia
2. Patient is unaware of his surroundings
3. Poor insight
4. Loss of words and utterance of stereotyped phrases
5. Aphasia (motor type)
6. Apraxia, may be earlier than agnosia
7. Apathy and indifference

BIBLIOGRAPHY:

1. Pick, A.: Apperzeptive Blindheit der Senilen. Arb. d. dtsch. Psychiat. Klin. in Prag, p. 43, 1908.
2. Best, F.: Augenveränderungen bei den Erkrankungen des Zentralnervensystems;-in Schieck, F. und Brückner, A.: *Kurzes Handbuch der Ophthalmologie,* vol. 6, Berlin, Julius Springer Verl., 1931.
3. Hassin, G. B. and Levitin, D,: Pick's Disease. Clinicopathologic study and report of a case, Arch. Neurol. & Psychiatry, *45:*814, 1941.
4. Wilson, S. A. K.; (edit. by Bruce): *Neurology,* vol. II, Baltimore, The Williams & Wilkins Co., 1940, pp. 906-918.

SYNDROME: Ascher
SYNONYMS: Blepharochalasis with struma and double lip
GEN. INFORMATION:

Rare occurrence. Questionable inheritance for the entire syndrome, though blepharochalasis is in general transmitted as a simple dominant gene. The syndrome has been noted in both sexes and it may be related to the development of the thyroid gland. Symptoms usually starting around puberty.

OCULAR FINDINGS:

Orbit ·	'Bulging' of orbital fat due to lack of tone of orbital septum: The protrusion of orbital fat will at least present upon pressure on the globe
Lids	Blepharochalasis (flaccid upper lid, with skin folds; it follows an atrophy of the dermis with secondary relaxing of the subcutaneous tissue (elastorrhexis)
Motility	
Lacr. App.	Protrusion of lacrimal gland due to same lack of tone of the orbital fascia which causes the bulging of the orbital fat
Vision	
Vis. Fields	
Intraoc. Ten.	
Ant. Segm. and Sclera	
Ocul. Media	
Retina and Choroid	
Optic Nerve	

OTHER CLINICAL FINDINGS:

1. Goiter
2. Reduplication of upper lip (acquired type). In the acquired type the border between the 'first' and 'second' lip is located some distance behind the normal lip margin with the skin. The second lip is caused by granulation or hypertrophy of mucous glands with otherwise normal mucosa. In the congenital type the border between the 'double' lip is located in the lip margin itself, *i.e.* more anteriorly.

BIBLIOGRAPHY:

1. Ascher, K. W.: Blepharochalasis mit Struma und Doppellippe, Kl. Mbl. Augenhk. *65*:86, 1920.
2. Eisenstodt, L. W.: Blepharochalasis with Double Upper Lip, Amer. J. ophthal. *32*:128, 1949.
3. François, J.: *Heredity in Ophthalmology,* St. Louis, C. V. Mosby Co., 1961.
4. Stehr, V. K.: Werb, K., Löblich, H. J.: Pathogenese und Therapie des Ascher-syndroms, Dtsch. Med. Wschr. *87*:1148, 1962.
5. Gorlin, R. J. and Pindborg, J. J.; *Syndromes of the Head and Neck,* New York, McGraw-Hill Book Co., (Blakiston Division), 1964.
6. Thiel, R.: *Atlas of Diseases of the Eye.* Vol. I., Amsterdam-London-New York, Elsevier Publishing Co. 1953.

SYNDROME: Axenfeld
SYNONYMS: Posterior embryotoxon
GEN. INFORMATION:
Dominant inheritance, however, sporadic cases have been reported. The syndrome is extremely variable in expression. Glaucoma apparent in adolescence or early adulthood. Prognosis is poor for long term retention of good visual function. Differential diagnoiss: Arcus senilis— 'gerontoxon'—(except no clear zone at the limbus in Axenfeld syndrome). Posterior embryotoxon, a descriptive term, is a congenital opacity at the level of Descemet's membrane arising as a congenital variation or anomaly of the size and position of the anterior border ring of Schwalbe (Hogan and Zimmerman). Embryologically it is caused by incomplete cleavage of iris and trabecular meshwork.

OCULAR FINDINGS:

Orbit	
Lids	
Motility	
Lacr. App.	
Vision	
Vis. Fields	
Ant. Segm. and Sclera	Posterior embryotoxon:long trabeculum, prominent Schwalbe's line, iris adhesions to Schwalbe's line and cornea with large abnormal iris processes or broad sheets of tissue of varying size and location. Anterior layer of iris may appear hypoplastic. Ectopia of the pupil not uncommon, polycoria occurs.
Ocul. Media	Ring-like opacity of the deep corneal layers extending several millimeters from the limbus in continuity with the sclera
Retina and Choroid	
Optic Nerve	

OTHER CLINICAL FINDINGS:
BIBLIOGRAPHY:
1. Axenfeld, Th.: Embryotoxon corneae posterius, Ber. dsch. Ophth. Ges. *42*:301, 1920
2. Vaughan, D., Cook, R. and Asbury, T.: *General Ophthalmology.* Los Altos, California, Lange Med. Publ., 1962, p. 229.
3. Hogen, M. J. and Zimmerman, L. E.: *Ophthalmic Pathology;* 2nd Ed., Philadelphia, W. B. Saunders Co., 1962.
4. Duke-Elder, *Sir* Stewart: *System of Ophthalmology,* Vol. III, Part 2, St. Louis, C. V. Mosby Co., 1963.

SYNDROME: Axenfeld-Schürenberg
SYNONYMS: Cyclic oculomotor paralysis
GEN. INFORMATION:
Congenital manifestation. Most frequently unilateral. The condition is detected by the parents usually during the first year of life.

OCULAR FINDINGS:

Orbit	
Lids	Ptosis during period of paralysis, during spasms the lids are raised
Motility	Cyclic oculomotor paralysis (paralysis alternating with spasm), during period of paralysis the affected eye is abducted, during phase of spasm deviation of the eye either inward or outward
Lacr. App.	
Vision	
Vis. Fields	
Intraoc. Ten.	
Ant. Segm. and Sclera	Fixed pupil with contraction during period of spasm
Ocul. Media	
Retina and Choroid	
Optic Nerve	

OTHER CLINICAL FINDINGS:
BIBLIOGRAPHY:
1. Axenfeld, T. and Schürenberg, L.: Beiträge zur Kenntnis der angeborenen Beweglichkeitsdefekte des Auges, Kl. Mbl. Augenhk. *39:* 64, 1901.
2. Latorre Morasso, S. and Aguilar, J. N.: Axenfeld-Schürenberg disease, Arch. de la Soc. Oft. Hisp.-Amer., *1:* 625, 1942. (Abstract, A. J. O., *27:* 1172, 1944.)

SYNDROME: Babinski-Nageotte
SYNONYMS: Medullary tegmental paralysis
GEN: INFORMATION:
Lesion in pontobulbar transitional region (corpus restiforme, Deiter's nucleus, sympathetic fibers). Ocular findings are located ipsilateral side of the lesion. Besides the involvement of the pyramidal tract, median fillet and cerebellar peduncle, Horner's trias is always part of this syndrome. The findings are similar to Cestan-Chenais syndrome and Wallenberg syndrome. In the latter hemiparesis is absent and there is nausea and difficulty in swallowing and speaking.

OCULAR FINDINGS:

Orbit	Enophthalmos*
Lids	Ptosis*
Motility	Nystagmus
Lacr. App.	
Vision	
Vis. Fields	
Intraoc. Ten.	
Ant. Segm. and Sclera	Miosis*
Ocul. Media	
Retina and Choroid	
Optic Nerve	*Horner's syndrome

OTHER CLINICAL FINDINGS:
1. Hemiparesis (contralateral)
2. Disturbance of sensibility (contralateral side of lesion)
3. Cerebellar hemiataxia (side of lesion)
4. Perhaps ipsilateral analgesia of the face, vocal chord and soft palate
5. Adiadochokinesis, lateral pulsion, dysmetria, (possible)

BIBLIOGRAPHY:
1. Babinski, J. F. F. and Nageotte, J.: Hémiasynergie, latéropulsion et myosis bulbaires avec hémianesthésie et hémiplégie crosées, Rev. neurol. (Paris) *10:*358, 1902.
2. Jaffe, N. S.: Localization of lesions causing Horner's syndrome, Arch. Ophth. *44:*710, 1950.
3, Hiller, F.: The vascular syndromes of the basilar and vertebral arteries and their branches, J. Nerv. & Ment. Dis., *116:*988, 1952.
4. Walsh, F. B.: *Clinical Neuro-Ophthalmology,* 2nd Ed., Baltimore, The Williams and Wilkins Co., 1957.

SYNDROME: Balint
SYNONYMS: Psychic paralysis of visual fixation syndrome
GEN. INFORMATION:
Bilateral lesion of the parieto-occipital region. The disease is rare. Relapses or remissions occur. Patients with this syndrome are unaware of objects otherwise familiar to them (Saraux et al.).

OCULAR FINDINGS:

Orbit	
Lids	
Motility	Psychic paralysis of visual fixation. Lack of full voluntary control of eye movements while random movements are normal. Oculomotor apraxia (Cogan and Adams)
Lacr. App.	
Vision	
Vis. Fields	
Intraoc. Ten.	
Ant. Segm. and Sclera	
Ocul. Media	
Retina and Choroid	
Optic Nerve	

OTHER CLINICAL FINDINGS:
1. Tonic and motor phenomena of upper limbs
2. Loss of body coordination (bilateral)
3. Optic ataxia

BIBLIOGRAPHY:
1. Balint, R.: Seelenlähmung des Schauens, optische Ataxie, räumliche Störung der Aufmerksamkeit, Mschr. Psychiat. Neurol. 25:51, 1909.
2. Holmes, G.: Looking and seeing, movements and fixations of the eye, Irish J. Med. Sc. 129:34. 1936.
3. Hécaen. H. and de Ajuriaguerra, J.: Balint's syndrome and its minor forms, Brain, 77:373, 1954.
4. Saraux, H., Esteve, P.; Graveleau, O. and Goupil, H.: Syndrome de Balint et apraxie oculo-motrice, Ann. Oculist. (Paris.) 195:456, 1962.
5. Cogan, D. G. and Adams, R. D.: A type of paralysis of conjugate gaze (ocular moter apraxia), Arch. Ophth. 71: 489, 1964.

SYNDROME: Barré-Liéou
SYNONYMS: Posterior cervical sympathetic syndrome
GEN. INFORMATION:
Irritation of the vertebral nerve causing circulatory disturbance in the area of the cranial nuclei. 5th and 8th nerve mainly involved. Trauma and arthritic changes involving 3rd and 4th crevical vertebrae may cause these symptoms. Cervical disk pathology may also be an etiological factor. The course is usually chronic, though some improvement may be seen. Occurrence more frequently in older patients. Trauma to the cervical spine has been found to be a cause of the clinical symptoms.

OCULAR FINDINGS:

Orbit	
Lids	Twitching of upper lid*
Motility	
Lacr. App.	
Vision	Reduced vision (transitory)
Vis. Fields	
Intraoc. Ten.	
Ant. Segm. and Sclera	
Ocul. Media	Corneal hypesthesia in association with persistant corneal ulcers confined to the lid fissure. This complication occurs mainly in association with chronic cervical arthritis when this is the cause of the symspathetic irritation.
Retina and Choriod	
Optic Nerve	

OTHER CLINICAL FINDINGS:
1. Headache, vertigo, mild dizziness
2. Vasomotor disturbances of face and facial pain
3. Laryngeal and pharyngeal paresthesia
4. Chronic cervical arthritis
5. Ear noises are frequent
6. Anxiety, depression
7. Impaired memory
8. Difficulty in thinking
9. Pain with movement of the neck

*Single observation

BIBLIOGRAPHY:
1. Barré, J. A.: Chronic vertebral arthritis and medullar disturbances; chronic vertebral arthritis and tumor of spinal cord, Paris med. 2:226, 1925.
2. Viallefont, H.: Ocular manifestations of the posterior cervical sympathetic syndrome, Arch. d'Opht. 50:630, 1933.
3. Roger, H.: Posterior cervical sympathetic syndrome of Barré-Liéou in traumatism of the cervical cord, Rev. oto-neuro-ophthl. 24:32, 1952

SYNDROME: Bassen-Kornzweig
SYNONYMS: A-ß-Lipoproteinemia
GEN. INFORMATION:

Genetically determined inability to absorb and transport lipids. Inherited most likely as an autosomal recessive gene.

Lab findings: Reduction of total serum lipids and serum phospholipids. Histologic examination of biopsies of the small intestinal mucosa has revealed in all instances unusual cytoplasm of the columnar cells covering the villi (Salt et al.), Cerebrospinal fluid protein usually elevated.

OCULAR FINDINGS:

Orbit	
Lids	Ptosis (may be present)*
Motility	Nystagmus, progressive external ophthalmoplegia*
Lacr. App.	
Vision	
Vis. Fields	
Intraoc. Ten.	
Ant. Segm. and Sclera	
Ocul. Media	
Retina and Choroid	Retinitis pigmentosa (usually atypical). The retinopathy is usually clinically not observable below the age of 10 to 14 years, but rather develops with age
Optic Nerve	Optic atrophy*

OTHER CLINICAL FINDINGS:

1. Steatorrhea
2. Hypocholesteremia
3. Acanthocytosis (thorny-shaped erythrocytes)
4. Neurologic disorder with ataxia (similar to Friedreich's ataxia)
5. Areflexia
6. Babinski sign
7. Muscle weakness (facial, lingual, proximal and distal)

*Less frequent

BIBLIOGRAPHY:

1. Bassen, F. E. and Kornzweig, A. L.: Malformation of the erythrocytes in a case of atypical retinitis pigmentosa, Blood, 5:381, 1950.
2. Salt, H. B.; Wolff, O. H.; Lloyd, J. K.; Fosbrooke, A. S.; Cameron, A. H. and Hubble, D. V.: On having no beta-lipoprotein. A syndrome comprising a-beta-lipoproteinemia, acanthocytosis and steatorrhea, Lancet, 2:325, 1960.
3. Becroft, D. M. O.; Costello, J. M. and Scott, P. J.:A-ß-Lipoproteinemia (Bassen-Kornzweig syndrome), Arch. Dis. Child. 40:40, 65.
4. Forsyth, C. L.; Lloyd, J. K. and Fosbrooke, A. S.:A-ß-Lipoproteinemia, Arch. Dis. Child. ,40:47, 1965.
5. Drachman, D. A.: Progressive external ophthalmoplegia-a finding associated with neurodegenerative disorders,—in Smith, J. L.: *Neuro-Ophthalmology,* Vol. IV, St. Louis, C. V. Mosby Co., 1968, p. 124.

SYNDROME: Batten-Mayau

SYNONYMS: Spielmeyer-Vogt Syndrome, Mayou-Batten disease, juvenile amaurotic family idiocy, cerebroretinal degeneration, pigmentary retinal lipoid neuronal heredodegeneration.

GEN. INFORMATION:

Etiology unknown, possible disturbance in lipoid metabolism, heredofamilial predisposition as a Mendelian recessive. Most common in Jewish families, but possible in any ethnic group. Onset between 5 and 8 years of life. Very poor prognosis, although quo ad vitam. Pathological findings: Cerebellar atrophy, complete destruction of all cerebellar layers. The disease may be diagnosed by demonstrating vacuoles in the lymphocytes of blood smears (3 to 40% of cells), a finding which has also been observed in lymphocytes obtained form conjunctival fluid (Norn *et al*). Vacuoles are present only in the cytoplasm, *not* in nucleus, which is of differential diagnostic importance against 'toxic vacuolation' in which vacuoles may be present in the nucleus as well.

OCULAR FINDINGS:

Orbit	
Lids	
Motility	
Lacr. App.	
Vision	Initially reduced progressive to total blindness
Vis. Fields	
Intraoc. Ten.	
Ant. Segm. and Sclera	
Ocul. Media	
Retina and Choroid	Fat deposition in the retina with gradual development of pigment disturbances resembling retinitis pigmentosa
Optic Nerve	Progressive primary optic atrophy .

OTHER CLINICAL FINDINGS:

1. Mental disturbances
2. Convulsions (later)
3. Apathy
4. Irritability
5. Ataxia, rigidity, tremor (possible)
6. Upper and lower motor neuron palsies
7. Terminal: complete paralysis and dementia
8. Rigidity

BIBLIOGRAPHY:

1. Batten, F.E. and Mayou, M.S.: Family cerebral degeneration with macular changes. Proc. Roy. Soc. Med. (Sect. Ophth) *8*:70, 1914.
2. Spielmeyer, W.: Ueber familiäre amaurotische Idiotien, Neurol. Zentralblatt *24*:620, 1905.
3. Vogt, H.: Ueber familiäre amaurotische Idiotie und verwandte Krankheitsbilder, Mschr. f. Psychiat. Neurol. *18*:161, 1905.
4. Hoffman, J.: Pigmentary retinal lipoid neuronal heredodegeneration (Spielmeyer-Vogt disease), neuro-ophthalmologic consideration, A. J. O., *42*:15, 1956.
5. Norn, M. S.: Vacuolated lymphocytes in the conjunctival fluid in juvenile amaurotic idiocy (Spielmeyer-Vogt's Lipoidosis), Acta Ophth. *42*:50, 1964.

4

SYNDROME: Behçet
SYNONYMS: Dermatostomato-ophthalmic syndrome, oculobuccogenital syndrome
GEN. INFORMATION:
Virus infection? The disease occurs in adults. It is a chronic disease, complete remission is rare. Pathological findings: multiple lesions with predilection of hypothalamus and brain stem in patients with CNS involvement. Laboratory tests have shown that in most patients with this syndrome the average value for riboflavin in the blood was lower than normal (6.5 vs 9.4% respectively). Histological evidence has been given that all lesions invoved have a common feature: fibrinoid degeneration of connective tissue and blood vessels, and excessive reformation of collagen fibers in later stages. Neurologic complications have been quoted with 10 to 25% of patients.

OCULAR FINDINGS:

Orbit	
Lids	
Motility	Muscle palsies (occasional), nystagmus (occasional)
Lacr. App.	
Vision	Gradual loss of vision with occasional complete blindness
Vis. Fields	
Intraoc. Ten.	
Ant. Segm. and Sclera	Conjunctivitis, hypopyon, iritis, recurrent uveitis, keratoconjunctivitis sicca
Ocul. Media	Keratitis, vitreous hemorrhages, vitreous degeneration
Retina and Choroid	Thrombophlebitis retinal veins (occasional), retinal hemorrhages, necrotic, degenerative, productive, and edematous lesions of retinal vessels may histologically be present
Optic Nerve	

OTHER CLINICAL FINDINGS:
1. Aphthous lesions of mucous membranes of the mouth and genitalia
2. Symptoms of CNS (cerebellar signs, convulsions, paraplegia)-occasional
3. Skin erythema (multiforme, bullosum)
4. Arthritis (occasional)
5. Urethritis
6. Glossitis
7. Increase in mucoprotein in blood plasma
8. Recurrent fever
9. Pleocytosis of cerebrospinal fluid

BIBLIOGRAPHY:
1. Behçet, H.. Über rezidivierende, aphthöse, durch ein Virus verursachte Geschwüre am Mund, am Auge und an den Genitalien, Derm. Wschr. *105:* 1152, 1937
2. Gray, G. S.: The triple complex syndrome of Behçet, Canad. M. A. J., *62:*597, 1950.
3. Eguchi, K.: Kato, T.; and Ujihara, H.: Metabolism of riboflavin in the Behçet's syndrome and other similar diseases, Jap. J. Ophth. *1:*22, 1957.
4. Kato, T.: A clinical study on Behçet's syndrome, Jap. J. Ophth. *2:*122, 1958.
5. Shikano, S.: A histopathological study on Behçet disease, Jap. J. Ophth *5:*54, 1961.
6. Wolf, S. M.; Schotland, D. L.; and Phillips, L. L.: Involvement of nervous system in Behçet's syndrome, Arch. Neurol. *12:*315, 1965.

SYNDROME: Behr
SYNONYMS: Optic atrophy-ataxia syndrome
GEN. INFORMATION:
Infantile form of heredofamilial optic atrophy and hereditary ataxia. Autosomal recessive. Regular dominant transmission in one family was observed by van Bogaert and André van Leeuwen (Bull. Acad. méd. belg. 7:218, 1942). Syndrome is rare. Temporary progression which after some years leads to a static condition. Both sexes are equally affected though the transmission of pure hereditary optic atrophy shows marked predominance of males. The spinocerebellar lesions characteristic of the hereditary ataxias show extensions to the hypothalamic and striatal level.

OCULAR FINDINGS:

Orbit	
Lids	
Motility	Nystagmus
Lacr. App.	
Vision	Central scotoma and occasional findings of peripheral field defects. Generally reduced vision related to the degree of optic atrophy
Vis. Fields	
Intraoc. Ten.	
Ant. Segm.	
and Sclera	
Ocul. Media	
Retina and	
Choroid	
Optic Nerve	Severe progressive temporal atrophy of the optic nerve. Bilateral retrobulbar neuritis. Symmetrical degeneration of both papillomacular bundles has been described (André-van Leeuwen and van Bogaert)

OTHER CLINICAL FINDINGS:
1. Pyramidal tract signs (increased tendon reflexes and positive Babinski sign)
2. Ataxia and disturbance of coordination
3. Mental deficiency
4. Vesical sphincter muscle weakness
5. Muscular hypertonia
6. Clubfoot

BIBLIOGRAPHY:
1. Behr, C.; Die komplizierte, hereditärfamiliäre Optikusatrophie des Kindesalters; ein bisher nicht beschriebener Symptomenkomplex, KI. Mbl. Augenhk, 47:138, 1909.
2. Franceschetti, A.: Le syndrome de Behr ses rapports avec la maladie de Leber et les hérédoataxies, Ophthalmologica, 107:17, 1944.
3. André-van Leeuwen, M. and van Bogaert, L.: Hereditary ataxia with optic atrophy of the retrobulbar neuritis type, and latent pallido luysian degeneration, Brain, 2:340, 1949.
4. François, J.: Heredity in Ophthalmology, St. Louis, C. V. Mosby Co., 1961.

SYNDROME: Benedikt
SYNONYMS: Tegmental syndrome
GEN. INFORMATION:
Lesion of the inferior nucleus ruber with obstruction of the third nerve. Arteriosclerotic occlusion of branches of the basilar artery, trauma and hemorrhages in the mid-brain, and neoplasm most common causes. Infiltrating tumors of the brain stem may cause fascicular lesions and involvement of infranuclear, nuclear and supranuclear structures. With the multiple involvement as frequently caused by nasopharyngeal tumors or glioma of the pons, the 6th and 7th nerve may become more often affected than the 3rd or 4th.

OCULAR FINDINGS:

Orbit	
Lids	
Motility	Paralysis oculomotor nerve (III) (homolateral), involves associated movements of convergence, elevation and depression of the eyes
Lacr. App.	
Vision	
Vis. Fields	
Intraoc. Ten.	
Ant. Segm. and Sclera	
Ocul. Media	
Retina and Choroid	
Optic Nerve	

OTHER CLINICAL FINDINGS:
1. Unilateral hyperkinesis
2. Paresis contralateral extremities
3. Coarse tremor contralateral upper extremity (greatly increased during movement)
4. Hemihypoesthesia
5. Absent deep sensibility
6. Ipsilateral ataxia

(contralateral side)

BIBLIOGRAPHY:
1. Benedikt, M.: Tremblement avec paralysie croiséè du moteur oculaire commune, Bull. méd,. Paris, *3:*547, 1889.
2. Walsh, F. B.: *Clinical Neuro-Ophthalmology,* 2nd Ed., Baltimore, The Williams & Wilkins Co., 1957.
3. Alfano, J. E.: Clinical lesions of the oculomotor nerve. III. Med. J. *112:*12 1957.
4. Waltman, S. R.: Ocular signs in mid-brain disease; (in Goy, A. J. and Burde, R. M. (eds.): Clinical Concepts in Neuro-Ophthalmology, Internat. Ophth. Clinics 7:807, 1967.

SYNDROME: Bielschowsky-Lutz-Cogan
SYNONYMS: Internuclear ophthalmoplegia
GEN. INFORMATION:

The syndrome is caused by a lesion in the medial longitudinal fasciculus. Cogan has demonstrated that the lesion is homolateral to the paralized internal rectus muscle. In his classification; (1) anterior internuclear ophthalmoplegia consists of paresis of convergence with paresis of homolateral int. rect. during lateral gaze toward opposite side of the lesion. (2) in posterior internuclear ophthalmoplegia convergence is *not* affected, while the homolateral int. rect. muscle is paralytic on lateral gaze. In Lutz's classification, the posterior internuclear ophthalmoplegia showed paralysis of one external rectus muscle only. Orlowski *et al.* have pointed to the complexities of the findings due to the extent of the disturbed functions of the medial longitudinal fasciculus.

OCULAR FINDINGS:

Orbit	
Lids	
Motility	Unilateral or bilateral palsy of the internal rectus muscle during conjugate lateral gaze but with or without normal function of this muscle during convergence, depending on the type of internuclear ophthalmoplegia (See: Gen. Inf. above). Dissociated nystagmus in the maximal abducted contralateral eye. The symptoms are caused by interruption of the medial longitudinal fasciculus connecting the nuclei of III, IV and VI
Lacr. App.	
Vision	
Vis. Fields	
Intraoc. Ten.	
Ant. Segm. **and Sclera**	
Ocul. Media	
Retina and **Choroid**	
Optic Nerve	

OTHER CLINICAL FINDINGS:
BIBLIOGRAPHY:

1. Bielschowsky, A.: Die Innervation der Musculi recti interni als Seitenwender. Ber. Deutsch. Ophth. Gesell., *30*:164, 1902.
2. Lutz, A.: Ueber die Bahnen der Blickwendung und deren Dissoziierung. Klin. Mbl. Augenhk. *70*:213, 1923.
3. Lutz, A.: Ueber einseitige Ophthalmoplegia internuclear is anterior. Graefes Arch. Ophth. *115*:695, 1925.
4. Cogan, D. G.; Kubik, C. S. and Smith, L.: Unilateral internuclear ophthalmoplegia: Report of eight clinical cases with one postmortem study, Arch. Ophth. *44*:783, 1950.
5. Cogan. D. G.: *Neurology of the Ocular Muscles, 2nd* Ed. Springfield, Charles C Thomas, 1956.
6. Orlowski, W. J.; Slomski, P. and Wojtowicz, St.: Bielschowsky-Lutz-Cogan Syndrome, Am. J.; Ophth. *59*:416, 1965

SYNDROME: Bloch-Sulzberger
SYNONYMS: Incontinentia pigmenti
GEN. INFORMATION:

Virus infection of the mother during pregnancy? Has been described as a familial disorder affecting primarily the ectoderm (Ref. 5). Manifestations are present at birth or shortly afterwards. The syndrome is almost exclusively found in females. Ocular defects occur in about 25% of patients with incontinentia pigmenti.

OCULAR FINDINGS:

Orbit	Orbital mass (metastatic ophthalmia-(Kawamura, 1954); retrolental fibroplasia, not identical with that seen after 'hyperoxia' in premature babies! (Ref. 5)-(Uebel, 1950; Watanabe, 1954); pseudo-glioma-(Bloch-Sulzberger, Franceschetti, Jadassohn, 1954)
Motility	Nystagmus (Huber, 1932),* strabismus
Lacr. App.	
Vision	
Vis. Fields	
Intraoc. Ten.	
Ant. Segm. and Sclera	Blue sclera (Sulzberger and Bloom, 1948)*
Ocul. Media	Cataract
Retina and Choroid	Pseudoglioma
Optic Nerve	Atrophy, papillitis *Single observations

OTHER CLINICAL FINDINGS:
1. Skin pigmentation in lines and whorls, usually preceded by inflammatory skin eruptions, though skin pigmentation may occur also without inflammation.
2. Alopecia in females
3. Dental anomalies with incomplete dentation

BIBLIOGRAPHY:

1. Bloch, B.: Eigentümliche bisher nicht beschriebene Pigment affection, Schweiz. med. Wschr. 7:404, 1926.
2. Sulzberger, M. B.: Ueber eine bisher nicht beschriebene congenitale Pigmentanomalie (incontinentia pigmenti), Arch. Derm. & Syph. (Berlin) 154: 19, 1928.
3. Findley, G. H.: On the pathogenesis of incontinentia pigmenti, Brit. J. Dermat., 64:141, 1952.
4. Harber, H.: The Bloch-Sulzberger syndrome, Brit. J. Dermat., 64:129, 1952.
5. Scott, J. G.; Friedmann, A. J.; Chitters, M. and Pepler, W. J.: Ocular changes in Bloch-Sulzberger syndrome (incontinentia pigmenti). Brit. J. Ophth. 39:276, 1955.
6. Lieb, W. A.: and Guerry, D.: Fundus changes in incontinentia pigmenti, A. J. O., 45:265, 1958.
7. Zweifach, P. H.: Incontinentia pigmenti: Its association with retinal dysplasia, Am. J. Ophth. 62:716, 1966.

SYNDROME: Bogorad
SYNONYMS: Paroxysmal lacrimation syndrome, crocodile tear syndrome
GEN. INFORMATION:
The syndrome often appears subsequent to facial palsy, but only if the lesion is located proximally to the geniculate ganglion (Ford: Arch. Neurol. & Psychiat., 1933,), during regeneration, fibers supposed to reinnervate the sublingual and submandibullar glands are in part interchanged with fibers innervating the lacrimal gland, hence, gustatory stimulation causes lacrimation. The syndrome has been observed after surgical complication (Boyer and Gardner: Arch. Neurol. & Psychiat., 1949), in Hunt's syndrome (Ford and Woodhall: Arch. Surg. 1938) and in vascular diseases.

OCULAR FINDINGS:

Orbit	
Lids	
Motility	
Lacr. App.	Unilateral lacrimation while eating or drinking due to misdirected nerve fibre regeneration
Vision	
Vis Fields	
Intraoc. Ten.	
Ant. Segm.	
and Sclera	
Ocul. Media	
Retina and	
Choroid	
Optic Nerve	

OTHER CLINICAL FINDINGS:
1. Excessive salivation (occasionally)
2. Diffuse facial muscle response or facial contracture may be associated with the lacrimation. It may occur when impulses formerly directed toward certain muscle groups are now widely distributed to various facial muscles (Gorlin *et al.*)

BIBLIOGRAPHY:
1. Bogorad, F. A.: Symptoms of Crocodile Tears, Vrăcu. delo. *11:*1328, 1928.
2. Russin, L. A.: Paroxysmal lacrimation during eating as a sequel of facial palsy: syndrome of crocodile tears, J. A. M. A.; *113:*(Part 2) 2310, 1939.
3. McGovern, F. H.: Paroxysmal lacrimation during eating following recovery from facial paralysis: Syndrome of Crocodile Tears, Am. J. Ophth. *23:*1388, 1954.
4. Chorobski, J.: Arch. Neurol. & Psychiat. *65:*299, 1951.
5. Gorlin, R. J. and Pindborg, J. J.: *Syndromes of the head and neck,* New York, McGraw-Hill Book. Co. (Blakiston Division), 1962.

43

SYNDROME: Bonnet-Dechaume-Blanc
SYNONYMS: Neuroretinoangiomatosis syndrome, Wyburn-Mason syndrome, Cerebroretinal arteriovenous aneurysm syndrome

GEN. INFORMATION:
Congenital manifestations. The condition is dominant. Unilateral or bilateral arteriovenous aneurysm of the midbrain with ipsilateral retinal angioma and skin nevi. The severity and extent of symptoms depends on the location of the cerebral aneurysm and the structures it may involve. When the abnormal vessels accompanying the aneurysm extend anteriorly from the midbrain they interfere with the optic tract on the affected side and tend to produce atrophy and gliosis. The incidence of intracranial arteriovenous aneurysm in cases where a similar lesion has been found in the retina is given with approximal 80% and in about 75% of established intracranial arteriovenous aneurysms a retinal aneurym can be expected. Differential diagnosis:Sturge-Weber syndrome, von Hippel-Lindau syndrome

OCULAR FINDINGS:

Orbit	Exophthalmos
Lids	Ptosis
Motility	Strabismus, nystagmus
Lacr. App.	
Vision	Loss of vision (any degree)
Vis. Fields	Hemianopsia due to lesion in optic tract or pulvinar
Intraoc. Ten.	
Ant. Segm. and Sclera	Reduced corneal reflex, sluggish pupils, anisocoria or other disturbances in pupil reaction
Ocul. Media	
Retina and Choroid	Retinal arteriovenous aneurysm, varicosity of retinal veins
Optic Nerve	Arteriovenous angiomas, papilledema and possible optic atrophy

OTHER CLINICAL FINDINGS:
1. Arteriovenous angiomas of the thalamus and mesencephalon
2. Facial vascular and pigmented naevi, usually in the trigeminal distribution
3. Psychic disturbances
4. Slow and scanning speech
5. Hydrocephalus
6. Headache, dizziness
7. Nausea, vomiting
8. Hemiplegia
9. Abnormal tendon reflexes.
10. A wide variety of neurological symptoms may be present.

BIBLIOGRAPHY:
1. Bonnet, P.; Dechaume, J. and Blanc, E.: L'anévrisme cirsoïde de la retine (anévrisme racémeux); ses relations avec l'anévrisme cirsoïde de la face et l'anévrisme cirsoïde du cerveau, Bull. et Mém. Soc. franc. d'opht. *51*:521, 1938; ibid. J. de méd. de Lyon, *18*:165, 1937.
2. Wyburn-Mason, R.: Arteriovenous aneurysm of mid-brain and retina, facial naevi and mental changes, Brain, *66*:163, 1943.
3. Fischgold, H.; Bregeat, P.; LeBesnerais, Y. and David, M.: Iconographie de l'angiomatose neurorétinienne (Syndrome de Bonnet, Dechaume et Blanc), Presse méd., *60*:1790, 1952.

SYNDROME: Bonnevie-Ullrich
SYNONYMS: Ullrich-Bonnevie syndrome, pterygolymphangiectasia syndrome
GEN. INFORMATION:
The syndrome occurs congenital. A hereditary factor has not been established. Etiology is not known. Females are more frequently affected (4:1). Whereas Ullrich pointed especially to the lymphangiectatic edema of feet and hands present at birth and subsiding during the first three years of life, this congenital feature has subsequently been mentioned only occasionally (Barlow and Levin). It has been suggested that this syndrome might be the same as the one described by Turner and Albright. This viewpoint has been expressed by Ullrich (1949) himself for the bilateral form of this condition, while the etiology of the asymmetric distribution explained by Bonnevie's 'wandering bleb mechanism' typifies these syndromes as to be different (Ref. 3) (See Turner's syndrome).

OCULAR FINDINGS:

Orbit	
Lids	Epicanthus, ptosis
Motility	Ocular paralyses
Lacr. App.	Caruncula lacrimalis and tear glands may be absent
Vision	
Vis. Fields	
Intraoc. Ten.	
Ant. Segm. and Sclera	
Ocul. Media	Congenital cataracts
Retina and Choroid	
Optic Nreve	

OTHER CLINICAL FINDINGS:
1. Hyperelastic skin
2. Cutaneous folds between mastoid and acromeon (Pterygium colli)
3. Cubitus valgus
4. Hypertrichosis
5. Facial paralysis
6. Edema of neck and limbs, mainly hands and feet
7. Skeletal abnormalities and retardation of growth
8. Ear deformities
9. Muscular hypotrophy

BIBLIOGRAPHY:
1. Ullrich, O.: Über typische Kombinationsbilder multipler Abartungen, Ztschr. f. Kinderhk. *49:*271, 1930.
2. Bonnevie, K.: J. Exp. Zool. *67:*443, 1934; ibid:Erbarzt, *2:*145, 1936.
3. Ullrich, O.: Turner's syndrome and Status Bonnevie-Ullrich, Am. J. Hum. Gen. *1:*179, 1949.
4. Keay, A. J. and Lewis, I. C.: The Bonnevie-Ullrich syndrome, Arch. Dis. Childh. *29:*424, 1954.
5. Barlow, J. and Levin, S. E.: Symmetrical form of status Bonnevie-Ullrich (Turner's syndrome), Brit. Med. J. *1:*890, 1955.
6. Stempfel, R. S., Jr.: Abnormalities of sexual differentiation, in:Gardner, L. I. (Edit.) *Endocrine and Genetic Diseases of Childhood,* Philadelphia, W. B. Saunders Co., 1969.

SYNDROME: Bourneville
SYNONYMS: Tuberous sclerosis, epiloia (Sherlock)
GEN. INFORMATION:
Heredofamilial. Transmitted as an irregular dominant. Although penetrance of gene is high, its power of expression may be very vaiable. Occurs usually in childhood but sometimes in adulthood. More frequent in females. Most patients die before age 24. Prognosis is poor. Institutional care is necessary. X-ray findings: nodules or masses demonstrable in ventriculograms. Sclerotic patches mainly on the surface on the lateral ventricles. Enlarged and sclerotic convolutions. Abnormal EEG (87%)

OCULAR FINDINGS:

Orbit	
Lids	
Motility	
Lacr. App.	
Vision	
Vis. Fields	
Intraoc. Ten.	Glaucoma (Renard)
Ant. Segm, and Sclera	Small pediculate whitish-gray tumors on palpebral conjunctiva (Luo)
Ocul. Media	Vitreous often cloudy, lens opacities, corneal opacities with subepithelial vascularization (Thomas et al.)
Retina and Choroid	Mushroom-like tumor of grayish-white color, yellowish-white plaques with small hemorrhages and cystic changes. Tumors derive from nerve fiber layer, occasionally from ganglion cell layer. (Histol.: most part fibrils, large round irregular cells with large nucleus and nucleolus.) Angioid streaks (single findings)
Optic Nerve	Involved in retinal changes. Papilledema as part of an intracranial hypertension syndrome. Sheets of glial tissue at the disc-Drusen

OTHER CLINICAL FINDINGS:
1. Epilepsy (manifest first 2 years of life) (grand mal, petit mal, Jacksonian)-93%
2. Mental changes from feeblemindedness to imbecility and idiocy-62%
3. Neurologic symptoms (simian hand, shortness and incurving little finger, misshaped ears, etc.)
4. Skin changes arranged usually about nose and cheeks (adenoma sebaceum) (diagnostic value)-83%
5. Congenital tumors of kidney (hypernephroma or tubular adenoma) and heart (rhabdomyoma)-53%
6. Spina bifida

BIBLIOGRAPHY:
1. Bourneville, D.: Contribution a l'étude de l'idiotie sclerose tubereuse des circonvulsions cerebrales: idiotie et epilepsie hemiplegique, Arch. Neurol. (Paris) 1:69, 1880/81.
2. Luo, E. H.: Conjunctival lesions in tuberous sclerosis, A. J. O., 23:1029, 1940.
3. Ross, A.; and Dickerson, W.: Tuberous sclerosis, Arch. Neurol. and Psychiat., 50:233, 1943.
4. Ballantyne, A. J. and Michaelson, I. C.: The Fundus of the Eye, Edinburgh, E. & S. Livingstone Ltd., 1962.

SYNDROME: Cartilaginous-arthritic-ophthalmic-deafness syndrome
SYNONYMS:
GEN. INFORMATION:
Etiology unknown. Only single observation has been reported. The arthritic changes differed from those present in rheumatoid arthritis in so far that there was little or no damage to the joint surfaces and no ankylosis. Onset of symptoms at the end of the sixth decade of life.

OCULAR FINDINGS:

Orbit	
Lids	
Motility	
Lacr. App.	
Vision	Progressive loss of vision
Vis. Fields	
Intraoc. Ten.	Hypotony may develop
Ant. Segm. and Sclera	Iridocyclitis with posterior synechiae, iris atrophy, scleritis
Ocul. Media	Cataract, keratitis
Retina and Choroid	
Optic Nerve	

OTHER CLINICAL FINDINGS:
1. Deafness
2. Rheumatoid arthritis (no ankylosis)
3. Multiple joint dislocation due to laxity of joint capsules
4. Hypertrophy as well as atrophy and degeneration of cartilage (particulary obvious on nose, ears, sternum and ribs)

BIBLIOGRAPHY:
1. Hilding, A. C.: Syndrome of cartilage pathology, destructive iridocyclitis, multiple joint dislocation: comparison with concurrent eye and joint diseases described in literature, Arch. Ophth., *48:*420, 1952.
2. Godfredsen, E.: Pathogenesis of concurrent eye and joint diseases, Brit. J. Ophth. *33:*261, 1949.

47

SYNDROME: Carotid artery-cavernous sinus fistula
SYNONYMS:
GEN. INFORAMTION:
Trauma is causing such fistula in about 75% with the remainder occurring spontaneously. Traumatic cases are seen more often in men and usually the defect is on the right. Spontaneous cases occur more frequently in women. Poor prognosis without treatment, except in cases where thrombosis of fistula provides permanent remission. Due to their anatomic position, the cranial nerves (II to VI) are frequently involved. The ophthalmic vein is greatly dilated. Differential diagnosis: Foix syndrome. X-ray examination shows erosions of the sella turcica, sphenoid, orbital walls. Arteriorgraphy may prove the fistula or aneurysm.

OCULAR FINDINGS:

Orbit	Progressive and usually pulsating exophthalmos. Exophthalmos on the contralateral side to the fistula may occur though its onset may vary within wide ranges. Distended pulsating superior orbital vein may be seen above the medial canthus
Lids	Veinous congestion
Motility	Ophthalmoplegia (to a varibale degree) depending on the extent of cranial nerve (II to VI) involvement
Lacr. App.	
Vision	
Vis. Fields	
Intraoc. Ten.	Secondary glaucoma in advanced cases
Ant. Segm. and Sclera	Congestion and thickening of the conjunctiva with severe chemosis
Ocul. Media	Corneal ulcerations due to exposure in the presence of severe conjunctival edema eversion of the lower lid and inability to close the eye. Loss of corneal sensation if Vth cranial nerve is involved intracranially
Retina and Choroid	Edema, engorgement of retinal veins, hemorrhages
Optic Nerve	Papilledema based on inadequate veinous drainage and usually of low grade. Optic atrophy in long standing cases.

OTHER CLINICAL FINDINGS:
1. Severe unilateral headache often preceding the exophthalmos
2. Buzzing noise experienced by patient in his head which disappears by compression of the involved carotid artery: In long-standing fistula this sign may fail due to compensatory circulatory channels which may have opened
Note: pulsating exophthalmos and bruits can be present in many other disease entities: The ocular findings vary considerably from one case to another

BIBLIOGRAPHY:
1. Abrahamson, J. and Bell, L.: Carotid-cavernous-fistula syndrome, A. J. O., *39*:521, 1955.
2. Dailey, E. J.; Holloway, J. A.; Murto, R. E. and Schlezinger, N. S.: Evaluation of ocular signs and symptoms in cerebral aneurysms, Arch. Ophth. *71*:463, 1964.
3. Hamby, W. B. and Dohn, D. F.: Carotid-cavernous fistulas: Report on thirty-six cases and discussion of their management, Clin. Neurosurg. *11*:150, 1964.
4. Lombardi, G.: *Radiology in Neuro-Ophthalmology,* Baltimore, The Williams & Wilkins Co., 1967, p. 48.

SYNDROME: Central nervous system deficiency
SYNONYMS:
GEN. INFORMATION:

Degenerative process with unknown etiology (dietary deficiency?). There is almost no improvement after normal diet is resumed. Mainly observed in prisoners who had long been on a deficient diet. No specific vitamin deficiency was found. Apparently no improvement of vision after return to normal diet.

OCULAR FINDINGS:

Orbit	
Lids	
Motility	
Lacr. App.	
Vision	Greatly reduced vision, particularly near vision, increasing over weeks or months but rarely progressing to complete blindness
Vis. Fields	Relative or absolute central or paracentral scotomata
Intraoc. Ten.	
Ant. Segm. and Sclera	
Ocul. Media.	
Retina and Choroid	
Optic Nerve	Bitemporal pallor of the discs

OTHER CLINICAL FINDINGS:
1. Incomplete bilateral deafness, never proceeding to complete deafness
2. Tinnitus
3. Numbness and tingling in the legs, rarely in the hands.
4. Loss of vibratory sense from pelvis downwards
5. Unsteadiness of gait in more severe cases.
6. Loss of postural sense in the toes
7. Abnormal tendon reflexes (both hyperactive or absent)
8. Laryngeal palsies and mental deterioration (Spillane and Scott)

BIBLIOGRAPHY:
1. Wilkinson, P. B. and King, A.: Amblyopia due to vitamin deficiency. Lancet, *1:528*, 1944.
2. Spillane, J. D. and Scott, G. I.: Obscure neuropathy in the middle east: Report on 112 cases in prisoners-of-war, Lancet, *2:261*, 1945.
3. Garland, H. G. : A central nervous deficiency syndrome, Proc. Roy. Soc. Med., *39:178*, 1946.

SYNDROME: Cestan-Chenais
SYNONYMS: Cestan's syndrome
GEN. INFORMATION:
The syndrome is a combination of Babinski-Negeotte and Avellis syndromes. Lesion in the lateral portion of the medulla oblongata. Ocular findings occur on ipsilateral side of lesion. Pathological findings: thrombosis of vertebral artery toward the medial side in relation to the posterior inferior cerebellar and anterior spinal branches.

OCULAR FINDINGS:

Orbit	Enophthalmos*
Lids	Ptosis*
Motility	Nystagmus
Lacr. App.	
Vision	
Vis. Fields	
Intraoc. Ten.	
And. Segm. and Sclera	Miosis*
Ocul. Media	
Retina and Choroid	
Optic Nerve	

OTHER CLINICAL FINDINGS:
1. Pharyngolaryngeal or glossopharyngeal paralysis (Avellis' syndrome), with lesion involving the nucleus ambiguus and spinothalmic tract.
2. Cerebellar hemiataxia ⎫ contralateral side of lesion
3. Disturbance of sensibility ⎭

*Horner's syndrome
BIBLIOGRAPHY:
1. Cestan, R. and Chenais, L.: Du myosis dans certaines lésions bulbaries en foyer hémiplégie du type Avellis associée au syndrome oculaire sympathique, Gaz. d. hop. 76:1229, 1903.
2. Hiller, F.: The vascular syndromes of the basilar and vertebral arteries and their branches, J. Nerv. & Ment. Dis. 116:988, 1952.

SYNDROME: Charcot-Marie-Tooth

SYNONYMS: Progressive neuritic muscular atrophy, progressive peroneal muscular atrophy

GEN. INFORMATION:

Dominant inheritance. Onset between 5 and 15 years or deferred until early middle life. The disease is very rare. Pathological findings: degeneration of muscular branches of the peroneal nerves first, followed by all motor fibers of the nerve trunks supplying the extremities. Changes in motor cells of spinal gray matter, pyramidal tracts and posterior columns. Clinically the muscular atrophy begins in the feet and legs until several years later the hands and arms become affected.

OCULAR FINDINGS:

Orbit	
Lids	
Motility	Nystagmus in all directions except vertically (Schneider and Abels)-(rare)
Lacr. App.	
Vision	Reduced if associated with optic nerve involvement
Vis. Fields	
Intraoc. Ten.	
Ant. Segm. and Sclera	Pupillary disturbances (very rare)
Ocul. Media	
Retina and Choroid	
Optic Nerve	Primary optic atrophy (rare)

OTHER CLINICAL FINDINGS:

1. Positive familial history
2. Atrophy of small muscles of hands and feet, slowly progressing to distal and then proximal arm and leg (very slow progression)
3. Fibrillary muscle twitchings (fasciculations) are common
4. Sensory disturbances may occur though they are most often absent
5. Vasomotor disturbances on distal parts of the limbs
6. Cramps are common

BIBLIOGRAPHY:

1. Charcot, J. M. and Marie, P.: Sur une forme particulière d'atrophie musculaire progressive, souvent familiale, débutant par les pieds et les jambes, et atteignant plus tard les mains, Rev. méd. 6:97, 1886.
2. Tooth, H. H.: The peroneal type of progressive muscular atrophy, London, H. L. Lewis & Co., Ltd., 1886.
3. Brodal, A.; Böyesen, S. and Frövic, A. G.: Progressive neuropathic (peroneal) muscular dystrophy (Charcot-Marie-Tooth disease); histopathological findings in muscle biopsy specimens in 14 cases, with notes on clinical diagnosis and familial occurrence, Arch. Neurol. & Psychiat. 70:1, 1953.
4. Walsh, F. B.: Clinical Neuro-Ophthalmology, 2nd Ed., The Williams & Wilkins Co., Baltimore, 1957, p. 763.

SYNDROME: Charcot-Wilbrand
SYNONYMS:
GEN. INFORMATION:
Occlusion of a portion of the posterior cerebral artery

OCULAR FINDINGS:

Orbit	
Lids	
Motility	
Lacr. App.	
Vision	Visual agnosia, loss of ability to revisualize images
Vis. Fields	
Intraoc. Ten.	
Ant. Segm. and Sclera	
Ocyl. Media	
Retina and Choroid	
Optic Nerve	

OTHER CLINICAL FINDINGS:

BIBLIOGRAPHY:
1. Charcot, J. M.: *Clinical Lectures on Diseases of the Nervous System,* Vol. III, London, The New Syndenham Society, 1889, Lects. 11-13.
2. Durham, R. H.: *Medical Syndromes,* New York, Paul B. Hoeber, Inc., 1960.
3. Tyler, H. R.: Cerebral disorders of vision, in Smith, J. L. (ed.) *Neuro-Ophthalmology,* Vol. IV, St. Louis, C. V. Mosby Co., 1968.

SYNDROME: Charlin
SYNONYMS: Nasal nerve syndrome, nasociliaris nerve syndrome
GEN. INFORMATION:
Neuritis of the nasal branch of the trigeminal nerve. Prognosis is good with therapy. Cocaine applied to the anterior ethmoidal nerve (in anterior portion of the nasal fossa) effects usually fast relief of ocular pain. The ocular pain may vary with either one or the other eye affected. There are three typical spots of pain according to the nerve distribution. (1) above and outside the nose; (2) above the inner canthus; (3) inferior angle of the medial tarsal ligament.

OCULAR FINDINGS:

Orbit	Severe ocular and orbital pain, mainly upper nasal-orbital angle: The degree of pain is in no proportion to the objective clinical ocular findings
Lids	Slight inflammatory swelling upper lid (occasional)
Motility	
Lacr. App.	
Vision	
Vis. Fields	
Intraoc. Ten.	
Ant. Segm. and Sclera	Photophobia, ciliary and conjunctival injection, pseudopurulent conjunctivitis, anterior uveitis, iritis, hypopyon
Ocul. Media	Keratitis, corneal ulcers
Retina and Choroid	
Optic Nerve	

OTHER CLINICAL FINDINGS:
1. Rhinorrhea
2. Rhinitis always on same side of the ocular involvement.
3. Severe pain of ala nasi

BIBLIOGRAPHY:
1. Charlin, C.: Le syndrome du nerf nasal, Ann. d'ocul., *168:*86, 1931.
2. Solotnitsky, I. N.: The syndrome of the nasal nerve (Charlin's symptom-complex). Acta Ophth. *14:*388, 1936.

5

SYNDROME: Chediak-Higashi
SYNONYMS: Anomalous leukocytic inclusions with constitutional stigmata
GEN. INFORMATION:
Occurs usually in albinoid siblings born of consanguinous parents. Lymphomatous development and infections resulting in early death. Typical ctyoplasmic inclusion bodies in many leucocytes An albino child with a blood dysplasia should therefore be examined keeping this possibility in mind, since the leukocytic findings are diagnostic of the syndrome. The syndrome is rare.

OCULAR FINDINGS:

Orbit	
Lids	Bilateral ptosis*
Motility	Bilateral 6th nerve palsy*
Lacr. App.	
Vision	
Vis. Fields	
Intraoc. Ten.	
Ant. Segm. and Sclera	Decreased iris pigmentation: Juvenile type ot ciliary body. Photophobia. Leukocytic inclusion bodies characteristic of the disease were found in the limbal area, iris and choroid. Anisocoria with absent pupil reaction.*
Ocul. Media	Edema of basal cells of corneal epithelium
Retina and Choroid	Small retinal vessels and decreased in number. Decreased pigmentation of choroid with immature lymphocyte infiltration
Optic Nerve	Elevated disc, papilledema

OTHER CLINICAL FINDINGS:
1. Anemia, neutropenia, thrombocytopenia
2. Recurrent infections
3. Hepatosplenomegaly
4. Lymphadenopathy
5. Oculo-cutaneous albinism
6. Xeroderma pigmentosum (single observation-Higashi)
7. Mental deficiency*

*Single case report (Donahue and Bain: Pediatrics 20:416, 1957)

BIBLIOGRAPHY:
1. Chediak, M.: Nouvelle anomalie leucocytaire de caractere constitutionale et familial, Rev. Hemat. 7:362, 1952.
2. Higashi, O.: Congenital gigantism of peroxidase granules, Tohoku J. Exp. Med. 59:315, 1954.
3. Stegmaier, O. C. and Schneider, L. A.: Chediak-Higashi syndrome, dermatologic manifestations, Arch. Derm. 91:1, 1965.
4. Johnson, D. L.; Jacobson, L. W.; Toyama, R. and Monohan, R. H.: Histopathology of eyes in Chediak-Higashi syndrome, Arch. Ophth. 75:84, 1966.

SYNDROME: Claude
SYNONYMS: Inferior nucleus ruber syndrome, rubrospinal cerebellar peduncle syndrome
GEN. INFORMATION:
Paramedian mesencephalic lesion starting in midbrain. Often occlusion of terminal branches of the paramedian arteries supplying the inferior portion of the nucleus ruber.

OCULAR FINDINGS:

Orbit	
Lids	
Motility	Paralysis ispilateral oculomotor and trochlear nerves (III, IV)
Lacr. App.	
Vision	
Vis. Fields	
Intraoc. Ten.	
Ant. Segm. and Sclera	
Ocul. Media	
Retina and Choroid	
Optic Nerve	

OTHER CLINICAL FINDINGS:
1. Ataxia contralateral limbs (occasionally)
2. Contralateral hemianesthesia

BIBLIOGRAPHY:
1. Claude, H.: Inferior nucleus ruber syndrome, Rev. neurol., *1*:311, 1912.
2. Hiller, F.: The vascular syndromes of the basilar and verteral arteries and their branches, J. Nerv. & Ment. Dis. *116*:988, 1952.

SYNDROME: Cockayne
SYNONYMS: Dwarfism wlth retinal atrophy and deafness
GEN. INFORMATION:

Autosomal recessive. Forty-seven chromosomes observed by Civantos, with an extra chromosome in the F group, interpreted as trisomy for chromosome number 20. A case with 46 chromosomes as determined by chromosomal analysis has been reported (Ref.4). Manifestations of the syndrome become apparent in the scond year ot life atter a normal infancy. Laboratory findings: nomal blood lipid levels (contrary to Gilford's progeria.) X-ray findings: marble epiphyses in some of the digits.

OCULAR FINDINGS:

Orbit	Enophthalmos ('sunken eyes')
Lids	
Motility	
Lacr. App.	
Vision	
Vis. Fields	
Intraoc. Ten.	
Ant. Segm. and Sclera	Poor pupillary response to mydriatics
Ocul. Media	Cataracts
Retina and Choroid	Pigmentary degeneration
Optic Nerve	Optic atrophy

OTHER CLINICAL FINDINGS:
1. Dwarfism (nanism) with disproportionally long limbs, large hands and feet
2. Kyphosis, deformed limbs, thickened skull
3. Intracranial calcifications
4. Mental retardation, prognathism
5. Deafness (often partial)
6. Precociously senile appearance
7. Sensitivity to sunlight with skin pigmentation and scarring
8. Hepatosplenomegaly

BIBLIOGRAPHY:
1. Cockayne, E. A.: Dwarfism with retinal atrophy and deafness, Arch. Childhood, *11*:1, 1961.
2. McKusick, V. A.: *Medical Genetics* 1958-1960 (765), St. Louis, C. V. Mosby Co., 1961.
3. Civantos, F.: Human chromosomal abnormalities, The Bull., Tulane Univ. Med. Fac., *20*:241, 1961.
4. Windmiller, J.; Whalley, P. J. and Fink, C. W.: Cockayne's syndrome with chromosomal analysis, Am. J. Dis. Child. *105*:204, 1963.

SYNDROME: Cogan
SYNONYMS: Nonsyphilitic interstitial keratitis
GEN. INFORMATION:
Etiology unknown. General hypersensitivity-reaction, systemic vascular disease (Fisher and Hellstrom: Arch. Path. 1961, a. o.), vasomotor disturbances, viral infection (Lindsay and Znidema: Laryngoscope, 1950) and several other connections with this syndrome have been reported. Young adults are most frequently affected but also older persons. The occurrence in a child (4 1/2 years) was reported by Stevens (Arch. Neurol. Psychiat., 1954). Sudden onset of manifestations is characteristic. The ocular findings are associated with vestibulo-auditory symptoms and are often bilateral. The condition extends over some months with minor variations in appearance and severity. Laboratory findings: elevated white blood cell count and mild eosinophilia may be present.

OCULAR FINDINGS:

Orbit	
Lids	Blepharospasm
Motility	
Lacr. App.	Lacrimation
Vision	Blurred vision
Vis. Fields	
Intraoc. Ten.	
Ant. Segm. **and Sclera**	Congested conjunctival vessels, subconjunctival hemorrhage. Little or no reaction in anterior chamber, but ciliary injection is present. Pain and photophobia
Ocul. Media	Interstitial keratitis (uni-or bilateral). Granular type infiltrates, patchy distribution deeper stroma. Later vascularization
Retina and **Choroid**	
Optic Nerve	

OTHER CLINICAL FINDINGS:
1. Vestibulo-auditory symptoms (similar to Ménière's syndrome)
2. Nausea, vomiting
3. Vertigo, tinnitus (abrupt onset)
4. Rapidly progressive deafness only rarely showing some improvement.
5. Loss of equilibration
6. Association with periarteritis nodosa described by Oliner

BIBLIOGRAPHY:
1. Cogan, D. G.: Syndrome of nonsyphilitic interstitial keratitis and vestibuloauditory symptoms, Arch. Ophth. *33:*144, 1945.
2. Cogan, D.: Nonsyphilitic interstitial keratitis with vestibuloauditory symptoms, Arch. Ophth., *42:*42, 1948.
3. Mogan, R. F. and Baumgartner, C. J.: Ménière's disease complicated by recurrent interstitial keratitis: Excellent results following cervical ganglionectomy, West. J. Surg. *42:*628, 1934.
4. Oliner, L.: Nonsyphilitic interstitial keratitis and bilateral deafness (Cogan's syndrome) associated with essential polyangitis (periarteritis nodosa) review of syndrome with consideration of possible pathogenic mechanism, New. Engl. J. Med., *248:*1001, 1953.
5. Eisenstein, B. and Taubenhaas, M.: Nonsyphilitic interstitial keratitis and bilateral deafness (Cogan's syndrome) associated with cardiovascular disease, New 'Engl. J. Med. *258:*1074. 1958

SYNDROME: Cone dysfunction syndrome
SYNONYMS:
GEN. INFORMATION:
Congenital male linked recessive inheritance. Male linkage with female carrier. Prognosis: stagnant, non progressive. Though there is evidence that the syndrome is due to malfunction of the general cone-system the precise nature of the defect is not completely known. Differential diagnosis: optic atrophy, albinism, cerebral pathway abnormalities, amblyopia without known etiology.

OCULAR FINDINGS:

Orbit	
Lids	
Motility	Nystagmus
Lacr. App.	
Vision	Decreased 20/50 to 20/200 or less, (1) no color vision, (2) reduced color vision, (3) rod and cone disfunction. Color vision might be affected with or without amblyopia
Vis. Fields	Peripheral field loss if rods and cones are involved
Intraoc. Ten.	
Ant. Segm. and Sclera	Photophobia
Ocul. Media	
Retina and Choroid	General fundus lesions, mainly macular involvement with depigmentation and degenerative changes. Normal number of cones in macular region with some disturbances in cone morphology has been reported by Larsen (Kl. Mbl. Augenhk. 1924), whereas Harrison *et al.* found a marked reduction in the number of cones in the retina of a ptaient with complete
Optic Nerve	achromatopsia. Absence of photopic flicker ERG

OTHER CLINICAL FINDINGS:

BIBLIOGRAPHY:
1. Goodman, G.; Ripps, H. and Siegal, I. M.: Cone dysfunction syndromes, Arch. Ophth., *70:*214, 1963.
2. Goodman, G. and Bornschein, H.: Comparative electroretinographic studies in congenital night blindness and total color blindness, Arch. Ophth., *58:* 174, 1957.
3. Harrison, R.; Haefnagel, D. and Hayward, J. N.: Congenital total color blindness: Clinicopathological report, Arch. Ophth. *64:*685, 1960.
4. Blackwell, H. R. and Blackwell, O. M.: Rod and cone receptor mechanisms in typical and atypical achromatopsia, Vision Res. *1:*62, 1961.
5. Goodman, G.; Ripps, H. and Siegel, I. M.: Sex-linked ocular disorders: Trait expressivity in males and carrier females, Arch. Ophth. *73:*387, 1965.

SYNDROME: Congenital epiblepharon-inferior oblique insufficiency
SYNONYMS:
GEN. INFORMATION:
Prognosis is good with treatment. Manifestations are present in infancy. The inversion of the lash line which occurs with epiblepharon is exaggerated by the inferior oblique insufficiency in a manner that causes the development of a spastic entropion (Swan). The condition is not rare (Swan reported 4 cases among 5000 hospital admissions). The most commonly accepted hypothesis of the pathogenesis of the epiblepharon is thought to be an anomalous muscle insertion with strands of the inferior rectus into the skin of the lower lid.

OCULAR FINDINGS:

Orbit	Narrow interpupillary distance, some ocular prominence
Lids	Epicanthus, epiblepharon exaggerated in downward gaze, spastic entropion with retroflexion of the eye lashes. Epiblepharon becomes less pronounced with growth and development. Usually bilateral but in some cases asymmetrical
Motility	Inferior oblique insufficiency usually unilateral. Generally little or no deviation except in the field of action of the affected muscle. The insuffiency is easy to overlook in infancy
Lacr. App.	Lacrimation due to conjunctival and corneal irritation
Vision	
Vis. Fields	
Intraoc. Ten.	
Ant. Segm. and Sclera	Persistant unilateral kerato-conjunctival irritation by the inverted ciliae (important sign to check for in this syndrome)
Ocul. Media	Keratitis and superficial corneal ulceration followed by corneal scarring due to retroflexion of the eye lashes (rare)
Retina and Choroid	
Optic Nerve	

OTHER CLINICAL FINDINGS:
1. Chubby cheeks

BIBLIOGRAPHY:
1. Swan, K. C.: The syndrome of congenital epiblepharon and inferior oblique insufficiency, A. J. O., *39* (S3): 130, 1954.
2. White, J. W.: A review of twenty-seven years with the obliques. Tr. Pac. Coast Oto-Ophth. Soc., *29:*112, 1941.
3. Duke-Elder, Sir Stewart: *System of Ophthalmology,* Vol. III, part 2, St. Louis, C. V. Mosby Co., 1963.

SYNDROME: Crouzon
SYNONYMS: Dysostosis cranio-facialis, oxycephaly, craniofacial dysostosis
GEN. INFORMATION:
Autosomal dominant inheritance. Manifestations are present at birth. X-ray examination reveals kyphosis basilaris, short anterior fossa, depressed middle fossa, deep occipital fossa, deep impressiones gyrorum, large sella turcica, ala parva and orbital margins very steep, shallow orbits, prematurely synostosed coronal, sagittal and lambdoidal sutures.

OCULAR FINDINGS:

Orbit	Bilateral exopthalmos (hypertelorism)** with possible luxation of the globe, wide interpupillary distance
Lids	Obliquity of palpebral fissures with outer canthus slanting downwards drooping lower lid due to relative mandibular prognathism
Motility	Nystagmus,** divergent strabismus**
Lacr. App.	Developmental abnormalities*
Vision	Loss of vision usually pronounced at age 6 to 7 years, in mild cases vision might remain good through life
Vis. Fields	Upper field defects due to anatomic changes with stretching and pressure upon the optic nerve on its lower part by entering the optic foramen
Intraoc. Ten.	
Ant. Segm. and Sclera	Sclera appears often bluish. Exposure keratitis* in extreme exophthalmos
Ocul. Media	Cataract*
Retina and Choroid	Medullated nerve fibers
Optic Nerve	Papilledema, secondary optic atrophy, optic nerve involvement (80%—Bertelsen, 1958) of differential diagnostic importance against other types of premature cranial synostoses

OTHER CLINICAL FINDINGS:
1. Prognathism
2. Maxillary hypoplasia with short upper lip**
3. Synostosis of coronal and lambda sutures**
4. Hydrocephalus internus
5. Syndactylism*
6. Short anteroposterior skull diameter
7. Parrot-beaked nose (psittacorhina)**
8. Widening temporal fossae**
9. Headaches
10. Convulsions*
11. Subnormal mentality
12. Some loss of hearing

*Less frequent   **Characteristic findings

BIBLIOGRAPHY:
1. Crouzon, O.: Dysostose cranio-faciale héréditaire, Bull. et. mém. Soc. Mde. des Hôp. Paris, *33:*545, 1912.
2. Greig, D. M.: Oxycephaly, Edinburgh M. J., *33:*189, 280, 357, 1926.
3. Mann, J.: A theory of the embryology of oxycephaly, Tr. Ophth. Soc. U. K., *55:*279, 1935.
4. Fairman, D. and Horrax, G.: Craniostenosis with notes on a modified operation for the brachycephalic form, J. Neurosurg., *6:*388, 1949.
5. Walsh, F. B.: *Clinical Neuro-Ophthalmology,* 2nd Ed., Baltimore, The Williams & Wilkins Co., 1957.
6. Gorlin, R. J. and Pindborg, J. J.: *Syndromes of the Head and Neck,* New York, Mc Graw-Hill Book Co., (Blakiston division), 1964.

SYNDROME: Cushing (1)
SYNONYMS: Adrenocortical syndrome, hyperadrenalism, pituitary basophilism, suprarenal syndrome.
GEN. INFORMATION:
Excessive secretion of adrenal cortical hormones due to primary or secondary
adrenal hyperplasia or induced by adrenal or extra-adrenal neoplastic tissue.
Multiglandular discorder. Most common in females of child bearing age. Pituitary
tumors clinically evident in 10 to 20%, characterized by aggresive growth, rapid
expansion and involving supra-and parasellar structures. 24% with pituitary
tumor develop ocular muscle palsies (*i.e.* about 2 to 4 times more frequently
than in the more common non-hormone-secretary chromophobe adenomas.)
Adrenalectomy may be followed by rapid growth of the pituitary tumor. In cases
where the syndrome is associated with pituitary tumors, more recent studies
indicate that chromophobe cells rather than basophils are involved. Though
ocular findings in the 'classical' syndrome are not frequent, their presence is of
great importance for the prognosis and management of the disease.

OCULAR FINDINGS:

Orbit	Proptosis (rare)
Lids	
Motility	Ocular muscle palsies (consequence of hemorrhagic infarction of the pituitary tumor with resultant cavernous sinus compression) and/or direct pressure or infiltration on the cavernous sinus by the expanding neoplasm.
Lacr. App.	
Vision	
Vis. Fields	Changes uncharacteristic and not necessarily of the bitemporal hemianopsia as seen with the typical chromophobe adenoma.
Intraoc. Ten.	
Ant. Segm. and Sclera	
Ocul. Media	
Retina and Choroid	
Optic Nerve	Optic nerve and/or chiasmal compression either uni-or bilateral

OTHER CLINICAL FINDINGS:
1. Hirsutism
2. Obesity-'buffalo hoop'
3. Hypertension
4. Diabetes
5. Skin pigmentation
6. Osteoparosis
7. Abdominal striae
8. Polyothemia and lymphopenia
9. Weakness
10. Nervousness, irritability
11. Dysmenorrhea
12. Increased urinary excretion of 11-oxysteroids and 17-ketosteroids

BIBLIOGRAPHY:
1. Cushing, H.: The basophil adenomas of the pituitary body and their clinical
   manifestations (pituitary basophilism), Bull. Johns Hopkins Hosp., *50:*137,
   1932.
2. Rovit, R. L. and Duane, T. D.: Eye signs in patients with Cushings Syndrome
   and pituitary tumors: Some observations related to chromophobe tumors
   and hyperadrenalism, Tr. Am. Ophth. Soc. *65:*52, 1967; Ibid: Arch Ophth.
   *79:*512, 1968.

SYNDROME: Cushing (2)
SYNONYMS: Angle tumor syndrome, cerebellopontine angle syndrome, pontocerebellar-angle tumor syndrome, acoustic neuroma syndrome.
GEN. INFORMATION:
Tumor inolving V, VI, VII, VIII cranial nerves and brain stem. Possible vascular lesion. Tumors occur in the majority of cases between 30 and 45 years of life. With the exception of the auditory nerve, which is usually completely paralyzed, the other cranial nerve palsies are frequently incomplete. Pressure upon the brain stem accounts for contralateral hemiparesis, increased reflexes and hemianesthesia. Pressure upon the cerebellum causes cerebellar signs (Walsh).

OCULAR FINDINGS:

Orbit	
Lids	Paresis orbicularis muscle (VII)
Motility	Paresis external rectus muscle (VI), mixed nystagmus with head tilt. Palsies of extraocular muscles are accounted for by increased intracranial pressure if the aqueduct of sylvius is closed by the growing tumor
Lacr. App.	
Vision	
Vis. Fields	
Intraoc. Ten.	
Ant. Segm. and Sclera	
Ocul. Media	Decreased corneal reflex, V (homolateral and early sign)
Retina and Choroid	
Optic Nerve	Bilateral papilledema (due to increased intracranial pressure)

OTHER CLINICAL FINDINGS:
1. Deafness (homolateral)
2. Labyrinth function disturbed or lost
3. Tinnitus
4. Hyperesthesia of the face
5. Facial nerve paresis, total paralysis is rare (homolateral)
6. Hoarseness
7. Difficulties in swallowing
8. Hiccoughs
9. Ataxia
10. Headaches

BIBLIOGRAPHY:
1. Cushing, H.: *Tumors of the Nervus Acusticus.* Philadelphia, W. B. Saunders Co., 1917.
2. Revilla, A. G.: Differential diagnosis of tumors of the cerebellopontile recess, Bull. Johns Hopkins Hosp. *38* (3): 187, 1948.
3. Brown, J.: Localizing cerebellar syndromes, J. A. M. A., *141*:518, 1949.
4. Tassman, J.: *The Eye Manifestations of Internal Diseases,* St. Louis, C. V. Mosby Co., 1951.
5. Walsh, F. B.: *Clinical Neuro-Ophthalmology,* Baltimore, The Williams & Wilkins Co., 1957, p. 1059.
6. Berg, E. F.: The ocular signs and symptoms of posterior fossa disorders, in Gay, A. J. and Burde, R. M.: Clinical concepts in neuro-ophthalmology, Internat. Ophth. Clinics, *7*:801, 1967.

SYNDROME: Cushing (3)
SYNONYMS: Chiasmal syndrome
GEN. INFORMATION:

Suprasellar meningioma, aneurysm in the anterior part of the circle of Willis and craniopharyngioma are the three most common lesions causing the syndrome besides primary intrasellar tumor. The syndrome occurs usually in adult patients. Possible posterior fossa lesion (Wagener and Cusick). X-ray examination shows a normal sella turcica or minimal changes in the tuberculum sellae and deformities of the clinoid process.

OCULAR FINDINGS:

Orbit	
Lids	
Motility	
Lacr. App.	
Vision	
Vis. Fields	Bitemporal hemianopsia (progressive): Visual fields at the onset of the disease usually not affected. The typical field defects may on the other hand be present long before optic atrophy becomes ophthalmoscopically visible. The fields may also be irregular instead of bitemporal and may affect one eye considerably more than the other
Ant. Segm. and Sclera	
Ocul. Media	
Retina and Choroid	
Optic Nerve	In early stages the optic disc may appear normal or only slightly pale, but later on the descending atrophy with sharp border-lined white optic disc becomes apparent.

OTHER CLINICAL FINDINGS:
BIBLIOGRAPHY:

1. Cushing, H. and Eisenhardt, L.: Meningiomas arising from tuberculum sellae, with syndrome of primary optic atrophy and bitemporal field defects combined with a normal sella turcica in middle-aged person, Arch. Ophth. *1*:1 and 168, 1929.
2. Cushing, H.: The chiasmal syndrome of primary optic atrophy and bitemporal field defects in adults with normal sella turcica, Arch. Ophth., *3*:505 and 704, 1930.
3. Wagener, H. and Cusick, P.: Chiasmal syndromes produced by lesions in posterior fossa, Arch. Ophth., *18*:887, 1937.
4. Schlezinger, N. S.; Alpers, B. J. and Weiss, B. P.: Suprasellar meningiomas associated with scotomatous field defects, Arch. Ophth. *35*:620, 1946.
5. Joy, H. H.: Suprasellar meningioma. Report of an atypical case, Am. J. Ophth. *35*:1139, 1952.
6. Lombardi, G.: *Radiology in Neuro-Ophthalmology*. Baltimore, The Williams & Wilkins Co., 1967.

SYNDROME: Dandy-Walker
SYNONYMS: Atresia of the foramen Magendie
GEN. INFORMATION:

Manifestations in infants. X-ray and pathological findings: Malformation and stenosiš of the foramina of Luschka and Magendie. Dilation of fourth ventricle. Anomaly of rostral portion of the vermis. The most frequent cause for the embryonal atresia is a bulging membrane attached to the margins of the foramen Magendie and occluding the foramens of Luschka. Depending on the elasticity and permeability of the membranes the syndrome is more or less severe. If it is more elastic it may form a diverticulum of the 4th ventricle which may herniate through the foramen magnum. If it is inelastic, the hindbrain itself may herniate (Arnold-Chiari syndrome) (Ref. 5). Since the clinical features of Dandy-Walker's syndrome, Arnold-Chiari's syndrome, cysts of the foramen of Magendie and syringomyelia are very similar, it has been suggested that they are merely expressions of the same disease, produced by failure of the outlets of the 4th ventricle to develop normally in the rhombic roof of the embryo (Gardner).

OCULAR FINDINGS:

Orbit	
Lids	Ptosis (Keet and Berman)
Motility	Sixth nerve paralysis (Keet and Berman)
Lacr. App.	
Vision	
Vis. Fields	
Intraoc. Ten.	
Ant. Segm. and Sclera	
Ocul. Media	
Retina and Choroid	
Optic Nerve	Papilledema

OTHER CLINICAL FINDINGS:
1. Hydrocephalus (varies in severity) with the enlargement of skull and thinning of the bone predominantly in occipital region
2. Loss of tendon reflexes
3. Basilar impression, scoliosis, hydromyelia

BIBLIOGRAPHY:
1. Dandy, W. E. and Blackfan, K. D.: Internal hydrocephalus. An experimental, clinical and pathological study, Am. J. Dis. Child, 8:406, 1914.
2. Dandy, W. E.: The diagnosis and treatment of hydrocephalus due to occlusions of the foramina of Magendie and Luschka, Surg. Gynec. Obstet. 32:112, 1921.
3. Walker, A. E.: A case of congenital atresia of the foramina of Luscka and Magendie. Surgical cure, J. Neuropath. & Exp. Neurol. 3:368, 1944.
4. Benda, C. E.: Dandy-Walker syndrome or so-called atresia of foramen Magendie, J. Neuropath. & Exp. Neurol. 13:14, 1954.
5. Gardner, W.; Abdullah, A. F. and McCormack, L. J.: The varying expressions of embryonal atresia of the fourth ventricle in adults, J. Neurosurg. 14:591, 1957.
6. Keet, P. C. and Berman, M. C.: Dandy-Walker syndrome, South Africa M. J., 35:6, 1961

SYNDROME: Degos
SYNONYMS: Malignant atrophic papulosis
GEN. INFORMATION:
Rare cutaneovisceral disease. Definite male preponderance. Death occurs generally few months after diffuse eruption of the skin lesions (range: days to 9 years). Multiple cerebral infarcts and/or thrombosis of small arteries with associated increase in cerebrospinal fluid protein and pleocytosis may account for optic nerve involvement. Biopsy of skin lesions have given the only confirmatory test for the diagnosis. Serum albumin is slightly decreased with increase in serum globulin. Elevation of CSF protein with pleocytosis.

OCULAR FINDINGS:

Orbit	
Lids	Atrophic skin of eye lids
Motility	Intermittent diplopia
Lacr. App.	
Vision	
Vis. Fields	
Intraoc. Ten.	
Ant. Segm. and Sclera	Conjunctiva may be atrophic. Telangiectasia of conjunctiva with microaneuryms
Ocul. Media	
Retina and Choroid	Peripheral choroiditis or small patches of atrophic choroiditis. Loss of retinal pigment epithelium and choroidal pigment in small areas peripherally
Optic Nerve	Papilledema has occured with progressive CNS involvement

OTHER CLINICAL FINDINGS:
1. Porcelain-white skin lesion (asymptomatic and diffuse)
2. Oral mucosa lesions may occur
3. Anorexia and/or weight loss
4. Gastrointestinal involvement (pain possible; x-ray studies probably not revealing)
5. Peritonitis (most frequent cause for death)
6. Numerous yellow-to-white subserous intestinal plaques over entire intestine at laparotomy.
7. Intermittent paresthesias with early CNS involvement
8. Signs of progressive cerebral and cerebellar atrophy.

BIBLIOGRAPHY:
1. Degos, R.; Delort, J. and Tricot, R.: Dermatite papulo-squameuse atrophiante, Bull. Soc. France Derm. Syph. 49:148, 281, 1942.
2. Feuerman, E. J.: Papulosis atrophicans maligna Degos, Arch. Derm. 94:440, 1966.
3. Howard, R. O.; Klaus, S. N.; Savin, R. C. and Fenton, R.: Malignant Atrophic Papulosis, Arch. Ophth. 79:262, 1968.

SYNDROME: Déjean
SYNONYMS: Orbital floor syndrome
GEN. INFORMATION:
Lesion involving the floor of the orbit. Extension of the lesion into the cranial cavity may occur.

OCULAR FINDINGS:

Orbit	Exophthalmos
Lids	
Motility	Diplopia due to displacement of the globe or restricted function of the inferior rectus and/or inferior oblique muscles
Lacr. App.	
Vision	
Vis. Fields	
Intraoc. Ten.	
Ant. Segm. and Sclera	
Ocul. Media	
Retina and Choroid	
Optic Nerve	

OTHER CLINCAL FINDINGS:
1. Severe pain in superior maxillary region
2. Numbness in area of 1st and 2nd branch of trigeminal nerve

BIBLIOGRAPHY:
1. Déjean, C.: Le syndrome du plancher de l'orbite, Bull. et mém. Soc. franc. d'ophth., *48:*473, 1935.
2. Spaeth, E. B.: Pathogenesis of unilateral exophthalmos, Review Arch. Ophth. *18:*107, 1937.
3. Meadows, S. P.: Orbital tumors. Proc. Roy. Soc. Med. (Neurol.) *38:*594, 1946.

SYNDROME: Déjerine-Klumpke
SYNONYMS: Lower radicular syndrome, Klumpke's syndrome
GEN. INFORMATION:

Lesion involving the inferior roots of the brachial plexus with nerves derived from the 8th cervical and 1st thoracic root. (Birth trauma, Pott's disease, hemorrhage, shoulder dislocation, myelitis, Pancoast's tumor, meningeal or spinal tumor). Prognosis depends on the etiology and corrective possibilities. Symptomatology is similar to that of superior pulmonary sulcus syndrome (Pancoast) and scalenus anticus syndrome (Naffziger).

OCULAR FINDINGS:

Orbit	Enophthalmos
Lids	Ptosis, narrowed palpebral fissure
Motility	
Lacr. App.	
Vision	
Vis. Fields	
Intraoc. Ten.	
Ant. Segm. and Sclera	Miosis
Ocul. Media	
Retina and Choroid	
Optic Nerve	

OTHER CLINCAL FINDINGS:
1. Paralysis and atrophy of the small muscles of forearm and hand (flexor carpi ulnaris, flexor digitorum, interossei, thenar, hypothenar)
2. Decreased sensation or increased sensibility on the inner side of the forearm
3. Severe pain may exist

BIBLIOGRAPHY:
1. Déjerine-Klumpke, A.: Contribution à l'etude des paralysies radiculaires du plexus brachial; paralysies radiculaires totales; paralysies radiculaires inférieures; de la participation des filets sympathiques oculopupillaires dans ces paralysies, Rev. méd., Paris, 5:591, 739, 1885.
2. Archambault, L. and Fromm, N. K.: Progressive facial hemiatrophy, Arch. Neurol. & Psychiat, 27:529, 1932.

SYNDROME: Déjerine-Roussy
SYNONYMS: Retrolenticular syndrome, thalamic syndrome, posterior thalamic syndrome, thalamic hyperesthetic anesthesia
GEN. INFORMATION:
Posterior thalamic lesion; lesion in ventral part of optic thalamus (hemorrhage, thrombosis, tumor). The classical syndrome ascribed by Walker to thrombosis of the thalamo-geniculate artery which supplies the posteroventral nucleus and lateroventral nucleus. Four essential factors were suggested (Ford): (1) Loss of superficial and deep sensibility on the opposite side of the body including face; (2) persisting pain in affected parts; (3) ataxia; (4) choreoathetotic movements (mainly arms). Walker, in addition, includes hemiplegia, vasomotor changes and hemianopsia

OCULAR FINDINGS:

Orbit Lids Motility Lacr. App. Vision Vis. Fields	
	Hemianopsia when the thalamogeniculate artery is thrombosed near its origin from the posterial cerebral artery since in that event there is involvement of the medial aspect of the lateral geniculate body. In case the posterior cerebral artery is thrombosed complete hemianopsia with macular sparing results
Intraoc. Ten. Ant. Segm. and Sclera Ocul. Media Retina and Choroid Optic Nerve	

OTHER CLINICAL FINDINGS:
1. Sensory disturbances
2. Hemiataxia
3. Hemiplegia (transient) } contralateral
4. Choreoathetotic movements
5. Spontaneous pain

7. Partial facial paresis
6. Bladder disturbance

BIBLIOGRAPHY:
1. Déjerine, J. and Roussy, G.: Le syndrome thalamique, Rev. Neurol., *14*:521, 1906.
2. Walker, A. E.: *The Primate Thalamus,* Chicago, University of Chicago Press, 1938.
3. Freeman, W.: Prefrontal lobotomy in treatment of pain, Postgrad. Med., 5:375, 1949.
4. Ford, F. R.: *Diseases of the Nervous System in Infancy, Childhood and Adolescence,* 3rd Ed. Springfield, Charles C Thomas, 1952, p. 147.
5. Walsh, F. B.: *Clinical Neuro-Ophthalmology,* Baltimore, The Williams & Wilkins Co., 1957.

SYNDROME: de Lange
SYNONYMS: Congenital muscular hypertrophy-cerebral syndrome
GEN. INFORMATION:

Congenital disorder. Etiology is not definitely known. The disorder may be transmitted as an autosomal recessive (Opitz *et al.*). No consistent chromosomal abnormalities and no common prenatal teratogenic stimuli have been observed. Pathological findings: True muscle hypertrophy, external hydrocephalus, polygyria, microgyria, cavitation of cerebral white matter and thalamus. Consistant clinical eye findings are synophrys (growing together of the eyebrows) and long eyelashes.

OCULAR FINDINGS:

Orbit	Antimongoloid slant of palpebral fissures, mild exophthalmos, microphthalmos*
Lids	Hypertrichosis of eyebrows, long eyelashes, telecanthus, ptosis, blepharophimosis
Motility	Nystagmus on lateral gaze, constant coarse nystagmus, strabismus, alternating exotropia, paresis orbicularis oculi*
Lacr. App.	
Vision	High myopia
Vis. Fields	
Intraoc. Ten.	
Ant. Segm. and Sclera	Anisocoria, partial absence of pupillary annulus minor, sluggish pupil reaction,* chronic conjunctivitis, blue sclera.
Ocul. Media	Corneal opacities associated with lack of tear formation*
Retina and Choroid	
Optic Nerve	Pallor of optic disc

OTHER CLINICAL FINDINGS:
1. Mental retardation (constant findings)
2. Growth retardation (constant findings)
3. Extrapyramidal motor disturbances
4. Multiple skeletal abnormalities with congenital muscular hypertrophy (symmetric)
5. Feeble, low pitched cry
6. Atypical facial appearance and sometimes large, misshapen head
7. Hirsutism, hypoplastic nipples

*Single observations

BIBLIOGRAPHY:
1. de Lange, C.: Sur un type nouveau de degeneration (typus Amstelodamensis), Arch. Med. Enf. *36:*713,1933.
2. de Lange, C.: Congenital hypertrophy of muscles, extrapyramidal motor disturbances and mental deficiency, clinical entity, Am. J. Dis. Child. *48:*243, 1934.
3. Opitz, J. M. *et al.*: Brachman—de Lange syndrome, Lancet, *2:*1019, 1964.
4. Nicholson, D. H. and Goldberg, M. F.: Ocular abnormalities in the de Lange syndrome, Arch. Ophth. *76:*214, 1966.

SYNDROME: Devic
SYNONYMS: Ophthalmoencephalomyelopathy, optical myelitis, neuromyelitis optica
GEN. INFORMATION:.
Etiology is unknown (toxic?, virus?, vascular?). Occurrence equally in both sexes and at any age but most fequently between 20 and 50 years. One or more remissions may occur over years. Mortality rate up to 50%. Recovery of vision in about 50% with remaining impairment of various degrees. Laboratory findings: spinal fluid protein elevated 2 to 3 times normal, moderate pleocytosis with increased lymphocytes. Pathological findings: Demyelinization of nerves with destruction of axis-cylinders, microglial proliferation, astrocytosis, perivascular lymphocytosis. These pathological findings and the extent of the lesions distinguish the pathology of Devic's disease from that of multiple sclerosis, of which some have believed it to be a form of (Ref. 3). Though the white matter is primarily involved, the gray matter may be affected as well.

OCULAR FINDINGS:

Orbit	
Lids	Ptosis (rare)—(Walsh)*
Motility	Ocular muscle palsy (rare)—abducens and oculomotor palsy (Walsh):* Paralysis of conjugate muscles (Mckee and Mc-Naughton: A. J. O., 1938)
Lacr. App.	
Vision	Progressive loss of vision to partial or complete blindness. Onset usually very sudden in one eye, followed by blindness in the other eye. Loss of vision is sometimes preceded by pain in or about the eye. The rapidity of visual loss is an important differential diagnostic sign against brain tumor
Vis. Fields	Variable and irregular visual field loss according to optic nerve involvement: Central scotomas most common
Intraoc. Ten.	
Ant. Segm. and Sclera	Narrowing of the pupil (Walsh)*
Ocul. Media	
Retina and Choroid	
Optic Nerve	Bilateral optic neuritis (unilateral involvement is rare), this may precede or follow the myelitis by months or years. Remissions are possible. There is often mild edema of the optic disc and occasionally pronounced swelling. In other cases no disc changes may be seen in the early phase until atrophic changes become visible. Optic atrophy

OTHER CLINICAL FINDINGS:
Prodromal signs:
1. Headache
2. Sore throat
3. Fever and malaise
4. Ascending myelitis with resulting pain, which may be severe
5. Numbness, weakness
6. Paralysis

*Findings were associated with cervical involvement of spinal cord or brain stem

BIBLIOGRAPHY:
1. Devic, E.: Myélite aiguë dorso-lumbaire avec nevrite optique; autopsie, Cong. franç. de méd. *1:*434, 1894–1895.
2. Allbutt, T. G.: On the opthalmoscopic signs of spinal disease, Lancet, *1:*76, 1870
3. Stansbury, F.: Neuromyelitis optica (Devic's disease) presentation of five cases, with pathologic study and review of literature, Arch. Ophth., *42:*292, 1949.
4. Walsh, F. B.: *Clinical Neuro-Ophthalmology,* Baltimore, The Williams & Wilkins Co., 1957, p.656
5. Hogan, M. J. and Zimmerman, L. E.: *Ophthalmic Pathology,* 2nd Ed., Philadelphia, W. B. Saunders Co., 1962.

SYNDROME: Dialinas—Amalric
SYNONYMS: Amalric—Dialinas syndrome, deaf-mutism—retinal degeneration syndrome
GEN. INFORMATION:
The syndrome belongs to the group of disease entities with the combination of retinal pigmentary disturbances and deafness as their outstanding findings but without severe general systemic disorders as seen in the syndromes of Hallgren, Cockayne, Alport, Laurence-Moon-Bardet-Biedl, a.o.. Three theories have been postulated to explain the relationship between deaf-mutism and retinal pigmentary anomalies: (1) A single gene is responsible for the various manifestations (Franceschetti, 1963; a.o.); (2) A single gene is responsible for deaf-mutism and retinitis pigmentosa and two other genes determining the appearance of both independently (Hammerschlag, 1910); (3) Two independent genes produce the manifestations simultaneously (Gedda, 1952).

OCULAR FINDINGS:

Orbit	
Lids	
Motility	
Lacr. App.	
Vision	*No* nightblindness
Vis. Fields	
Intraoc. Ten.	
Ant. Segm. and Sclera	
Ocul. Media	Atypical retinitis pigmentosa with small scattered fine pigmented deposits in the macular region with some accumulations and accompained by small white and yellow spots. The vascular choroidal plexus can easily be identified beneath the retinal pathology. These changes are not associated with night blindness or abnormalities of the ERG
Retina and Choroid	
Optic Nerve	

OTHER CLINICAL FINDINGS:
Deaf mutism

BIBLIOGRAPHY:
1. Dialinas, N. P.: Les altérations oculaires chez les sourds-muets. Génét Hum. *8*:225, 1959.
2. Amalric, P.: Nouveau type de dégénérescence tapéto-rétinienne au cours de la surdimutité, Bul. Soc. Ophtal. France *196*:211, 1960
3. Amalric, P. and Bessou, P.: Nouvelles preuves de la transmission héréditaires des dégénérescences rétiniennes "a minima" associees à la surdimutité, Rev. Oto-Neuro-Opht., *36*:109, 1964.
4. Hammerschlag, V.: Zur Kenntnis der hereditär degenerativen Taubstummheit, Z. Ohrenheilk. *61*:225, 1910.
5. Gedda, L.: Sordomotismo e genetica, Minerva med., *19*:433, 1952.
6. Franceschetti, A.; François, J. and Babel, J.: *Les hérédodégénérescenses choro-rétiniennes,* Vol. 2, Paris, Masson et cie. 1963.
7. Charamis, J.; Tsamparlakis, J.; Palimeris, G. and Koliopoulos, J.: Deaf-Mutism and ophthalmic Lesions, J. Ped. Ophth. *5*:230, 1968.

SYNDROME: Double Whammy
SYNONYMS: Voluntary propulsion of the eyes
GEN. INFORMATION:

The term propulsion does not apply to exophthalmos due to certain diseases, but rather has to be reserved for the ability of actively displacing the globe forward while retracting the upper and lower lid behind the equator of the eye ball. Involuntary propulsion on the basis of trauma was described by Friedenwald in infants following forceps delivery.

The term 'double whammy syndrome' was introduced by Berman (1966).

OCULAR FINDINGS:

Orbit	
Lids	
Motility	Voluntary dislocation of either eye separately or both simultaneously. The phenomenon is explained by contraction of the superior and inferior obliques and simultaneous relaxation of all rectus muscles. While the globes are luxated forward, the upper and lower lid slip behind the equator and fixate the eye balls in this position by slight contraction of the orbicularis muscle. To replace the eyes, they were rotated laterally at which time the adducted eye slipped back and at gaze to the opposite side the other eye retracted (Berman).
Lacr. App.	
Vision	
Vis. Fields	
Intraoc. Ten.	
Ant. Segm. and Sclera	
Ocul. Media	
Retina and Choroid	
Optic Nerve	Apparently no damage to optic nerve even after years of practicing the voluntary propulsion.

OTHER CLINICAL FINDINGS:
BIBLIOGRAPHY:

1. Friedenwald, H.: Luxation and avulsion of eye ball during birth. Amer. J. Ophth. *1*:9, 1918.
2. Ferrer, H.: Voluntary propulsion of both eye balls. Amer. J. Ophth. *11*:883, 1928.
3. Smith, J. A.: Voluntary propulsion of both eye balls. JAMA. *98*:398, 1932.
4. Lyle, D. J. and McGavic, J. S.: The cause of voluntary forward luxation of the eye ball. Amer. J. Ophth. *19*:316, 1936.
5. Berman, B.: Voluntary propulsion of the eye balls. Arch. Int .Med., *117*: 648, 1966.
6. Walsh, T. J. and Gilman, M.: Voluntary propulsion of the eyes. Am. J. Ophth. *67*:583, 1969.

SYNDROME: Down

SYNONYMS: Mongolism, 21 Trisomy syndrome, mongoloid idiocy.

GEN. INFORMATION:

Trisomy of chromosome 21, probably results from maternal primary nondisjunction related to age dependent factors(Berg). In the majority of patients with this syndrome an additional small acrocentric chromosome exists. According to Neu and Kajii, there is some uncertainty as to whether the chromosome involved is actually a number 21 or 22. A number of cases of G-group trisomy have been reported without the symptoms of Down's syndrome, and it was suggested that in those the extra chromosome present is a 22,—or the chromosome not involved in Down's syndrome. This extra chromosome was, however, not definitely identified as a number 22 and could have been a Y chromosome in certain cases or material from an autosome.

OCULAR FINDINGS:

Orbit	Hypertelorism
Lids	Small and oblique eyelid fissures, epicanthus, blepharitis, ectropion
Motility	Nystagmus, convergent strabismus
Lacr. App.	
ViSion	High myopia (30%), hyperopia, colorblindness
Vis. Fields	
Intraoc. Ten.	
Ant. Segm. and Sclera	Yellow spots on the iris, hypoplasia of the iris, blepharo-conjunctivitis
Ocul. Media	Lens opacities (50%), keratoconus (may be acute) (Ref. 4), corneal hydrops, corneal ectasia, corneal edema, leukoma
Retina and Choroid	
Optic Nerve	

OTHER CLINICAL FINDINGS:

1. Mental retardation
2. Skeletal abnormalities (especially skull and long bones)
3. Overextension of joints
4. Deformed and low set ears
5. Short 5th finger
6. Transverse palmar crease
7. Fissured tongue
8. Salivation
9. Irritation and aggressiveness
10. Heart anomalies

BIBLIOGRAPHY:

1. Down, J. L. H.: Observations on ethnic classifications of idiots, Clin. lect. & Rep. Lond. Hosp. *111*:259, 1866.
2. Down, J. L. H.: Marriages of consanguinity in relation to degeneration of race, Lond. Hosp. clin. Lect. Rep. *3*:224, 1866.
3. Rados, A.: Conical cornea and mongolism, Arch. Ophth. *40*:454, 1948.
4. François, J.: *Heredity in Ophthalmology,* St. Louis, C. V. Mosby Co., 1961.
5. Slusher, M. M.; Laibson, P. R.; and Mulberger, R. D.: Keratoconus in Down's syndrome, Am. J. Ophth. *66*:1137, 1968.
6. Berg. W. R.: Autosomal Abnormalities (p. 608) in Gardner, L. I.:*Endocrine and Genetic Diseases of Childhood,* Philadelphia, W. B. Saunders Co., 1969: Ibid: Neu, R. L. and Kajii, T.: Other Autosomal Abnormalities, p. 652

SYNDROME: Duane
SYNONYMS: Retraction syndrome, Stilling's syndrome, Turk-Stilling syndrome
GEN. INFORMATION:
The disease is autosomal dominant. More frequent in females. Manifestations are congenital. This syndrome has long been considered to be due to fibrosis of the lateral rectus muscle or abnormal check ligaments. It has now been firmly established that it is due to faulty innervation. EMG shows anomalous cocontraction or paradoxial innervation of the lateral and medial recti. It is felt that the pathologic change is central, probably a supranuclear lesion. The congenital aberrant innervation affects III and VII nerves.

OCULAR FINDINGS:

Orbit	
Lids	Narrowing of palpebral fissure on adduction, widening on abduction
Motility	Primary global retraction: Deficiency of medial and lateral recti motility (most frequently unilateral and left eye). Limitation of abduction in affected eye is usually complete, but if incomplete, there is fuller movement in the upper and lower fields, due to the abducting power of superior and inferior oblique muscles. Retraction of the globe with attempted adduction varies from 1 to 10 mm
Lacr. App.	
Vision	Not affected
Vis. Fields	
Intraoc. Ten.	
Ant. Segm. and Sclera	Pupillary changes (Aebli)
Ocul. Media	
Retina and Choroid	
Optic Nerve	

OTHER CLINICAL FINDINGS:
1. Associated Klippel-Feil syndrome
2. Malformation of face, ears, teeth

BIBLIOGRAPHY:
1. Duane, A.: Congenital deficiency of abduction, associated with impairment of abduction, retraction movements, contractions of the palpebral fissure and oblique movements of the eye Arch. Ophth. *34:*133, 1905.
2. Aebli, R.: Retraction syndrome, Arch. Ophth. *10:*602, 1933.
3. Costa Fernandes, R.: Duane's syndrome, Rev. brasil. oftal., *10:*333, 1953 (Abstract, A. J. O., *36:*146, 1953).
4. Blodi, F. C.; Van Allen, M. W. and Yarbrough, J. C.: Duane's syndrome: A brain-stem lesion: an electromyographic study, Tr. Amer. Acad. Ophth. Otolaryng. *68:*802, 1964; Ibid: Arch. Ophth. *72:*171, 1964.
5. Huber, A. *et al.:* Zum Problem des Duane-Syndroms, Graefe Arch. Ophth. 167:169, 1964.

SYNDROME: Eaton-Lambert
SYNONYMS: Myasthenic syndrome, ocular myoclonus, myoclonic syndrome
GEN. INFORMATION:
Predominant in males, usually over 40 years of age. Frequently associated with intrathoracic tumor, especially oat cell Ca. EMG shows greatly reduced amplitude upon a single maximal shock, although the strength of these muscles on voluntary contraction is mostly normal. At repetitive stimulation at rates of 1 to 10/sec, there is further decline in response, similar to that in myasthenia gravis. But a marked facilitation of the response (up to 10 × the initial amplitude) occurs during repetitive stimulation at higher rates. This method seems to be very reliable in the differentiation of myasthenia gravis and this myasthenic syndrome.

OCULAR FINDINGS:

Orbit	
Lids	
Motility	Decreased amplitude of version in all directions of gaze. Positive Bell's phenomenon, ocular myoclonus
Lacr. App.	
Vision	Decreased visual acuity
Vis. Fields	
Intraoc. Ten.	
Ant. Segm. and Sclera	Corneal haziness and abrasion, decreased corneal sensitivity. Conjunctival injection, miotic pupil
Ocul. Media	
Retina and Choroid	
Optic Nerve	

OTHER CLINICAL FINDINGS:
1. Weakness, fatigue
2. Peripheral paresthesia
3. Dryness of mouth
4. Marked sensitivity to d-tubocurarine
5. Poor response to neostigmin

BIBLIOGRAPHY:
1. Eaton, L.M. and Lambert, E. H.: Electromyography and electric stimulation of nerves in diseases of the motor units: observations on myasthenic syndrome associated with malignant tumors, J. A. M. A. *163:*1117, 1957.
2. Lambert, E. M.; Eaton, L. M.; and Rooke, E. D.: Defect of neuromuscular conduction associated with malignant neoplasms, Am. J. Physiol. *187:*612, 1956.
3. Wise, R. P.: Myasthenic syndrome, Anesthesiology, *27:*870, 1966.
4. McQuillen, M. P.; Cantor, H. E.; and O'Rourke, J. R.: Myasthenic syndrome associated with antibiotics, Arch. Neurol. *18:*402, 1968.
5. Retzlaff, J. A.; Kearns, T. P.; Howard, F. M., Jr. and Cronin, M. L.: Lancaster Red-Green Test in evaluation of edrophonium effect in myasthenia gravis, Am. J. Ophth., *67:*13, 1969.
6. Tiltarelli, R.; Giagheddu, M. and Spadetta, V.: Typical ophthalmoscopic picture of "Cherry-Red-Spot" in an adult with the myoclonic syndrome, Brit. J. Ophth. *50:*414, 1966.

SYNDROME: Ehlers-Danlos
SYNONYMS: Fibrodysplasia elastica generalisata, cutis hyperelastica
GEN. INFORMATION:
Present at birth. Transmitted as a regular or irregular autosomal dominant condition with relative low penetrance. In certain cases inheritance may be recessive. Two groups: (1) cutaneous, (2) articular. Pathological findings: Systematized elastic mesenchymal affection and aplasia of collagen bundles of the dermis, hypodermis and articular ligaments. The syndrome is one of the three primary disorders of elastic tissue, the other two are psudoxanthoma elastium (Groenblad-Strandberg syndrome) and senile elastosis. More recently it has been questioned that in these diseases the elastic tissue is selectively involved, but that most likely collagen fibers may be affected as well. (McKusick, 1960)

OCULAR FINDINGS:

Orbit	
Lids	Hyperelasticity of palpebral skin. Easy eversion of upper lid. Ptosis. Epicanthal folds (frequent)
Motility	Hypotony of extraocular muscles. Strabismus
Lacr. App.	
Vision	
Vis. Fields	.
Intraoc. Ten.	Occasionally increased.
Ant. Segm. and Sclera	Microcornea, thinning of cornea with keratoconus. Thinning of sclera (blue sclerae)
Ocul. Media	Subluxation of lens
Retina and Choroid	Degeneration of Bruch's membrane, angiod streaks, chorio-retinal hemorrhages, retinitis proliferans with secondary detachment, macular degeneration
Optic Nerve	

OTHER CLINICAL FINDINGS:

Cutaneous type
1. Cutaneous hyperelasticity
2. Thin skin, atrophic, fragile
3. Pseudomolluscoid tumors

Articular type
1. Excessive articular laxity
2. Luxations

BIBLIOGRAPHY:
1. Ehlers, E.: Cutus laxa, Neigung zu Hoemorrhagien in der Haut, Lockerung mehrerer Artikulationen, Dermat. Zschr. *8:*173, 1901.
2. Danlos, H.: Un cas de cutis laxa avec tumeurs par contusion chronique des caudes et des genoux, Bull. Soc. franç. dermat. et syph., *19:*70, 1908.
3. Johnson, S. A. M. and Falls, M. O.: Ehlers-Danlos syndrome, Arch. Derm. & Syph., *60:*82, 1949.
4. McKusick, V. A.: *Heritable Disorders of Connective Tissue,* St. Louis, C. V. Mosby Co., 1960, p. 213.
5. Green, W. R.; Friedman-Kieu, A. and Banfield, W. G.: Angioid Streaks in Ehlers-Danlos Syndrome, Arch. Ophth. *76:*197, 1966.
6. Pemberton, J. W.; Freeman, H. M. and Schepens, C. L.: Familial retinal detachment and the Ehlers-Danlos Syndrome, Arch. Ophth. *76:*817, 1966.

SYNDROME: Eilis-van Crefeld
SYNONYMS: Chondroectodermal dysplasia
GEN. INFORMATION:
Inherited as an autosomal recessive trait. Parental consanguinity in about 25%
of patients. X-ray findings: Plump diaphyseal end of humerus and femur.
Shortened radius and ulna with proximal part of the ulna and distal part of the
radius exceptionally large. Fibula very short. Anomalies of metacarpal and
phalangeal bones. Dental anomalies are most frequent finding of this syndrome

OCULAR FINDINGS:

Orbit	
Lids	
Motility	Internal strabismus
Lacr. App.	
Vision	
Vis. Fields	
Intraoc. Ten.	
Ant. Segm.	Iris coloboma (McGregor; Proc. Roy. Soc. Med., 1954)
and Sclera	
Ocul. Media	Congenital cataract
Retina and	
Choroid	
Optic Nerve	

OTHER CLINICAL FINDINGS:
1. Bilateral polydactyly
2. Short and plump limbs
3. Genu valgum
4. Talipes (equinovarus, calcaneovalgus)
5. Thoracic constriction
6. Fusion of middle part of upper lip to maxillary gingival margin
7. Dental anomalies: numbers, shape, spacing
8. Congenital heart defect in about 50% of patients
9. Dystrophic fingernails
10. Genital anomalies
11. Mental retardation at various degrees in about 30%

BIBLIOGRAPHY:
1. Ellis, R. W. B. and van Crefeld, S.: A syndrome characterized by ectodermal dysplasia, polydactyly, chondro-dysplasia and congenital morbus cordis, Arch. Dis. Childhood, *15*:65, 1940.
2. Metrakos, J. D. and Fraser, F. C.: Evidence for a hereditary factor in chondroectodermal dysplasia (Ellis-van Crefeld syndrome), Am. J. Human Genet. *6*:260, 1954.
3. Ellis, R. W. B. and Andrew, J. D.: Chondroectodermal dysplasia, J. Bone & Joint Surg. *44*-B:626, 1962.

SYNDROME: Empty sella syndrome
SYNONYMS:
GEN. INFORMATION:
Further progression of ocular findings and symptoms after treatment of pituitary tumors either by surgery, x-ray, etc. is usually interpreted as recurrence of tumor. On rare occasions upon surgical exploration no such new tumor growth may be found. X-ray findings: Enlarged sella turcica. On occasion a pneumoencephalogram may reveal air in the sella.

OCULAR FINDINGS:

Orbit	
Lids	
Motility	
Lacr. App.	
Vision	Reduced visual acuity and possible blindness
Vis. Fields	Hemianopsia, quadranopsia or irregular field defects, central scotoma may also be present
Intraoc. Ten.	
Ant. Segm. and Sclera	
Ocul. Media	
Retina and Choroid	
Optic Nerve	Pale optic discs. It has been suggested that the further deterioration of visual function could be attributed to x-ray damage with atrophy in cases this is applicable or to scar formation with traction on and 'strangulation' of the chiasm and optic nerve directly or vascular strangulation with resulting ischemia

OTHER CLINICAL FINDINGS:
Acromegalic features and other general sytemic manifestations depend on the type of the primary tumor the patient had and are not part of the 'empty sella syndrome' which is responsible for the progression of ocular pathologic condition.

BIBLIOGRAPHY:
1. Colby, M. Y., Jr. and Kearns, T. P.: Radiation therapy of pituitary adenomas with associated visual impairment, Proc. Staff Meet., Mayo Clin., *37:*15, 1962.
2. Hartog, M.; Doyle, F.; Fraser, R. and Joplin, G. F.: Partial pituitary ablation with implants of Gold—198 and Yttrium—90 for acromegaly, Brit. med. J. *2:*396, 1965.
3. Morello, G. and Frera, C.: Visual damage after removal of hypohyseal adenomas: Possible importance of vascular disturbances of the optic nerves and chiasma, Acta neurochir. *15:*1, 1966.
4. Lee, W. M. and Adams, J. E.: The Empty Sella Syndrome, J. Neurosurg. *28:*351, 1968.

SYNDROME: Erb-Goldflam
SYNONYMS: Myasthenia gravis, pseudoparalytic syndrome
GEN. INFORMATION:
Rare familial occurrence. Ratio of incidence in (female vs. male subjects) about 3:2. Onset at all ages possible. Defect at myoneural junction with involvement or disturbance of the acetylcholine metabolism. Prostigmin reverses muscular symptoms. Thymona reported in 10 to 15%, malignant or benign tumors of the thymus were found in up to 50% in autopsies. (See also: Eaton-Lambert syndrome). Tonography recorded during intravenous administration of Tensilon showed increase in intraocular pressure in patients with myasthenia gravis, while this test was negative in all other control subjects (Glaser).

OCULAR FINDINGS:

Orbit	
Lids	Ptosis (unilateral or bilateral); ptosis may shift from one eye to the other, which, when present, is pathognomonic for the disease
Motility	Strabismus, ophthalmoplegia externa*
Lacr. App.	
Vision	Diplopia, blurred vision
Vis Fields	
Intraoc. Ten.	
Ant. Segm.	
and Sclera	
Ocul. Media	
Retina and	
Choroid	
Optic Nerve	

OTHER CLINICAL FINDINGS:
1. Masticatory muscle weakness
2. Dysphonia
3. Dysphagia
4. General muscle weakness after
   only mild exercise
5. Good response to neostigmin
6. Respiratory stress may occur
7. Paresthesias*

*Occasionally

BIBLIOGRAPHY:
1. Grob, D.: Course and management of myasthenia gravis, J. A. M. A., *153:* 529, 1953.
2. Duke-Elder, Sir Stewart: *System of Ophthalmology,* Vol. VII, St. Louis, C. V. Mosby Co., 1962. p. 565.
3. Glaser, J. S.: Tensilon Tonography in the diagnosis of myasthenia gravis, Invest. Ophth. *6:*135, 1967.
4. Osserman, K. E.: Ocular myasthenia gravis, Invest. Ophth. *6:*277, 1967.
5. Erb. W.: Zur Casuistik der bulbaren Lähmungen III. Ueber einen neuen wahrscheinlich bulbären Symptomenkomplex, Arch. f. Psychiat. *9:*336, 1878.
6. Erb. W. H.: Über einen eigenthümlichen bulbären (?) Symptomenkomplex, Arch. Psychiat. Nervenkr. *9:*172, 1879.
7. Goldflam, S. V.: Über einen scheinbar heilbaren bulbärparalytischen Symptomenkomplex mit Betheiligung der Extremitäten, Dtsch. Z. Nervenheilk. *4:*312, 1893.
8. Cogan, D. G.: Myasthenia gravis, Arch. Ophth. *74:*217, 1965.

SYNDROME: Espildora-Luque
SYNONYMS: Ophthalmic-Sylvian syndrome
GEN. INFORMATION:
Embolism of the ophthalmic artery with reflectory spasm of the middle cerebral artery.

OCULAR FINDINGS:

Orbit	
Lids	
Motility	
Lacr. App.	
Vision	Unilateral blindness (caused by ophthalmic artery embolism)
Vis. Fields	
Intraoc. Ten.	
Ant. Segm.	
and Sclera	
Ocul. Media	
Retina and	
Choroid	
Optic Nerve	

OTHER CLINICAL FINDINGS:
Temporary hemiplegia contralateral side of amaurosis (caused by reflex spasm of the middle cerebral artery)

BIBLIOGRAPHY:
Espildora-Luque, C.: Ophthalmic Sylvian Syndrome, Arch. de Oft. Hisp.—Amer., *34:*616, 1934 (Abstract, A. J. O., *18:*402, 1935).

SYNDROME: Fabry-Anderson

SYNONYMS: Angiokeratoma corporis diffusum syndrome, diffuse angiokeratosis

GEN. INFORMATION:
Most likely lipoid storage disorder. Inheritance by x-linked recessive trait. Some signs of the syndrome have been observed in a few heterozygous females (Weicksel:Dtsch. Med. Wschr., 1925)

OCULAR FINDINGS:

Orbit	
Lids	Swelling of eye lids
Motility	
Lacr. App.	
Vision	
Vis. Fields	
Intraoc. Ten.	
Ant. Segm.	Varicositis of palpebral and bulbar conjunctiva
and Sclera	
Ocul. Media	Corneal opacities
Retina and	Increased tortuosity of retinal vessels and aneurysmal dilatations
Choroid	
Optic Nerve	

OTHER CLINICAL FINDINGS:
1. Angiokeratoma of the skin with small, grouped papular lesions mainly over scrotum, thighs, buttocks, sacral area, umbilical area, and hips.
2. Elevated blood pressure
3. Disturbance in sweat secretion
4. Pain in arms and legs
5. Enlarged heart
6. Albuminuria
7. Prominent lower jaw and lips.

BIBLIOGRAPHY:
1. Anderson, W.: A case of 'Angiokeratoma', Brit. J. Dermat. *10:*113, 1898.
2. Fabry, J.: Ein Beitrag zur Kenntnis der Purpura haemorrhagica nodularis (purpura papulosa haemorrhagica Hebrae), Arch. Dermat. u. Syph. *43:*187, 1898.
3. Franceschetti, A. and Thier, C. J.: Über Hornhautdystrophien bei Genodermatosen unter besonderer Berücksichtigung der Palmoplantarkeratosen, von Graefes Arch. Ophth. *162:*610, 1961.

SYNDROME: Feer

SYNONYMS: Swift-Feer syndrome, infantile acrodynia, acrodynia, Pink Disease

GEN. INFORMATION:

Etiology is unknown (infectious?) involving the vegetative nervous system. Mercury has been suggested as etiological factor. This assumption is based on the increased urinary excretion of mercury, the similarity of symptoms in this syndrome and those seen in adults with mercury poisoning and the frequent history of contact with mercury containing drugs o.a. of children with this syndrome. In cases without mercury contact, a double deficiency of vitamin B and essential fatty acids has been postulated (Barret: M. J. Austral., 1957). Onset in early childhood (4 months to 4 years). Both sexes are qeually affected. The prognosis is relatively good, complete recurrence usually within several months, but sometimes lasting over years, with recurrences. Approximately 5 to 10% mortality. Ocular findings occur in approximately 50% of the cases (Walsh). Histopathology: Chronic inflammatory changes of spinal cord and nerve roots, peripheral neuritis. In skin sections acanthosis with papillomatosis, parakeratosis and necrobiotic changes in spinous and basal cell layers.

OCULAR FINDINGS

Orbit	Proptosis
Lids	
Motility	
Lacr. App.	
Vision	Lacrimation
Vis. Fields	
Intraoc. Ten.	
Ant. Segm. and Sclera	Pronounced photophobia, severe conjunctival itching, conjunctival injection with occasional marked signs of inflammation.* Keratoconjunctival irritation is very prominent, however, they may be only very mild or barely perceptible in some cases
Ocul. Media	Severe keratitis (occasionally)
Retina and Choroid	
Optic Nerve	Choked disc (rare), mild optic neuritis (rare)

OTHER CLINICAL FINDINGS:

1. Restlessness*
2. Irritability*
3. Sleeplessness
4. Continuous profuse sweating*
5. Cyanosis of fingers, toes, nose
6. Muscle hypotony*
7. Reduced motility
8. Rectal prolapse
9. Tremor

10. Rapid pulse (tachycardia)*
11. Elevated blood pressure
12. Trophic disturbances possible with loss of healthy teeth, mucous membrane ulcers, gangrenous ulcers of fingers.
13. Exanthema of palms and soles with exfoliation of large skin flaps.*
14. Stomatitis*

*Most typical findings

BIBLIOGRAPHY:

1. Feer, E.: Eine eigenartige Neurose des vegetativen Systems beim Kleinkinde, Ergebn. inn. Med. u. Kinderh. 24:100, 1923.
2. Swift, H.: Erythroedema. Trans. Austral. Med. Congr. (10th), New Zealand, 1914.
3. Crawford, S.: Juvenile acrodynia. Arch. Dermat. & Syph. 26:215, 1932.
4. Feer, E.: Lehrbuch der Kinderheilkunde, Jena., G. Fischer, Verl., 1948, p. 483.
5. Walsh, F.: Clinical Neuro-Ophthalmology, 2nd Ed., Baltimore, The Williams & Wilkins Co., 1957, p. 728.
6. Duke-Elder, Sir Stewart: Systems of Ophthalmology, Vol. VIII, Part 2, St. Louis, C. V. Mosby Co., 1965.

SYNDROME: Felty

SYNONYMS: Chauffard-Still syndrome, primary splenic neutropenia with arthritis, rheumatoid arthritis with hypersplenism

GEN. INFORMATION:

The etiology of this syndrome is not fully understood. Infection has been generally accepted as cause, though allergy has been considered by some. The disease follows a chronic course and onset usually in middle-aged patients. Arthritis is mostly the first finding with fingers and toes first affected followed later on by involvement of larger joints. Laboratory findings: Leukopenia, mainly granulocytes, lymphocytes usually normal. Pathological findings: Hyperplastic bone marrow. Endothelial proliferation of the spleen.

OCULAR FINDINGS:

Orbit	
Lids	
Motility	
Lacr. App.	
Vision	
Vis. Fields	
Intraoc. Ten.	
Ant. Segm. **and Sclera**	Scleritis,* scleromalacia perforance (Ref. 2)
Ocul. Media	Keratitis*
Retina and **Choroid**	
Optic Nerve	

OTHER CLINICAL FINDINGS:

1. Rheumatoid arthritis
2. Splenomegaly
3. Leukopenia
4. Anemia (mild)
5. Lymphadenopathy*
6. Low grade fever*
7. Leg ulcers*
8. Achylia*
9. Oral lesion with ulcers and atrophy

*Occasional findings

BIBLIOGRAPHY:

1. Felty, A. R.: Chronic arthritis in the adult associated with splenomegaly and leukopenia, Bull. Johns Hopkins Hosp. 35:16, 1924.
2. Anderson, B. and Margolis, G.: Scleromalacia, Am. J. Ophth. 35:917, 1952.
3. Ostriker, P. J.; Ostriker, M. and Lasky, M. A.: Keratitis and skleritis associated with Felty's syndrome, Arch Ophth. 54:858, 1955.

SYNDROME: Fisher
SYNONYMS: Ophthalmoplegia-ataxia-areflexia syndrome
GEN. INFORMATION:
Acute idiopathic polyneuritis. Prognosis is good. Complete recovery as a rule over several weeks (7 to 12). High elevation of protein in cerebrospinal fluid in late stages have indicated a close relation to Guillain-Barré type of polyneuropathy (Fisher)

OCULAR FINDINGS:

Orbit	
Lids	Moderate ptosis
Motility	Symmetrical, complete external and almost complete internal ophthalmoplegia
Lacr. App.	
Vision	Diplopia
Vis. Fields	
Intraoc. Ten.	
Ant. Segm. and Sclera	Sluggish pupil reaction to light
Ocul. Media	
Retina and Choroid	
Optic Nerve	

OTHER CLINICAL FINDINGS:

1. Dizziness
2. Severe ataxia (cerebellar type)
3. Loss of tendon reflexes
4. Chest pains
5. Difficulties in chewing
6. Diminished or absent sense of vibration
7. Numbness of fingers (transient)

BIBLIOGRAPHY:
1. Fisher, M.: An unusual variant of acute idiopathic polyneuritis (Syndrome of ophthalmoplegia, ataxia and areflexia), New Engl. J. Med., 255:57, 1956.
2. Collier, J.: Peripheral neuritis: Morison lectures, Edinburgh Med. J. 39:601; 672; 679; 1932.
3. Barber, H. S.: Polyradiculoneuritis in east anglia, Lancet, 2:548, 1940.

SYNDROME: Foix
SYNONYMS: Cavernous sinus syndrome, hypophyseal-sphenoidal syndrome
GEN. INFORMATION:
Tumor lateral sinus wall or sphenoid bone, intracranial aneurysm, cavernous and lateral sinus thrombosis, inflammatory lesions. Differential diagnosis: Carotid artery—cavernous sinus fistula syndrome.

OCULAR FINDINGS:

Orbit	Proptosis
Lids	Lid edema
Motility	Paresis or paralysis III, IV, VI.
Lacr. App.	
Vision	
Vis. Fields	
Intraoc. Ten.	
Ant. Segm. and Sclera	Chemosis, paresis or paralysis V (ophth. branch)
Ocul. Media	
Retina and Choroid	
Optic Nerve	Optic atrophy

OTHER CLINICAL FINDINGS:
1. Postauricular edema (possible)
2. Less distended external jugular vein on affected side
3. Maxillary division of the 5th cranial nerve often affected, causing trigeminal neuralgia

BIBLIOGRAPHY:
1. Foix, C.: Syndrome de la paroi externe du sinus caverneux, Rev. neurol., *37/38*:827, 1922.
2. Goldman, M. and Adams, R.: Fibrosarcoma of sphenoid bone, producing syndrome of lateral wall of cavernous sinus-case report, J. Neuropath & Exp. Neurol., *5*:155, 1946.
3. Huber, A.: Über das Syndrom des Sinus Cavernosus, Ophthalmologica, *121*: 118, 1951.
4. Alfano, J. E.: (in Vail, D. T. edit.) Neuro-Ophthalmology, Internat. Ophth. Clinics, *1*:651-737, 1961.
5. Rucker, C. W.: The causes of paralysis of the third, fourth and sixth cranial nerves, Am. J. Ophth. *61*:1293, 1966.

7

SYNDROME: Foster Kennedy
SYNONYMS: Basal-frontal syndrome, Gowers-Paton-Kennedy syndrome
GEN. INFORMATION:
Tumor in the base of the frontal lobe or sphenoidal meningioma (aneurysm, abscess, sclerosis, etc. possible). Prognosis depends on the type of lesion. Differential diagnosis: General paresis, bromide intoxication, space-taking lesions of the frontal lobe. Ischemic optic neuropathy and idiopathic optic neuritis can cause sudden losses of vision associated with papilledema. The suddeness of visual loss distinguishes such cases from the more gradual loss seen with frontal lobe tumors (Schatz and Smith)

OCULAR FINDINGS:

Orbit	
Lids	
Motility	
Lacr. App.	
Vision	
Vis. Fields	Central scotoma may be present on side of optic atrophy, enlarged blind spot and peripheral contraction of field (opposite eye)
Intraoc. Ten.	
Ant. Segm. and Sclera	
Ocul. Media	
Retina and Choroid	
Optic Nerve	Homolateral descending optic atrophy due to compression of the ipsilateral optic nerve at the optic foramen, and contralateral papilledema due to increased intracranial pressure.

OTHER CLINICAL FINDINGS:
1. Anosmia

BIBLIOGRAPHY:
1. Kennedy, F.: Retrobulbar neuritis as an exact diagnostic sign of certain tumors and abscesses in frontal lobes, Amer. J. Med. Sci., *142:*355, 1911.
2. Kennedy, F.: A further note on the diagnostic value of retrobulbar neuritis in expanding lesions of the frontal lobes: with a report of this syndrome in a case of aneurysm of the right internal carotid artery, J. A. M. A., *67:*1361, 1916.
3. Yaskin, H. E. and Alpers, B. J: Foster Kennedy syndrome with posttraumatic arachnoiditis of optic chiasm and base of frontal lobes, Arch. Ophth. *45:*70, 1951.
4. Masters, S.: Foster Kennedy syndrome, A. J. O., *36:*983, 1953.
5. Schatz, N. J. and Smith, J. L.: Non-tumor causes of Foster Kennedy syndrome, J. Neurosurg., *27:*37, 1967.
6. Cogan, D. G.: *Neurology of the Visual System,* 2nd Ed., Springfield, Charles C Thomas, 1967.

SYNDROME: Foville
SYNONYMS: Foville's peduncular syndrome
GEN. INFORMATION:

Foville's syndrome belongs to the brain stem syndromes. Pontine area tumor, hemorrhage, tuberculoma, multiple sclerosis, or unilateral obstruction of paramedian branches may cause the clinical manifestations. Lesions deep in pons, near center, with impairment of postural sensibility of opposite side of the body. Lesion lateral portion of pons with damage to spinothalamic tract, crossed analgesia, with or without impairment of sensibility of N. *V.* on side of lesion.

OCULAR FINDINGS:

Orbit	
Lids	
Motility	Paralysis VI through involvement of the nucleus and supranuclear pathways. Paralysis of conjugate movement to the side of the lesion. Thus, inability to abduct the eye and deviation of the eyes away from the lesion (or toward it if the lesion is irritative). Convergence is preserved; During recovery possible nystagmus with large oscillations and gaze directed toward affected side
Lacr. App.	
Vision	
Vis. Fields	
Intraoc. Ten.	
Ant. Segm. and Scleja	
Ocul. Media	
Retina and Choroid	
Optic Nerve	

OTHER CLINICAL FINDINGS:
1. Peripheral facial palsy
2. Contralateral hemiplegia

BIBLIOGRAPHY:

1. Foville, A. L. F.: Note sur une paralysie peu connue des certains muscles de l'oeil, et sa liaison avec quelques points de l'anatomie et la physiologie de la protubérance annulaire, Bull. Soc. Anat. Paris, *33:* 393, 1858.
2. Freeman, W.; Ammerman, H. M. and Stanley, M.: Syndromes of pontic tegmentum; report of 3 cases, Arch. Neurol. & Psychiat. *50:*462, 1943.
3. Melkild, A. and Mörstad, K.: Foville's syndrome as a complication of phaeochromocytoma, Acta. med. Scandinav., *159:*471, 1957.

SYNDROME: Franceschetti

SYNONYMS: Franceschetti-Zwalen-Klein syndrome, Treacher Collins syndrome, mandibulo-facial dysostosis, Mandibulofacial syndrome, Eyelid-malor-mandible syndrome

GEN. INFORMATION:
Genetic origin, transmitted in an irregular dominant mode, incomplete penetrance and variable expressivity. Occurrence in several generations of the same family not infrequent (Franceschetti *et al.*). Arrested development in early fetal life with defective ossification of facial bones derived from the visceral mesoderm. Another theory was suggested by which the syndrome results from incorrect development or failure of development of the stapedial artery (McKenzie and Craig: Arch. Dis. Childh., 1955). Miscarriage or death shortly after birth are common (Böök and Fraccaro: Acta Benet., 1955). It may occur also in atypical or incomplete forms.

OCULAR FINDINGS:

Orbit	Microphthalmia
Lids	Oblique position of eyes with lateral downward slope of palpebral fissure,** temporal lower lid coloboma** (approx. 75%), lack of cilia middle third of lower lid (about 50%), absence of Meibomian glands (Mann and Kilner: Brit. J. Ophth., 1943)
Motility	
Lacr. App.	Absent puncta of lower lids* (Nonay: Conf. Neurol., 1951)
Vision	
Vis. Fields	
Intraoc. Ten.	
Ant. Segm. and Sclera	Iris coloboma (occasionally)
Ocul. Media	
Retina and Choroid	
Optic Nerve	

OTHER CLINICAL FINDINGS:
1. Fish-like face with sunken cheek bones, receding chin, large wide mouth**
2. Absent or malformed external ears with auricular appendages,** absent external auditory canal and hearing defect
3. High palate and possible harelip
4. Hypoplastic zygomatic arc with absence of normal malar eminences**
5. Abnormal dentation
6. Prolonged hairline on the cheek**
7. Clubfoot*
8. Synostosis of joints*
9. Chest asymmetry*
10. Mental deficiency*

*Occasional findings   **Characteristic findings

BIBLIOGRAPHY:
1. Collins, E.T.: Cases with symmetrical congenital notches in the outer part of each lid and defective development of the malar bones, Tr. Ophth. Soc. U. Kingdom, *20:*190, 1900.
2. Franceschetti, A. and Zwahlen, P.: Un Syndrome nouveau, la dysostose mandibulo-faciale, Bull. schweiz. Akad. med. Wissensch. *1:*60, 1944.
3. Franceschetti, A. and Klein, D.: Mandibulo-faciale dysostosis; new hereditary syndrome, Acta Ophth. *27:*143, 1949.
4. Harrison, S. H.: Treacher Collins syndrome, Brit. J. Plastic Surg., *3:*282, 1950.
5. McKusick, V. A.: *Medical Genetics* 1958-1960, St. Louis, C. V. Mosby Co., 1961, p. 764.
6. Duke-Elder, Sir Stewart: *System of Ophthalmology,* Vol. VIII, Part 2, St. Louis, C. V. Mosby Co., 1963.

SYNDROME: Frankl-Hochwart
SYNONYMS: Pineal-neurologic-ophthalmic syndrome
GEN. INFORMATION:

Pineal tumor. The symptoms of the syndrome are often caused by pressure on portions of the brain. Pineal neopasms usually occur in early adulthood and are occasionally associated with endocrine disturbances

OCULAR FINDINGS:

Orbit	
Lids	
Motility	Limitation of upward gaze
Lacr. App.	
Vision	
Vis. Fields	Concentric field constriction
Intraoc. Ten.	
Ant. Segm. and Sclera	
Ocul. Media	
Retina and Choroid	
Optic Nerve	Papilledema

OTHER CLINICAL FINDINGS:

1. Bilateral deafness
2. Ataxia
3. Hypopituitarism
4. Headache ⎱ caused by increased
5. Vomiting ⎰ intracranial pressure

BIBLIOGRAPHY:

1. Gross, R. E.: Neoplasms producing endocrine disturbances in childhood, Am. J. Dis. Child. *59:*579, 1940.
2. Tassman, J.: *The Eye Manifestations of Internal Diseases,* 3rd. Ed., St. Louis, C. V. Mosby Co,. 1951.
3. Newton, T. H.: Neuroradiologic evaluation of lesions affecting the third ventricle and adjacent structures, in Smith, J. L. (ed.) *Neuro-Ophthalmology,* Vol. 3, St. Louis, C. V. Mosby Co., 1967.

SYNDROME: Frenkel
SYNONYMS: Ocular contusion syndrome, anterior-segment traumatic syndrome
GEN. INFORMATION:
Minor blunt trauma to the anterior segment of the globe. Some of the iris changes are only visible with focal retroillumination. The associated pathological findings in the iris root, lens equator, ciliary body and viterous have been described as possibly been caused by the relative movement of constituent parts against each other.

OCULAR FINDINGS:

Orbit	
Lids	
Motility	
Lacr. App.	
Vision	Slight reduced vision usually caused by mimimal macular edema which is easily overlooked
Vis. Fields	
Intraoc. Ten.	
Ant. Segm. and Sclera	Sluggish pupil reaction (direct, consensual and in convergence): D-shaped traumatic mydriasis with poor reaction to mydriatics and miotics in the sector corresponding to the 'straight' border (iridoplegia) and dehiscences of the iris pigment layer in the same sector (epidialysis) is a frequent finding. Irisdialysis and 'notching' of the pupillary border. Iris involvement in this syndrome has been listed with 50% of all cases*
Ocul. Media	Fine pigment precipitates on the corneal endothelium are only rarely seen in contrast to heavy pigment deposits on the vitreous surface (56% of cases*): Subulxation of the lens, transient posterior cortical lens opacities, permanent anterior or posterior capsular opacities, coronary opacities, late anterior cortical rosette, late total traumatic cataract, and Vossius' ring following hyphema. Lenticular involvement was said to be present in 60% of the cases*
Retina and Choroid	Peripheral pigment disturbance resembling atypical retinitis pigmentosa (58%)* Macular edema and minor foveal and parafoveal yellowish small patches (Berlin's edema) are regarded as contre coup effect
Optic Nerve	

OTHER CLINICAL FINDINGS:

*Frequency of occurrence quoted from Davidson (Ref. 2)

BIBLIOGRAPHY:
1. Frenkel. H.: Sur la valeur medico-legale du syndrome traumatique du segment anterieur, Arch. d'Opht., *48:*5, 1931.
2. Davidson, M.: Minor sequelae of eye contusion, A. J. O., *19:*757, 1936.
3. Paton, D. and Goldberg, M. F.: *Injuries of the Eye, the Lids and the Orbit: Diagnosis and Management,* Philadelphia, W. B. Saunders Co., 1968.

SYNDROME: Fröhlïch
SYNONYMS: Dystrophia adiposogenitalis
GEN. INFORMATION:
Chromophobe adenoma of the pituitary; Rathke pouch tumors; Craniopharyngeomas; suprasellar tumors (hypophyseal duct); encephalitis, trauma, etc. More frequent in Jews. Manifestations occur in childhood, most often during puberty, rarely in postadolescent period. Prognosis depends on early recognition and cause. Laboratory findings show increased sugar tolerance, reduction or absence of urinary gonadotropins (FSH) in both sexes. X-ray findings: enlargement or destruction of sella turcica or suprasellar calcification (80 to 90%). Ventriculography may reveal internal hydrocephalus.

OCULAR FINDINGS:

Orbit	
Lids	
Motility	
Lacr. App.	
Vision	Impaired scotopic vision
Vis. Fields	Bitemporal hemianopsia (occasionally with increased intracranial pressure)
Intraoc. Ten.	
Ant. Segm. and Sclera	
Ocul. Media	
Retina and Choroid	Impaired scotopic vision (dark adaptation), Landau and Bromberg
Optic Nerve	Papilledema, atrophy (with increased intracranial pressure)

OTHER CLINICAL FINDINGS:
1. Adioposity
2. Genital hypoplasia
3. In female: menstruation fails to appear or may cease in postpuberal period
4. In male: voice remains high pitched, undescended testes, absent facial hair, feminine pubic line
5. Open epiphyses (occasionally)
6. Possible retarded growth
7. Occasional mental infantilism
8. Polyuria
9. Polydypsia

BIBLIOGRAPHY:
1. Fröhlich, A.: Ein Fall von Tumor der Hypophysis cerebri ohne Akromegalie, Wien. klin. Rdsch. *15*:883 and 906, 1901.
2. Armstrong, C. N.: Three cases of supra pituitary tumour presenting Fröhlich's syndrome, Brain, *45*:113, 1922.
3. Landau, J. and Bromberg, Y. M.: Impaired scotopic vision in adiposogenital dystrophy, Brit. J. Ophthal., *38*:155, 1955.
4. Walsh, F. B.: *Clinical Neuro-Ophthalmology,* 2nd Ed., Baltimore, The Williams & Wilkins Co., 1957.
5. Reichlin, S.: Neuroendocrinology, in R. H. Williams (ed.): *Endocrinology,* Philadelphia, W. B. Saunders Co., 1968, p. 1005.

SYNDROME: Fuchs (1)
SYNONYMS: Heterochromic cyclitis syndrome
GEN. INFORMATION:
Etiology is unknown. Mild infective cyclitis most likely cause. During active periods of cyclitis there is increased protein content within the anterior chamber (Auvert and Lavat: Ann. Oculist. (Par.), 1952) with increased capillary permeability of the ciliary body (Amsler and Huber: Ophthalmologica, 1946). Histologic findings may consist of a lack of chromatophores in the iris, a connective tissue overgrowth in the stroma, hyalinization of vessel walls and infiltration with lymphocytes and plasmacells.

OCULAR FINDINGS:

Orbit Lids Motility Lacr. App.	
Vision	Not impaired except for the common development of a complicated cararact
Vis. Fields	
Intraoc. Ten.	Secondary glaucoma exists in about 5 to 15 % in unilateral, and in 22 to 33% in bilateral cases (Velicky: Csl. Ofthal., 1964; Huber)
Ant. Segm. and Sclera	Unilateral heterochromia; cyclitis with absence of synechiae, little or no ciliary injection no discomfort or pain. The iris architecture with typical trabeculae is lost. Some ragged and defective appearance of the deep pigmentary layer at the pupillary margin
Ocul. Media	Secondary cataract. Mild flare and cells in anterior chamber. Vitreous opacities. Small white discrete keratic precipitates with fine filaments between these precipitates. Corneal epithelium may be slightly edematous
Retina and Choroid Optic Nerve	Peripheral choroiditis occasionally

OTHER CLINICAL FINDINGS:
It has been suggested that 5 groups of heterochromia may exist: (1) Simple heterochromia; (2) atrophic; (3) sympathetic; (4) abiotrophic and (5) cyclitic
BIBLIOGRAPHY:
1. Fuchs, E.: Über Komplikationen der Heterochromie, Z. Augenhk. *15:*191, 1906.
2. Kimura, S. J.: Hogan, M. J. and Thygeson, P.: Fuchs' syndrome of heterochromic cyclitis, Arch. Ophth., *54:*179, 1955.
3. Huber, A.: Glaucoma as a complication in heterochromia of Fuchs', Ophthalmologica, *142:*66, 1961; ibid. *141:*122, 1961.
4. Lerman, S. and Levy, Ch.: Heterochromic iritis and secondary neovascular glaucoma, Am. J. Ophth. *57:*479, 1964.
5. Duke-Elder, Sir Stewart: *System of Ophthalmology,* Vol. IX, St. Louis, C. V. Mosby Co., 1966.

SYNDROME: Fuchs (2)
SYNONYMS: Mucocutaneous ocular syndrome
GEN. INFORMATION:
Etiology is unknown. The prognosis is good, complete recovery usually within 4 weeks without remission. The syndrome is often thought of as being identical with 'Erythema Multiforme Exudativum', which itself has been regarded frequently as a synonym of Stevens-Johnson syndrome. The described symptoms and the clinical manifestations in published reports have been regarded as merely different grades of severity and expressions of the same disease entity. Proppe (Arch f. Derm.) suggested to combine all the described disease complexes under the name of mucocutaneous-ocular syndrome of Fuchs. (see also Stevens-Johnson's syndrome.)

OCULAR FINDINGS:

Orbit	
Lids	
Motility	
Lacr. App.	
Vision	
Vis. Fields	
Intraoc. Ten.	
Ant. Segm.	Severe conjunctivitis with bullous lesions or ulcerations
and Sclera	
Ocul. Media	
Retina and	
Choroid	
Optic Nerve	

OTHER CLINICAL FINDINGS:
1. Headache
2. Macular eruptions of skin, as well as vesicular lesions
3. Swelling of the face
4. Cyanosis
5. Ulcers of mucous membranes
6. Stomatitis
7. Fever

BIBLIOGRAPHY:
1. Fuchs, E.: Herpes iris conjunctivae, Kl. Mbl. Augenhk *14:*333, 1876.
2. Costello, M. J. and Vandow, J. E.: Erythema multiforme. New York J. Med. *48:*2481, 1948.
3. Proppe, A.: Die Baadersche Dermatostomatitis, die Ektodermosis erosiva pluriorificialis Fiesinger und Rendu, das Stevens-Johnsonsche Syndrom und die Conjunctivitis et Stomatitis pseudomembranacea als Syndroma mucocutaneo-oculare acutum Fuchs, Arch. Dermat. u. Syph., *187:*392, 1949.
4. Robinson, H. M. and McCrumb, F.R.: Comparative analysis of the mucocutaneous-ocular syndromes, Arch. Dermat. & Syph., *61:*539, 1950.
5. Thies, O.: The mucocutaneous ocular syndrome of Fuchs', Kl. Mbl. Augenhk., *119:*486, 1951 (Abstract, A. J. O., *35:*749, 1952).

SYNDROME: Gänsslen
SYNONYMS: Familial hemolytic icterus, hematologic-metabolic bone disorder
GEN. INFORMATION:
The disease occurs mainly in caucasians. Heredity by dominant transmission with irregular penetrance. X-ray findings: Osteoporosis, thinned cortex of bones, "tower skull". Laboratory findings: decreased osmotic resistance of erythrocytes, microspherocytosis and reticulocytosis. Life expectancy may be prolonged with splenectomy.

OCULAR FINDINGS:

Orbit	Increased interpupillary distance, microphthalmos (occasionally)
Lids	Epicanthus, narrowing of palpebral fissure, lid hemorrhages
Motility	
Lacr. App.	
Vision	Myopia, dyschromatopsia
Vis. Fields	
Intraoc. Ten.	
Ant. Segm. and Sclera	Heterochromia irides, scleral icterus, conjunctival hemorrhages
Ocul. Media	Congenital cataract
Retina and Choroid	Retinal pallor and edema in advanced stages. Dilated retinal arteries and veins. Round retinal hemorrhages in deeper retinal layers, retinal exudates and macular star. Retinal detachment is rare and prognosis is good with absorption of subretinal exudate. Abnormal fundus pigmentation (occasionally)
Optic Nerve	

OTHER CLINICAL FINDINGS:

1. Splenomegaly
2. Hemolytic crises
3. Dental deformities
4. Brachydactyly
5. Polydactyly
6. Congenital hip luxation
7. Protrusion of frontal and parietal bones
8. Oxycephaly (approx. 50% of cases)
9. Deformities of the outer ear and otosclerosis
10. Hypogenitalism
11. Infantilismus

BIBLIOGRAPHY:
1. Gänsslen, M.: Uber hämolytischen Ikterus, Dt. Arch. Klin, Med., *140:*210, 1922, 1925
2. Weber, F.P.: A hemolytic jaundice family, Internat. Clin., *3:*148, 1931.
3. Gänsslen, M.: *Handbuch der Erbbiologie,* Berlin, Julius Springer, 1940.
4. Francois, J.: *Heredity in Opthalmology,* Sy. Louis, C. V. Mosby Co., 1961.
5. Thiel, R.: *Atlas of Diseases of the Eye,* Vol. 2, Amsterdam-London-New York, Elsevier Publ. Comp., 1963, p. 491.

SYNDROME: Gaucher
SYNONYMS: Glucocerebroside storage disease
GEN. INFORMATION:
Disorder with storage of glucocerebroside in the reticuloendothelial system. Autosomal recessive inheritance with occasionally dominant inheritance (Hsia *et al.*). Frequently found in Jewish families. Onset at any age, usually sudden in the infantile form. The prognosis and course of the disease is determined by the time of onset. The acute infantile form results in death usually before age two years. The disease belongs to the group of lipid storage disturbances such as ganglioside (Tay-Sachs), sphingomyelin (Niemann-Pick), ceremide-trihexoside (Fabry), a. o. Pathol. Find.: Typical Gaucher cells with one or more small dense nuclei eccentrically located in the large cell body. The cytoplasm is opaque and granular. The cells are found in liver, spleen, lymph nodes, lung, bone marrow. Neurophagia may be present in nuclei of basal cell ganglia and brain stem (Banker *et al.*).

OCULAR FINDINGS:

Orbit	
Lids	
Motility	Strabismus*
Lacr. App.	
Vision	
Vis. Fields	
Intraoc. Ten.	
Ant. Segm. and Sclera	Pinguecula of brown-yellowish color and wedge-shaped configuration**
Ocul. Media	
Retina and Choroid	Infiltration of the macula (isolated finding in which the generalized clinical features were akin to Gaucher's disease) Ref. 4
Optic Nerve	

OTHER CLINICAL FINDINGS:

Infantile form:*
1. Generalized hypertonia
2. Opisthotonus
3. Dysphagia, vomiting
4. Laryngeal spasm, dyspnea
5. Cachexia (final stage)

Chronic form:**
1. Hepatosplenomegaly
2. Lymphadenopathy (usually late)
3. Mild to moderate anemia
4. Yellowish-brown patchy skin pigmentation
5. Pathological fractures (occasionally) Osteolytic lesions and osteomyelitis

BIBLIOGRAPHY:
1. Gaucher, P. C. E.: De l'épithélioma primitif de la rate, hypertrophie idiopathique de la rate sans leucémie, Paris, Thèse, 1882.
2. Banker, B. Q.; Miller, J. Q. and Crocker, A. C.: The neurological disorder in infantile Gaucher's disease, Tr. Am. Neurol. A., *86:*43, 1961.
3. Hsia, D. Y.; Naylor, J. and Bigler, J. A.: The genetic mechanism of Gaucher's disease: in Aronson, S. M. and Volk, B. W. (Eds.): *Cerebral Sphingolipidoses,* New York, Academic Press, 1962, p. 327.
4. Cogan, D. G. and Federman, D. D.: Retinal involvement with reticuloendotheliosis of unclassified type, Arch. Ophth. *71:*489, 1964.
5. Crakushansky, G.: The lipidoses, in Gardner, L. I. (Ed.) *Endocrine and Genetic Diseases of Childhood,* Philadelphia, W. B. Saunders Co., 1969, p. 956.

SYNDROME: Goldenhar
SYNONYMS: Oculoauriculovertebral dysplasia
GEN. INFORMATION:
There seems to be no inheritance of the syndrome. The dermoid is usually flat and solid and bilateral. The vertebral anomalies are of great variety with cuneiform vertebrae, synostoses between two or more vertebrae, spina bifida, scoliosis, a. o. In spite of these multiple anomalies, neurological symptoms are infrequent.

OCULAR FINDINGS:

Orbit	
Lids	Lid coloboma, usually unilateral, involving the temporal half of the upper lid. Antimongolian slant of lid fissure
Motility	
Lacr. App.	
Vision	
Vis. Fields	
Intraoc. Ten.	
Ant. Segm. and Sclera	Epibulbar dermoid or lipodermoids (may also occur together in one eye). While the dermoid is usually located at the corneoscleral junction of the lower temporal quadrant, lipodermoids are more frequently found in the upper temporal quadrant. Iris coloboma (occasional)
Ocul. Media	
Retina and Choroid	
Optic Nerve	

OTHER CLINICAL FINDINGS:
1. Frontal bulging of the skull
2. Receding chin
3. Malar hypoplasia (mild)
4. Deafness and absence of external auditory meatus (occasionally)
5. Micrognathia and macrostomia (frequent)
6. Auricular appendices (single or multiple)
7. Multiple vertebral anomalies
8. Preauricular fistulas
9. Hemifacial microsomia (occasionally)
10. Mental retardation (about 10% of patients)

BIBLIOGRAPHY:
1. Goldenhar, M.: Associations malformations de l'oeil et de l'oreille, en particulier le syndrome dermoide épibulbaire-appendices auriculaires-fistula auris congenita et ses relations avec la dysostose mandibulo-faciale, J. Génét. hum. *1*:243, 1953.
2. Sinhar, P. N. and Mishra, S.: Corneal dermoid, Am. J. Ophth. *33*:1137, 1950.
3. Mahneke, A.: Epibulbar dermoids; preauricular appendices combined with unilateral malformation of the face, Acta Ophth. *34*:412, 1956.

SYNDROME: Goldscheider
SYNONYMS: Weber-Cockayne syndrome, epidermolysis bullosa
GEN. INFORMATION:

The syndrome is rare. Weber-Cockayne syndrome, inherited as an autosomal dominant trait, is actually a milder form without scar formation, whereas Goldscheider's syndrome, inherited either autosomal dominant or recessive, shows dystrophic changes with scarring. A polydysplasic form of the recessively inherited disease is lethal, usually causing death within the first 3 months of life (Ref. 2). Parental consanguinity is relatively frequent.

OCULAR FINDINGS:

Orbit	
Lids	Blepharitis
Motility	
Lacr. App.	
Vision	
Vit. Fields	
Intraoc. Ten.	
Ant. Segm. **and Sclera**	Shrinkage of conjunctiva, pseudomembrane formation, symblepharon, conjunctivitis, bullous keratitis and subepithelial blisters which lead to erosions with subsequent ulcerations and corneal opacities or even perforation. The sclera may be similarily involved
Ocul. Media	
Retina and **Choroid**	
Optic Nerve	

OTHER CLINICAL FINDINGS:

1. Vesicular and bullous skin lesions and similar lesions of mucous membranes which occur spontaneously or after mild trauma. The bullous lesions contain a sterile fluid but secondary infection when they rupture is a frequent complication. Keloid scars and kontraction after healing are common in the dystrophic forms, whereas in the mild form the lesions heal without scarring but maybe leaving some skin pigmentation
2. Growth and mental retardation may be present in the group of recessive inheritance
3. Stenosis of the larynx due to scarring may occur

BIBLIOGRAPHY:

1. Goldscheider, A.: Hereditäre Neigung zur Blasenbildung, Monatsh. prakt. Dermat., *1*:163, 1882.
2. Silver, H. K.: Epidermolysis bullosa hereditaria letalis, Arch. Dis. Child. *32*:216, 1957.
3. Sorsby, A.: *Modern Ophthalmology,* Vol. 2, Washington, Butterworths, 1963.
4. Duke-Elder, Sir Stewart: *System of Ophthalmology,* Vol. VIII, Part 1, St. Louis, C. V. Mosby Co., 1965.

SYNDROME: Gorlin-Chaudhry-Moss
SYNONYMS:
GEN. INFORMATION:
From the first reported few cases it is not possible to determine whether all the observed anomalies could have been caused by a single pleiotropic gene or by multiple, closely linked, genes.

OCULAR FINDINGS:

Orbit	Microphthalmia, hypertelorism, depressed supraorbital ridges
Lids	Inability to open or close lids fully, due to incomplete lid development, antimongoloid, oblique palpebral fissures, sparse eye lash development, lid defect (notching)
Motility	Horizontal nystagmus at extreme lateral gaze, limited upper gaze
Lacr. App.	
Vision	Astigmatism (secondary to corneal scars), marked hyperopia
Vis. Fields	
Intraoc Ten.	
Ant. Segm. and Sclera	Normal pupillary reaction to light but poor with accommodation
Ocul. Media	Corneal scars (exposure keratitis?)
Retina	
Retina and Choroid	
Optic Nerve	

OTHER CLINICAL FINDINGS:

1. Craniofacial dysostosi
2. Saddled appearance of upper face
3. High arched, narrow palate
4. Dental anomalies (size, number, position)
5. Hypertrichosis
6. Hypoplasia of labia majora
7. Patent ductus arteriosus
8. Normal mental development
9. Fatigue
10. Frontal headache

BIBLIOGRAPHY:
Gorlin, R. J.: Chaudhry, A. P. and Moss, M. L.: Craniofacial dysostosis, patent ductus arteriosus, hypertrichosis, hypoplasia of labia majora, dental and eye anomalies, J. Pediat., *56:*778, 1960.

SYNDROME: Gorlin-Goltz
SYNONYMS: Multiple basel cell nevi syndrome
GEN. INFORMATION:
Autosomal dominant inheritance with poor penetrance was suggested (Ref. 1). Onset of skin lesions in childhood and mainly about puberty. Microscopically the skin lesions follow a wide variety of pattern (superficial, solid or cystic, pigmented or not, lattice-like, etc.). Absence of significant urinary excretion of phosphorus following intravenous parathormone injection may be of diagnostic aid (Block and Clendenning).

A number of cases with this syndrome have been reported since the first description of the clinical findings by Jarisch in 1894. However, the first comprehensive study of this entity, the recognition and appreciation that the multiple clinical symptoms and findings are part and parcel of one inherited syndrome was given by Gorlin and Goltz.

OCULAR FINDINGS:

Orbit	Prominence of supraorbital ridges, causing the eyes to appear sunken. Hypertelorism, dystopia canthorum
Lids	Papulous nevoid basal cell carcinomas of upper lids
Motility	Internal strabismus
Lacr. App.	
Vision	"Congenital blindness" (Oliver: Arch. Dermat., 1960)
Vis. Fields	
Intraoc. Ten.	Glaucoma
Ant. Segm. and Sclera	
Ocul. Media	Congenital cataract, corneal leukoma
Retina and Choroid	Choroidal coloboma*
Optic Nerve	Optic nerve coloboma*　　　　　　　*(Observed in same patient)

OTHER CLINICAL FINDINGS:
1. Multiple basal cell nevi involving primarily nose, upper eyelids, cheeks, trunk, neck, arms
2. Cysts of the jaws of various sizes
3. Rib anomalies (usually bifid) and may involve more than one rib
4. Kyphoscoliosis and fusion of vertebrae
5. Short 4th metacarpals (isolated finding)
6. Mental retardation or schizophrenia (occasional)
7. Medulloblastoma
8. Mild degree of frontal and temporoparietal bossing
9. Broad nasal root

BIBLIOGRAPHY:
1. Gorlin, R. J. and Goltz, R. W.: Multiple nevoid basal cell epithelioma, jaw cysts and bified rib: A syndrome, New England J. Med., 262, 908, 1960.
2. Jarisch,: Zur Lehre von den Hautgeschwülsten, Arch. f. Dermat. u. Syph., 28:163, 1894.
3. Yunis, J. and Gorlin, R. J.: Chromosomal study in patients with cysts of the jaw, multiple nevoid basal cell carcinoma and bifid rib syndrome, Chromosoma, 14:140, 1963.
4. Gorlin, R. J.; Vickers, R. A.; Kelln, E. and Williamson, J. J.: The Multiple Basal Cell Nevi Syndrome: An analysis of a syndrome consisting of multiple nevoid basal-cell carcinoma, jaw cysts, skeletal anomalies, medulloblastoma, and hyporesponsiveness to parathormone, Cancer, 18 (1):89, 1965.

SYNDROME: Gradenigro
SYNONYMS: Temporal syndrome, Lannois-Gradenigro syndrome
GEN. INFORMATION:
Extradural abscess of the petrosus portion of the temporal bone. Causes: trauma, meningitis, hemorrhage (meningeal) are possible. Mastoiditis with extradural abscess. Prognosis is good. Differential diagnosis: Syphilitic meningitis, tuberculous meningitis, cerebellopontine angle tumor, cholesteatoma.

OCULAR FINDINGS:

Orbit	
Lids	
Motility	Ipsilateral paralysis (VI): The VI nerve becomes involved as it passes through Dorello's canal, intracranially. Spasm of homolateral internal rectus, transient involvement of III and IV occasionally present
Lacr. App.	
Vision	Diplopia
Vis. Fields	
Intraoc. Ten.	
Ant. Segm. **and Sclera**	Heavy pain in area of ophthalmic branch (V); photophobia; lacrimation; reduced sensitivity (corneal)
Ocul. Media	
Retina and **Choroid**	
Optic Nerve	Optic nerve involvement occasionally present.

OTHER CLINICAL FINDINGS:
1. Inner ear infection with deafness
2. Mastoiditis
3. Facial paresis possible
4. Temperature may be elevated
5. Signs of meningitis possible

BIBLIOGRAPHY:
1. Gradenigro, G.: A special syndrome of endocranial otitic complications, Ann. Otol. Rhin. & Laryng., *13:*637, 1904.
2. Meltzer, P. E.: Gradenigro's syndrome, Arch. Otolaryng. *13:*89, 1931.
3. Walsh, F. B.: Clinical Neuro-Ophthalmology, 2nd Ed., Baltimore, The Williams & Wilkins Co., 1957.
4. Alfano, J. E.: Clinical lesions of the IIIrd, IVth and VIth cranial nerves. (in Vail, D. T., edit.) Neuro-Ophthalmology, Internat. Ophth. Clinics, *1:*689, 1961.
5. Joffe, W. S.: Cranial nerve disease (in Gay, A. J. and Burde, R. M. (eds.)) Clinical Concepts in Neuro-Ophthalmology, Internat. Ophth. Clinics, 7*:*823, 1967.

SYNDROME: Greig
SYNONYMS: Ocular hypertelorism syndrome, hypertelorism
GEN. INFORMATION:
Etiology is unknown. The condition is rare. Defect occurs in early embryonic development (spontaneous and familial occurrence). In one instance, the syndrome was transmitted as an autosomal dominant trait over 5 generations with 11 out of 24 members of the same family affected (Bojlen and Brems: Acta path. et biol. scand., 1938) Fuller and Weber found in 2 siblings a male with sex chromatin anomaly-XXXY complex possibly-; and a female with probably XXX chromosome. Manifestations are present at birth. Abnormal development of the ala parva of the sphenoid bone and various other anomalies may be present. X-ray findings: Widely spaced orbits, increased number and site of ethmoidal cells.

OCULAR FINDINGS:

Orbit	Wide spacing of orbits, hypertelorism, enophthalmos (occasionally)
Lids	Epicanthus, deformities of eye lids and brows, defects of the palpebral fissure
Motility	Bilateral 6th nerve paralysis, convergent squint
Lacr. App.	
Vision	High astigmatism, binocular fusion sometimes absent because of extreme hypertelorism.
Vis. Fields	Visual field defects
Intraoc. Ten.	
Ant. Segm. and Sclera	
Ocul. Media	
Retina and Choroid	
Optic Nerve	Optic atrophy by tension on the optic nerve. Optic canal may be narrowed (Berliner and Gartner: Arch Ophth., 1940)

OTHER CLINICAL FINDINGS:
1. Skull may show mild malformations: Bitemporal eminences, decreased anteroposterior diameter
2. Harelip, high arched palate, cleft palate
3. Broad and flat nasal root
4. Mental impairment (frequent)
A number of other anomalies have been reported in association with this syndrome

BIBLIOGRAPHY:
1. Greig, D. M.: Hypertelorism. A hitherto undifferentiated congenital craniofacial deformity, Edinburgh M. J. *31*:560, 1924.
2. Brown, A. and Harper, R. K.: Craniofacial dysostosis: The significance of ocular hypertelorism, Quart. J. Med., *15*:171, 1946.
3. Meisenbach, A.: Bilateral paralysis of external rectus muscle in hypertelorism, report of a case with convergent strabismus, A. J. O., *33*:83, 1950.
4. Fuller, R. W. and Weber, A. N.: Hypertelorism in association with sex chromatin abnormality in two siblings, Am. J. Ment. Deficincy, *66*:844, 1961-62.
5. Gorlin, R.J. and Pindborg, J.J.: *Syndromes of the Head and Neck*, New York, Mc Graw-Hill Book Co. (Blakiston Division), 1964.

8

SYNDROME: Groenblad-Strandberg
SYNONYMS: Systemic elastodystrophy, pseudoxanthoma elasticum, ellas-torrhexis
GEN. INFORMATION:
Familial, autosomal recessive inheritance, consanguinity of parents relatively frequent (about 20%—Schloz: Arch. Ophth., 1941). May be partially sex-limited to females (Berlyne *et al.*: Quartl J. Med., 1961). Dominant inheritance was also suggested (Coffman and Sommers: Circulation, 1959). All ages involved, but usually manifest in youth and early middle age. Prognosis good. Affection of collagen, characterized by fibroid degeneration of the basic substance of connective tissue. The connective tissue fibers of the midcutis are thickened, fragmented, curled, and granulated with basophilic affinity to H. and E. stain and positive staining with elastic tissue stains. Calcium often present in degenerated fibers. Arterial sclerosis with parietal calcification.

OCULAR FINDINGS:

Orbit	
Lids	
Motility	
Lacr. App.	
Vision	Normal, unless the macula is involved
Vis. Fields	
Intraoc. Ten.	
Ant. Segm. and Sclera	
Ocul. Media	Subepithelial degeneration of corneal limbal area
Retina and Choroid	'Angioid streaks' of the retina, caused by pathologic condition within Bruch's membrane, clinically appear as a network of brownish-red to gray lines or streaks. They may be of various width and extend from a whitish ring surrounding the disc in a starlike fashion peripherally to the equator of the globe. Macular hemorrhages and transudates not infrequent (similar to Kuhnt-Junius macular degeneration). Choroidal sclerosis and atrophy at the posterior pole. Defects in the elastic layer of choroidal and ciliary arteries
Optic Nerve	

OTHER CLINICAL FINDINGS:
1. Pseudoxanthoma elasticum with thickening, softening, and relaxation of the skin: Skin changes are symmetrical in skin folds near large joints (axilla, elbow, inguineal region, lower abdomen, neck)
2. Flattening of the pulse curve and peripheral vascular disturbances (Plang)
3. Gastrointestinal hemorrhages (Kaplan and Hartman)
4. Intracranial aneurysm (Dixon)
5. Association with sickle cell disease (von Sallmann, Geeraets, Guerry, and Paton)
6. Association with Paget Disease (Woodcock, Shafer *et al.*)

BIBLIOGRAPHY:
1. Groenblad, E.: Angioid streaks, pseudoxanthoma elasticum, Acta. Ophth., 7:329, 1929.
2. Stegmaier, O.: Pseudoxanthoma elasticum (associated with angioid streaks of the retina), Arch. Dermat. & Syph. 70:530, 1954.
3. Darier, J.: Pseudoxanthoma elasticum, Monatsh. prakt. Derm. 23:609, 1896.
4. Böck, J.: Zur Klinik und Anatomie der gefässähnlichen Streifen im Augenhintergrund, Ztschr. f. Augenhk., 95:1, 1938.
5. Hagedoorn, A.: Angioid streaks, Arch. Ophth., 21:746, 1939.
6. Shaffer, B.; Copelan, H. W. and Beerman, H.: Pseudoxanthoma elasticum Arch. Dermat., 76:622, 1957.
7. Geeraets, W. J. and Guerry, D.: Angioid streaks and sickle cell disease, A. J. O., 49:450, 1960.

SYNDROME: Guillain-Barrè
SYNONYMS: Landry's paralysis, acute infectious neuritis, acute polyradiculitis
GEN. INFORMATION:
Etiology is unknown. Occurs in children and adults (16 to 50 years of age). Prognosis: About 20% mortality. Beside this the course is benign, recovery usually between several weeks to 3 months. Laboratory findings: hyperalbuminosis of cerebrospinal fluid without cellular reaction. Pathological findings: chromatolysis (Collier) of anterior horn cells and cells of Clark's column. Possible slight hyperemia of the spinal cord and few hemorrhages in the gray matter.

OCULAR FINDINGS:

Orbit	
Lids	Facial nerve paralysis with paralytic ectropion of the lower eyelid
Motility	Ocular nerves may be involved to various extents including complete external ophthalmoplegia
Lacr. App.	
Vision	
Vis. Fields	
Intraoc. Ten.	
Ant. Segm. and Sclera	Fixed and dilated pupils have been described (Barber)
Ocul. Media	
Retina and Choroid	
Optic Nerve	Optic neuritis (Glenn); Papilledema, it has been explained on the basis of elevated cerebrospinal fluid pressure due to blockage of drainage channels by excessive protein (Feldman *et al.*): Recurrent papilledema has also been described (Popek: Abstr., Exerpta Med. XII, 13:242, 1959)

OTHER CLINICAL FINDINGS:
1. Polyneuritis involving facial peripheral motor nerves and spinal cord
2. Facial diplegia
3. Bladder incontinence
4. Tendon reflexes absent
5. Variable degree of paralysis, usually
   beginning in lower extremities
6. Involvement of respiratory muscles possible
7. Parasynthesias (symmetric)
8. No elevated temperature
9. No pain

BIBLIOGRAPHY:
1. Guillain, G.; Barré, J. A. and Strohl, A.: Sur un syndrome de radiculonéurite avec hyperalbuminose du liquide céphalo-rachidien sans réaction cellulaire. Remarques sur les caractères cliniques et graphiques des réflexes tendineux, Bull. et mém. Soc. méd. hôp. Paris 40:1462, 1916.
2. Barber, H. S.: Polyradiculoneuritis in east anglia, Lancet, 2:548, 1940.
3. Ford, F. R. and Walsh, F. B.: Guillain-Barré syndrome with increased intracranial pressure and papilledema, Bull. Johns Hopkins Hospital, 73:391, 1943.
4. Feldman, S.; Landau, J. and Halpern, L.: Papilledema in Guillain-Barré syndrome, Arch. Neurol. Psychiat., 73:678, 1955
5. Joynt, R. J.: Mechanism of production of papilledema in the Guillain-Barré syndrome, Neurology, 8:8, 1958.

SYNDROME: Hallermann—Streiff
SYNONYMS: Dyscephalic-mandibulo-oculo-facial syndrome, oculomandibulodyscephaly
GEN. INFORMATION:
Rare syndrome. Familial occurrence and consanguinity between parents have been reported. Male and females equally affected. Cytogenetic studies have revealed a normal modal number chromosomes and in the karyotypes some discrepancy in size of two members of a pair of the 13 to 15 (D) group. (Carones, 1961). Normal sex chromatin was reported in a case of Falls and Schull (1960).

OCULAR FINDINGS:

Orbit	Microphthalmos (bilateral), severe unilateral proptosis*
Lids	
Motility	Nystagmus, strabismus
Lacr. App.	
Vision	
Vis. Fields	
Intraoc. Ten.	
Ant. Segm. and Sclera	
Ocul. Media	Cataracts (congenital), spontaneous resorption of the cataracts occurs)
Retina and Choroid	Chorioretinal atrophy,**peripapillary choroidal atrophy**
Optic Nerve	Bilateral optic atrophy*

OTHER CLINICAL FINDINGS:
1. Malformations of skull (brachycephaly), facial skeleton and jaws
2. Erupted teeth at birth
3. Dwarfism
4. Mental retardation
5. Diminished hair growth
6. Hyperextensibility of joints
7. Osteosclerosis*
8. Marble bones*

*(Consul et al.)   **Isolated findings

BIBLIOGRAPHY:
1. Hallermann, W.: Vogelgesicht und Cataracta congenita. Kl. Mbl. Augenhk. *113:*315, 1948.
2. Streiff, E. B.: Dysmorphic mandibulo-faciale (tête d'oiseau) et altérations oculaires, Ophthalmologica (Basel) *120:*79, 1950.
3. François, J.: A new syndrome. Dyscephalia with bird face and dental anomalies, nanism, hypotrichosis, cutaneous atrophy, microphthalmia, and congenital cataract, Arch. Ophth. *63:*409, 1958.
4. François, J.: Syndromes with congenital cataract (XVI Jackson Memorial Lecture), Trans. Am. Acad. Ophth. *64:*433, 1960.
5. Hoefnagel, D. and Benirschke, K.: Dyscephalia mandibulo-oculo-facialis: (Hallermann-Streiff syndrome), Arch. Dis. Child. *40:*57, 1965.

SYNDROME: Hallgren
SYNONYMS: Retinitis pigmentosa-deafness-ataxia syndrome
GEN. INFORMATION:
The syndrome is due to a single autosomal recessive gene with complete penetrance in both sexes. A pleiotropic effect causes retinitis pigmentosa and deafness
in all cases and mental deficiency, psychosis and vestibular ataxia in various pro-
portions. Mortality among the affected individuals is not increased, whereas
fertility is greatly reduced. Males and females are equally affected. (See also:
Usher's syndrome.)

OCULAR FINDINGS:

Orbit	
Lids	
Motility	Nystagmus (10%)—horizontal, undulating type
Lacr. App.	
Vision	Nightblindness present at preschool age, complete blindness at age 40 to 50 (approx. 40%), at age 60 to 70 (75%)
Vision	
Intraoc. Ten.	
Ant. Segm.	
and Sclera	
Ocul. Media	
Retina and	Cataract—(capsular, cortical, polar, zonular)—35% of all cases
Choroid	Retinitis pigmentosa, retinal atrophy, ERG confirmatory for the retinal involvement also in cases with lack of ophthal- moscopic narrow retinal vessels. Foveal reflex absent, dis- cernable pigmentary degeneration, (retinitis pigmentosa sine pigmento)
Optic Nerve	Optic atrophy

OTHER CLINICAL FINDINGS:
1. Congenital deafness (complete or at least very severe auditory impairment
2. Mental deficiency (25%), oligophrenia
3. Vestibulo-cerebellar ataxia (90%)
4. Schizophrenia-like symptoms (25%)
5. Skeletal anomalies (short stature, genu valgum, kyphosis, club foot)—occasional findings

BIBLIOGRAPHY:
1. Hallgren, B.: Retinitis pigmentosa combined with congenital deafness with
   vestibulocerebellar ataxia and neural abnormality in a proportion of cases:
   A clinical and geneticostatistical study, Acta psychiat. Scand. Supplements,
   138: 1–101, 1959/1960
2. v. Graefe, A.: Vereinzelte Beobachtungen und Bemerkungen No. 6,
   Exceptionelles Verhalten des Gesichtsfeldes bei Pigmentierung der Netzhaut,
   v. Graefe's Arch. f. Ophth. *4:*250, 1858.
3. Lidenov,H.: The etiology of deaf-mvtism, Diss., Copenhagen, 1945.

SYNDROME: Hand-Schüller-Christian
SYNONYMS: Lipoid granuloma, xanthomatous granuloma syndrome, Schüller-Christian-Hand syndrnme
GEN. INFORMATION:

Etiology is unknown. Male preponderance 2:1. Onset in childhood (before age of 6). Prognosis is chronic with remissions. Tendency to healing and fibrosis. Mortality up to 50%. High incidence of vasopressin deficiency. Hypercholesteremia, hyperplastic reticulum cells, irregular skull defects with sharp borderlines (up to 5 cm in diameter). Lipoid cell infiltration of lungs and pleura. Granulomatous lesions of the RES with lipoid cell hyperplasia and proliferation of histiocytes.

OCULAR FINDINGS:

Orbit	Exopthalmos (might be unilateral) (30% of cases); ocular pulsation may occur in cases of orbital roof defects with transmittance of brain pulsation
Lids	Xanthelasma and xanthomatous tumors, ecchimosis, swelling of upper and lower lid, blepharitis
Motility	Internal ophthalmoplegia may occur. Nystagmus has been reported (Davison)
Lacr. App.	
Vision	
Vis Fields	
Intraoc. Ten.	
Ant. Segm. and Sclera	
Ocul. Media	Partial fatty degeneration of the cornea (Jaensch)
Retina and Choroid	Hemorrhages and exudates
Optic Nerve	Papilledema; xanthomatous deposits about the disc (Jaensch); optic atrophy following papilledema or due to intracranial or intraorbital pressure

OTHER CLINICAL FINDINGS:

1. Xanthoma of the skin
2. Diabetes insipidus (50% of cases)
3. Skull defects
4. Lung fibrosis
5. Secondary cardiac insufficiency
6. Defects in mandibula, long bones, pelvis, ribs and spine possible
7. Ulcers of gingivae
8. Lymph adenopathy
9. Hepatosplenomegaly
10. Growth and sexual retardation

BIBLIOGRAPHY:

1. Hand, A.: Polyuria and tuberculosis, Arch Pediat. *10:*673, 1893; Ibid.: Amer. J. Med. Sc. *162:*509, 1921; Ibid.: Proc. Phil. Path. Soc. *16:*282, 1893.
2. Schüller, A.: Wien. med. Wschr. *71:*510, 1921.
3. Christian, H. A.: Defects in membraneus bones, expohthalmos and diabetes insipidus; New York, Paul B. Hoeber, Inc. Vol. I, p. 390, 1919.
4. Davision, C.: Xanthomatosis and the CNS, Arch. Neurol. and Psychiat. *30:*75, 1933.
5. Jaensch, P.A.: Seltene Augenveründerungen bei Schüller-Christianscher Krankheit, Klin. Mbl. Augenhk., *92:*158, 1934.
6. Avery, M. E.; McAfee, J. G.; and Guild, H. G.: The course and prognosis of reticuloendotheliosis (eosinophilic granuloma, Schüller-Christian disease and Letterer-Siwe disease), Am. J. Med. *22:*636, 1957.

SYNDROME: Heerfordt
SYNONYMS: Uveoparotid fever, unveoparotitic paralysis
GEN. INFORMATION:
Females more often affected than men. The disease occurs mainly in young adults. (See also Schaumann's syndrome). Sarcoidosis is most widely accepted as the cause for the clinical and pathological findings of this disorder. Though lymph node biopsies have been reported as having shown reticuloendotheliosis and tuberculous granulation tissue.

OCULAR FINDINGS:

Orbit	
Lids	Lid granulations may rarely occur
Motility	
Lacr. App.	
Vision	
Vis. Fields	
Intraoc. Ten	
Ant. Segm. and Sclera	Bilateral uveitis (granulomatous), iridocyclitis. Onset suddenly or more gradually and rather little discomfort and pain. Usually both eyes become involved, though frequently not at the same time. Posterior synechiae are common and iris nodules occur in about 35% of cases. The conjunctiva may occasionally be involved
Ocul. Media	Vitreous opacities
Retina and Choroid	
Optic Nerve	Optic neuritis (isolated findings)

OTHER CLINICAL FINDINGS:

1. Parotid glands swelling (6 weeks' to 2 years' duration)
2. Submaxillary and sublingual glands might be involved
3. Nervous system involvement with facial paralysis (up to 50%) and not infrequently bilateral (Ref. 2). The paralysis usually disappears within a few months, though it has persisted in some patients (Schönholzer: Schweiz. med. Wschr., 1914)
4. Peripheral polyneuritis (not uncommon)
5. Lymphadenopathy, splenomegaly
6. Cutaneous and subcutaneous nodules
7. Slight fever

BIBLIOGRAPHY:

1. Heerfordt, C. F.: Über eine "Febris uveoparotidea subchronica" in der Glandula parotis und der Uvea des Auges lokalisiert und häufig mit Paresen cerebrospinaler Nerven kompliziert, Graefes Arch. f. Ophth., 70:254, 1909.
2. Savin, L. H.: An analysis of the signs and symptoms of 66 published cases of the uveoparotid syndrome, with details of an additional case, Tr. Ophth. Soc. U. Kingdom, 54:549, 1934.
3. Granström, K. O.; Gripwall, E.; Kristofferson, C. E. and Lindgren, A. G. H.: A case of uveoparotid fever (Heerfordt) with autopsy findings, Acta med. scand. 126:307, 1946.
4. Duke-Elder, Sir Stewart: System of Ophthalmology, Vol. 9, St. Louis, C. V. Mosby Co. 1966.

SYNDROME: Heidenhain

SYNONYMS: Presenile dementia-cortical degeneration syndrome

GEN. INFORMATION:

The fatal disease is rare. Prognosis is poor, rapidly progressive deterioration with death after few months. Mainly occipital cortical degeneration including the calcarine region (status spongiosus) with relative little cerebral involvement of the parietal cortex. Histological findings: disturbed architecture and proliferation of protoplasmic and fibrous astrocytes. Shrinkage and pigment atrophy of the small nerve cells (Heidenhain).

OCULAR FINDINGS:

Orbit	
Lids	
Motility	
Lacr. App.	
Vision	Rapid loss of vision (cortical blindness)
Vis. Fields	
Intraoc. Ten.	
Ant. Segm. and Sclera	
Ocul. Media	
Retina and Choroid	No pathologic condition of the fundus
Optic Nerve	•

OTHER CLINICAL FINDINGS:

1. Presenile dementia
2. Dysarthria
3. Ataxia
4. Athetotic movements
5. General rigidity without signs of pyramidal disorder

BIBLIOGRAPHY:

1. Heidenhain, A.: Klinische und anatomische Untersuchungen über eine eigenartige organische Erkrankung des Zentralnervensystems im Praesenium, Z. ges. Neurol. Psychiat. *118:*49, 1928.
2. Meyer, A.; Leigh, D. and Bagg, C. E.: A rare presenile dementia associated with cortical blindness (Heidenhain's syndrome), J. Neurol. Neurosurg. & Psychiat., *17:*129, 1954.
3. Jones, D. P. and Nevin, S.: Rapidly progressive cerebral degeneration (subacute vascular encephalopathy) with mental disorder, focal disturbances and myoclonic epilepsy, J. Neurol., Neurosurg. & Psychiat. *17:*148, 1954.

SYNDROME: Hemifacial Microsomia
SYNONYMS: Unilateral facial agenesis, otomandibular dysostosis
GEN. INFORMATION:

Apparently no inheritance. The left side of the face seemed to have been some-what more frequently involved (Gorlin and Pindborg) though it was stated that the statistical significance of this observation was doubtful. Asymmetry of the face is usually the most obvious finding. The eye on the affected side appears to be situated lower. The cause for the deformities has been suggested to occur at an approximate 20 to 25 mm stage of fetal life.

OCULAR FINDINGS:

Orbit	Microphthalmos, congenital cystic ophthalmia
Lids	Palpebral fissure lower on affected side
Motility	Strabismus
Lacr. App.	
Vision	
Vis. Fields	
Intraoc. Ten.	
Ant. Segm. and Sclera	Iris coloboma
Ocul. Media	
Retina and Choroid	Choroidal coloboma
Optic Nerve	

OTHER CLINICAL FINDINGS:

1. Microtia
2. Macrostomia (about 30%)
3. Failure of development of mandibular ramus and condyle
4. External auditory meatus may be absent
5. Single or numerous ear tags
6. Hypoplasia of facial muscles one side.
7. Pulmonary agenesis (ipsilateral side)

BIBLIOGRAPHY:

1. François, J. and Haustrate, L.: Anomalies colobomateuses du globe oculaire et syndrome du premier arch, Ann. ocul. *187*:340, 1954.
2. Theier. C. J.: Symptomenkomplexe im Rahmen der mandibulo-fazialen Dysplasien, Klin. Mbl. Augenhk. *135*:378, 1959.
3. Gorlin, R. J. and Pindborg, J. J.: *Syndromes of the Head and Neck,* New York, McGraw-Hill Book Co. (Blakiston Division), 1964.

SYNDROME: Hennebert
SYNONYMS: Luetic-otitic-nystagmus syndrome
GEN. INFORMATION:

Congenital syphilis. Manifestations in childhood. When a fistula in the labyrinth exists, compression of the external auditory meatus will produce nystagmus of a wide amplitude (diagnostic of fistula). Such labyrinthine fistula are not uncommon in congenital syphilitics. Out of 40 syphilitic children nystagmus was present in 13 of which 8 presented positive fistula symptoms while they were doubtful in the remaining 5 (Asherson).

OCULAR FINDINGS:

Orbit	
Lids	
Motility	Spontaneous nystagmus of otitic origin and giddiness with exaggeration of the nystagmus when the column of air in the auditory canal is compressed.
Lacr. App.	
Vision	
Vis. Fields	
Intraoc. Ten.	
Ant. Segm. and Sclera	
Ocul. Media	Interstitial keratitis*
Retina and Choriod	Disseminated syphilitic chorioretinitis may be present.*
Optic Nerve	

OTHER CLINICAL FINDINGS:

1. Vertigo
2. Fistula in the labyrinth
3. Deafness
4. Other clinical manifestations of congenital syphilis may be present such as 'saddle' nose, Hutchington's teeth, etc.*

*Although these findings are frequently found, they do not form a constant part of this syndrome

BIBLIOGRAPHY:

1. Asherson, N.: Spontaneous nystagmus in congenital syphilis, Arch. Dis. Childhood, 5:331, 1930.
2. Ford, F. R.: *Diseases of the Nervous System in Infancy, Childhood and Adolescence,* Springfield, Charles C Thomas, 1952.
3. Walsh, F. B.: *Chinical Neuro-Ophthalmology,* Baltimore, The Williams & Wilkins Co., 1957.

SYNDROME: Herrick
SYNONYMS: Dresbach's syndrome; sickle cell disease; drepanocytic anemia
GEN. INFORMATION:
With few exceptions, only in members of the Negro race. Poor prognosis. Laboratory findings: sickle-shaped erythrocytes. Hemoglobin electrophoresis shows atypical hemoglobin types S, C and combinations of those with normal hemoglobin. X-ray examination reveals narrowing of the medullary space with increased density of the cortex of long bones. "Hair-on-End" appearance of the skull (due to extension of the marrow through the outer table of the bone. Path. Findings: Intracranial hemorrhages, cardiac hypertrophy, thrombosis, liver cirrhosis, infarction of the spleen.

OCULAR FINDINGS:

Orbit	
Lids	
Motility	
Lacr. App.	
Vision	
Vis. Fields	
Intraoc. Ten.	Secondary glaucoma
Ant. Segm. and Sclera	Stasis and telangiectasis of conjunctival vessels, scleral icterus
Ocul. Media	Vitreous hemorrhages, complicated cataract
Retina and Choroid	Hemorrhages, exudates, neovascularization, retinitis proliferans, microaneurysms, thrombosis of retinal venules, ischemia, vascular sheathing, chorioretinal degeneration, central vein occlusion, angioid streaks, retinopathy with 'black sunburst sign' in SS patients and 'sea fan sign' in patients with SC hemoglobin (Welch and Goldberg)
Optic Nerve	Papilledema (rare)

OTHER CLINICAL FINDINGS:
1. Severe anemia with hemolytic crises
2. Bone and joints aches
3. Hemarthrosis
4. Jaundice
5. Hepatosplenomegaly
6. Enlarged lymph nodes
7. Cardiomegaly

BIBLIOGRAPHY:
1. Herrick, J. B.: Peculiar elongated and sickle-shaped red corpuscles in a case of severe anemia, Arch. Int. Med. 6:517, 910.
2. Goodman, G.; Sallmann, L. von; Holland, M. G.: Ocular manifestations of sickle cell disease, Arch. Ophth., 58:655, 1957.
3. Lieb, W. A.; Geeraets, W. J.; and Guerry, D. III: Sickle cell retinopathy, Acta. Ophth., Suppl. 58, 1959.
4. Geeraets, W. J.; and Guerry, D.: Angioid streaks in sickle-cell disease, Am. J. Ophth. 49:450, 1960. Elastic Tissue degeneration in sickle cell disease, Am. J. Ophth. 50:213, 1960.
5. Paton, D.: Conjunctival signs of sickle cell disease, Arch. Ophth. 66:90, 1961.
6. Conrad, W. C. and Penner, R.: Sickle cell trait and central retinal artery occlusion, Am. J. Ophth. 63:465, 1967.
7. Welch, R. B. and Goldberg, M. F.: Sickle-Cell Hemoglobin and its Relation to Fundus Abnormality, Arch. Ophth. 75:353, 1966.

SYNDROME: Homocystinuria
SYNONYMS:
GEN. INFORMATION:
Rare disease. Hereditary disorder of amino acid metabolism. The trait is transmitted as a Mendelian recessive. Plasma homocystine and methionine levels elevated. Urinary excretion of homocystine elevated. Nitro-prusside test of urine positive. Stickiness of platelets. It is the third inborn type of disordered metabolism of amino acid of particular interest to ophthalmology (cystinosis and Lowe's syndrome being the other two)

OCULAR FINDINGS:

Orbit	
Lids	
Motility	
Lacr. App.	
Vision	
Vis. Fields	
Intraoc. Ten.	
Ant. Segm. and Sclera	Aniridia (single observation) Ref. 4
Ocul. Media	Dislocated or subluxated lenses, spherophakia, congenital cataract
Retina and Choroid	Retinal detachment and retinal cyst (single observation) Ref. 4
Optic Nerve	Optic atrophy

OTHER CLINICAL FINDINGS:
1. Mental retardation
2. Genu valgum
3. Sparseness of hair
4. Thromboembolism
5. Arachnodactyly

BIBLIOGRAPHY:
1. Gibson, J. B.; Carson, N. A. J. and Neill, D. W.: Pathological findings in homocystinuria, J. Clin. Path. *17:*427, 1964.
2. Arnott, E. J.; and Greaves, D. P.: Ocular involvement in homocystinuria, Brit. J. Ophth. *48:*688, 1964.
3. Cogan, D.: Dislocated lenses and homocystinuria, Arch. Ophth. *74:*446, 1965.
4. Presley, G. D. and Sidbury, J. B.: Homocystinuria and ocular defects, Am. J. Ophth. *63:*1723, 1967.

SYNDROME: Horner

SYNONYMS: Bernard-Horner syndrome, cervical sympathetic paralysis syndrome, Claude-Bernard-Horner syndrome, Horner's oculopupillary syndrome.

GEN. INFORMATION:

Paralysis of cervical sympathetic. Hypothalamic lesion with first neuron involved, or lesion in the pons or cervical portion of cord. Trauma with hemorrhage, cervical rib, osteochondroma of first rib, postoperatively after thoracoplasty, extrapleural pneumolysis, resection of phrenic nerve, cervicodorsal sympathectomy, after goiter, Pancoast tumor, esophagus carcinoma, aortal aneurysm, etc. The syndrome is present in Babinski-Nageotte, Cestan-Chenais, Dejerine-Klumple, Pancoast, Raeder and Wallerberg syndromes.

OCULAR FINDINGS:

Orbit	Enophthalmos
Lids	Ptosis or narrowing of palpebral fissure
Motility	Excessive secretion of tears
Lacr. App.	
Vision	
Vis. Fields	
Intraoc. Ten.	Ocular hypotony
Ant. Segm. and Sclera	Miosis, degree of miosis depends on site of the lesion and is most pronounced when roots of VII and VIII cranial nerves and the 1st thoracic nerve are involved. Lack of iris pigmentation (children>adults). Pupil does not dilate with cocaine
Ocul. Media	
Retina and Choroid	
Optic Nerve	

OTHER CLINICAL FINDINGS:

1. Anhidrosis ipsilateral side of face and neck
2. Transitory rise in facial temperature
3. Hemifacial atrophy

BIBLIOGRAPHY:

1. Horner, F.: Ueber eine Form von Ptosis, Klin. Mbl. Augenhk. 7:193, 1869.
2. Jaffe, N.: Localization of lesions causing Horner's syndrome, Arch. Ophth., 44:710, 1950.
3. Jaffe, N.: Horner's syndrome, A. J. O., 34:1181, 1951.
4. Durham, D. G.: Congenital heredity in Horner's syndrome, Arch. Ophth., 60:939, 1958.
5. Adler, F. M.: Physiology of the Eye, St. Louis, 4th Ed., C. V. Mosby Co., 1965.
6. Burde, R. M.: The pupil; in Gay, A. J. and Burde, R. M. (eds.): Clinical concepts in Neuroophthalmology, Intnat. Ophth. Clinics. 7:839, 1967.

SYNDROME: Hunt
SYNONYMS: Ramsay Hunt syndrome, geniculate neuralgia, herpes zoster auricularis
GEN. INFORMATION:
Herpes of the geniculate, or sensory, ganglion. The course of the disease if often prolonged, it may be mild or severe and is self-limited. Peripheral ganglions of 8th, 9th and 10th cranial nerves may be involved as well. On the other hand it has been reported that in this syndrome the geniculate ganglion not always had been involved when the symptoms of this syndrome were rpesent. (Danny-Brown: Arch. Neurol. & Psychiat., 1944). Pain is severe and frequently precedes the skin and mucosal lesions and may persist for some time after the lesions have disappeared.

OCULAR FINDINGS:

Orbit	
Lids	
Motility	
Lacr. App.	Diminished lacrimation
Vision	
Vis. Fields	
Intraoc. Ten.	
Ant. Segm. and Sclera	
Ocul. Media	Absence of motor conreal reflex on affected side, whereas the consensual reflex of the non-involved eye remains normal
Retina and Choroid	
Optic Nerve	

OTHER CLINICAL FINDINGS:

1. Herpes zoster lesion external ear and oral mucosa
2. Severe pain external auditory meatus and pinna
3. Diminished hearing, tinnitus
4. Vertigo
5. Facial palsy
6. Loss or diminished superficial and deep facial reflex
7. Zoster lesions may involve scalp, face, neck
8. Loss of taste anterior two-thirds of tongue (occasionally)
9. Diminished salivation
10. Hoarseness

BIBLIOGRAPHY:
1. Hunt, J.R.: On herpetic inflammations of the geniculate ganglion: a new syndrome and its complications, J. Nerv. & Ment. Dis. N.Y. *34:*73, 1907.
2. Engström, H. and Wohlfahrt, G.: Herpes Zoster of the seventh, eighth, ninth and tenth cranial nerves, Arch. Neurol & Psychiat., *62:*638, 1949.
3. Wilson, A.: Geniculate Neuralgia; Report of a case relieved by intracranial section of the nerve of Wrisberg, J. Neurosurgery *7:*473, 1950.

SYNONYMS: Systemic mucopolysaccharidosis Type (MPS) II
GEN. INFORMATION:
Genetic disorder. Sex linked recessive. Absence of lumbar gibbus. Clinically less severe than Hurler's syndrome (MPS I) with a longer life span (into adulthood). Similar as in MPS I (Hurler's syndrome), chondroitin sulfate B and heparitin sulfate are excreted in excess in urine. (See also: Sanfillipo-Good, Morquio-Brailsford and Scheie's syndromes)

OCULAR FINDINGS:

Orbit	
Lids	
Molitity	
Lacr. App.	
Vision	Decreased (see retina below), nightblindness may exist
Vis. Fields	Fields may be constricted
Intraoc. Ten.	
Ant. Segm. and Sclera	Deposition of abnormal mucopolysaccharides in the corneal stroma is minimal. Large concentrations are present in the corneal endothelium, the epithelial structures of the iris and ciliary body and in the thickened sclera. Thickened pigment epithelium of the iris
Ocul. Media	Splitting or absence of Bowman's membrane in the periphery. Usually no corneal clouding, though slight stromal haze may be present
Retina and Choroid	Pigmentary degeneration of the retina. Nightblindness, narrowed retinal vessels and central choroidal sclerosis. ERG reduced and no scotopic response. EOG extinguished (Gills *et al.*)
Optic Nerve	Pale disc (Gills *et al.*)

OTHER CLINICAL FINDINGS:
1. Dwarfism
2. Stiff joints
3. Hepatosplenomegaly
4. Gargoyle-like facies
5. Perceptive type of deafness

BIBLIOGRAPHY:
1. Hunter, L.: A rare disease in two brothers, Proc. Roy. Soc. Med. *10*:104, 1917.
2. Gills, J. P.; Hobson, R.; Hanley, W. B. and McKusick, V. A.: Electroretinography and fundus oculi findings in *Hurler's* and allied mucopolysaccharidoses, Arch. Ophth. *74*:596, 1965.
3. McKusick, V. A.: The Genetic Mucopolysaccharidoses, Medicine (see Ref. 2)
4. Goldberg, M.F. and Duke, J. R.: Ocular histopathology in Hunter's syndrome, Arch. Ophth. *77*:503, 1967.

SYNDROME: Hurler
SYNONYMS: Pfaundler-Hurler syndrome, gargoylism, dysostosis multiplex, chondroosteo-dystrophy,systemic mucopolysaccharidosis type (MPS) I.
GEN. INFORMATION:
Sporadic, familial, autosomal recessive. Beside corneal opacities and enlargement of the head at birth, other symptoms become apparent at the end of the first year. Prognosis: death occurs usually before age 20 years. X-ray findings: wide sella turcica, thorax deformities, short and broad phalanxes, delayed epiphyseal development. Analitative and quantitative examination of urinary MPS excretion is essential for accurate diagnosis and classification. Gross excess of chondroitin sulfate B and heparitin sulfate in urine. (See also: Hunter, Sanfillipo-Good, Morquio-Brailsford and Scheie's Syndromes.)

OCULAR FINDINGS:

Orbit	Proptosis, hypertelorism
Lids	Slight ptosis, thick enlarged lids
Motility	Internal strabismus
Lacr. App,	
Vision	
Vis. Fields	
Intraoc. Ten.	Glaucoma*
Ant. Segm.	
and Sclera	
Ocul. Media	Diffuse haziness of the corneae at birth progressive to milky opacity. Lipid-like infiltration in the cornea below the epithelium throughout the stroma. No vascularization. Absence of Bowman's membrane (Wagner)
Retina and Choroid	Retinal pigmentary changes may exist. Macula edema and absence of foveal reflex described (Walsh); ERG responses subnormal without scotopic component and more marked in older patients (Gills *et al.*)
Optic Nerve	Optic atrophy (Davis and Currier), redness of optic disc (Slot and Burgess)

OTHER CLINICAL FINDINGS:
1. Dorsolumbar kyphosis
2. Normal development greatly retarded
3. Head deformities with depressed nose bridge
4. Short cervical spine
5. Spina bifida*
6. Wide clavicles
7. Abnormal protuberans
8. Short limbs
9. Late dentation
10. Macroglossia
11. Enlarged liver and spleen
12. Infantilism

*Rare
BIBLIOGRAPHY:
1. Hurler, G.: Ueber einen Typ multipler Abartungen, vorwiegend am Skelletsystem Zt. Kinderhk. *24:*220, 1919.
2. Berliner, M. L.: Lipinkeratitis of Hurler's syndrome, clinical and pathologic report, Arch. Ophth. *22:*97. 1939.
3. Meyers, S. J. and Okner, H. B.: Dysostosis multiplex with special reference to ocular findings, A. J. O., *22:*713, 1939.
4. Wagner, F.: Beitrag zur Frage der Dysostosis Multiplex (Pfaundler-Hurler) mit Fehlbildung der Bowmanschen Membrane, Ztschr. Kinderh., *69:*179, 1951.
5. Gills, J. P.; Hobson, R.; Hanley, W. B. and McKusick, V. A.: Electroretinography and fundus oculi findings in Hurler's disease and allied mucopolysaccharidoses, Arch. Ophth. *74:*596, 1965.
6. McKusick, V. A.: The genetic mucopolysaccharidoses, Medicine (See Ref. 5)

SYNDROME: Hutchinson
SYNONYMS: Adrenal cortex neuroblastoma with orbital melastasis
GEN. INFORMATION:

Infraorbital neuroblastoma. The often stated theory of multicentric neuroblastoma formation with a primary, intraorbital tumor development as the cause of Hutchinson's syndrome, is of little significance. Histopathological studies have shown numerous tumor cell embolisms which indicate a metastatic tumor growth after hematogenous dissemination (Ref. 4). The eye frequently presents the first noticable indication of the disease. The syndrome occurs in infants and up to 6 years of age. Poor prognosis with life expectancy of few months to one year.

OCULAR FINDINGS:

Orbit	Exophthalmos
Lids	Lid hematoma
Motility	Extraocular muscle palsy
Lacr. App.	
Vision	
Vis. Fields	
Intraoc. Ten.	
Ant. Segm. and Sclera	Subconjunctival hemorrhages (hyposphagma)
Ocul. Media	
Retina and Choroid	Choroidal metastatic tumor (Ref. 2)
Optic Nerve	Papilledema, optic atrophy from neuroblastoma

OTHER CLINICAL FINDINGS:
1. Severe anemia
2. Increased sedimentation rate
3. Urinary excretion of 3-methoxy-4-hydroxy mandelic acid
4. Occasionally abdominal tumor palpable

BIBLIOGRAPHY:
1. Hutchinson, R.: Suprarenal sarcoma in children with metastasis in the skull, Quart. J. Med. *1*:33, 1907/8
2. Bothman, L. and Blankstein, S. S.: The eye in adrenal sympathicoblastoma (Neuroblastoma), Arch. Ophth. *27*:746, 1942.
3. Cox, R. A.: Proptosis due to neuroblastoma of the adrenal cortex (Hutchinson's syndrome), Arch. Ophth. *39*:713, 1948.
4. Pesch, K. J.: Zur Pathogenese des Hutchinson-Syndromes, Klin. Mbl. Augenhk. *145*:376, 1964.

SYNDROME: Jacod
SYNONYMS: Negri-Jacod's syndrome; petrosphenoidal space syndrome.
GEN. INFORMATION:
Lesion involving nerve II through VI. Most frequent maligant nasopharyngeal tumor originating in lateropharyngeal area. With lesions located on the floor of the middle cranial fossa, nerves which pass through the foramen ovale, foramen rotundum and through the sphenoidal fissure become involved giving rise to ophthalmoplegia in which the III, IV and VI cranial nerves may be involved as well as the optic nerve.

OCULAR FINDINGS:

Orbit	
Lids	
Motility	Ophthalmoplegia
Lacr. App.	
Vision	Unilateral blindness, depending on optic nerve involvement
Vis. Fields	
Intraoc. Ten.	
Ant. Segm.	
and Sclera	Trigeminal neuralgia (ophthalmic branch)
Ocul. Media	
Retina and	
Choroid	
Optic Nerve	Descending optic atrophy if IInd nerve becomes involved

OTHER CLINICAL FINDINGS:
1. Trigeminal neuralgia: at the beginning the 1st and 2nd division of V are involved; later the 3rd division is affected as well
2. Uni- or bilateral enlargement of cervical lymph nodes (30%)

BIBLIOGRAPHY:
1. Jacod, M.: Sur la propagation intracrânienne des sarcomes de la trompe d' Eustache syndrome du carrefour pétro-sphénoidale paralysie des, 2,3,4,5, et 6 paires crâniennes, Rev. neurol., *38*:33, 1921.
2. Godtfredsen, E.: Ophthalmo-neurological symptoms in malignant naso-pharyngeal tumors, Brit. J. Ophth., *31*:78, 1947.
3. Ormerod, F. C.: Malignant disease of the nasopharynx, J. Laryng. & Otol. *65*:778, 1951.
4. Riggs, H. E.: Cranial nerve syndromes associated with nasopharyngeal malignancy, Arch. Neurol. & Psychiat. *77*:473, 1957.

SYNDROME: Jadassohn-Lewandowski
SYNONYMS: Pachyonychia congenita
GEN. INFORMATION:

The syndrome is inherited by an autosomal dominant pattern with low penetrance, though not observed in all reported cases (Kumer and Loos:Wien. Kl. Wschr., 1935). These authors grouped the syndrome in 3 types. Type I: Symmetrical keratoses of hand and feet and follicular keratoses of the body. Type II: same as Type I, plus leukokeratosis oris (typus Riehl), and Type III: same as Type I, plus corneal changes. Pathological findings: Mainly thickening of the skin with plugged follicles and ducts of sweat glands by cornified derbis. Intracellular vacuolization of oral mucosa and pronounced parakeratosis are frequent findings.

OCULAR FINDINGS:

Orbit	
Lids	
Motility	
Lacr. App.	
Vision	
Vis. Fields	
Intraoc. Ten.	
Ant. Segm. and Sclera	
Ocul. Media	Dyskeratosis of the cornea
Retina and Choroid	
Optic Nerve	

OTHER CLINICAL FINDINGS:

1. Keratosis and hyperhidrosis of palms and soles, whereas the remaining skin is usually rather dry
2. Bullous lesions may occur with secondary infections mainly during warm seasons
3. Leukokeratosis of oral mucosa (mainly tongue)
4. Follicular keratosis
5. Granulosis rubra nasi
6. Congenital pachyonychia (The nails may not only be thickened but may be lost with aggravation at regrowth and frequent inflammation)
7. Follicular papules over knees and elbows in younger age not infrequent

BIBLIOGRAPHY:

1. Jadassohn, J. and Lewandowski, K.: in Neisser, A. and Jacobi, E.: *Ikonographia Dermatologica,* Berlin, Urban & Schwarzenberg, 1906, p. 29.
2. Burns, F. S.: A case of generalized congenital keratoderma with unusual involvement of the eyes, ears and nasal and buccal mucous membranes, J. Cutan. Dis. *33:*255, 1915.
3. Diasio, F. A.: Pachyonychia congenita Jadassohn, Arch Dermat. & Syph., *30:*218, 1934.
4. Jackson, A. D. M. and Lawler, S. .: Pachyonychia congenita: A report of six cases in one family, Ann. Eugenics, *16:*142, 1951/52

SYNDROME: Johnson
SYNONYMS: Adherence syndrome, adherent lateral rectus syndrome
GEN. INFORMATION:

Manifestation of congenital delayed development. Most frequent in children below age 3 years, thereafter of decreasing frequency. Spontaneous disappearance possible. These ocular findings are important in all cases of double elevator palsy, Duane's and Moebius' syndromes, which might be related. The condition is present in children less than 3 years of age and occasionally between 3 and 5 years and is usually bilateral. There are 2 principle types of disturbances: (1) Adhesions between sheaths of external rectus and inferior oblique with resulting limits in abduction. (2) Adhesions between sheaths of superior rectus and superior oblique with resulting limits in elevation. *a.* Adhesions between sheaths of superior rectus and superior oblique where they cross. *b.* Adhesions between sheaths of superior rectus and superior oblique far forward with limitation of downward movements and head tilt is usually present.

OCULAR FINDINGS:

Orbit	
Lids	
Motility	Forced muscle duction test may prove presence or absence of adherence versus paralysis
Lacr. App.	
Vision	
Vis. Fields	
Intraoc. Ten.	
Ant. Segm. and Sclera	
Ocul. Media	
Retina and Choroid	
Optic Nerve	

OTHER CLINICAL FINDINGS:
BIBLIOGRAPHY:

1. Johnson, L. V.: Adherence syndrome (pseudoparalysis lateral or superior rectus muscles), Arch. Ophth., *44:*870, 1950.
2. Walsh, F. B.: *Clinical Neuro-Ophthalmology,* Baltimore, The Williams & Wilkins Co., 1957.

SYNDROME: Klinefelter
SYNONYMS: Gynecomastia-aspermatogenesis syndrome
GEN. INFORMATION:

Occurrence in 1% of retarded males. Phenotypically males with positive female sex chromatin. A minority has sex-chromatine-negative nuclei as have normal males, whereas the majority has sex-chromatine positive nuclei as have normal females. Laboratory findings: Increased urinary gonadotropins. Karyotype shows 47 chromosomes, 44 autosomes and 3 sex chromosomes with the complement XXY (Jacobs and Strong). The two X-chromosomes in the XXY patient come from the mother and is most likely caused by non-disjunction of the X-chromosomes during oogenesis.

OCULAR FINDINGS:

Orbit	
Lids	
Motility	
Lacr. App.	
Vision	
Vis. Fields	
Intraoc. Ten.	
Ant. Segm.	
and Sclera	
Ocul. Media	
Retina and	Color blindness more rare (1%) in comparison to normal male
Choroid	population (8%) (Polani): This may be explained by the presence of two X chromosomes where the normal X chromosome suppresses the effect of the color blind gene on the other X chromosome
Optic Nerve	

OTHER CLINICAL FINDINGS:

1. Testicular hypoplasia. (Path: Testes show fibrosis and hyalinization of seminiferous tubules)
2. Sterility
3. Gynecomastia
4. Eunchoid physique
5. Mental retardation (mild)

BIBLIOGRAPHY:

1. Klinefelter, H. F., Jr.: Syndrome characterized by gynecomastia, aspermatogenesis without A-Leydigism and increased excretion of follicle-stimulating hormone, J. Clin. Endocrinol. 2:615, 1942.
2. Stern, C.: Color blindness in Klinefelter's syndrome, Nature *183*:1452, 1959.
3. Jacobs, P. A. and Strong, J. A.: A case of human intersexuality having a possible XXY sex determining mechanism, Nature, *183*:302, 1959.
4. Polani, P. E.: The Sex Chromosomes in Klinefelter's Syndrome in Gonadal Dysplasia, in *Molecular Genetics and Human Disease,* Ed. by Gardner, L. I., Springfield, Charles C Thomas, 1961.
5. Francois, J. and Matton-Van Leuwen, M. T.: Chromosome abnormalities and ophthalmology, J. Ped. Ophth., *1*:5, 1964.

SYNDROME: Klippel-Feil
SYNONYMS: Congenital brevicollis, synostosis cervical vertebrae.
GEN. INFORMATION:
Autosomal recessive inheritance but Gorlin *et al.* pointed to a possible autosomal dominance with poor penetrance and variable expression, based on published reports of familial occurrence. Manifestations present at birth, but often not recognized until considerably later. Females more commonly affected (65%— Gorlin *et al.*). Two etiological theories have been offered: (1) Defect in maternal intestinal tract and fetal foregut (Wimbourne: J. Path. & Bact., 1961); (2) Faulty segmentation of the mesodermal somites between 3rd and 7th gestational week (Shoul and Ritvo: A. J. Roent., 1952). Prognosis: progressive paraplegia may develop late in life. X-ray findings: Malformation of cervical and thoracic vertebrae with fusion or reduced number.* Spina bifida occulta in cervical region, defect of occipital bone. Atlas and axis show deformities.

OCULAR FINDINGS:

Orbit	
Lids	
Motility	Convergent strabismus (Bauman, J. A. M. A., 1932) a. o., hypertropia combined with torticollis. Horizontal nystagmus (occasional)
Lacr. App.	
Vision	
Vis. Fields	
Intraoc. Ten.	
Ant.Segm. and Sclera	
Ocul. Media	
Retina and Choroid	Chorioretinal atrophy (isolated finding)
Optic Nerve	

OTHER CLINICAL FINDINGS:
1. Platybasia*
2. Congenital upward displacement of scapula (Sprengel's deformity)
3. Brevicollis,* torticollis
4. Immobility of neck (painless)*
5. Mirror movement (Erskine: 1946) a.o.
6. Low posterior hairline*
7. Relative elevation of thorax
8. Deafness
9. Paralysis (Mosberg: J. Nerv. & Ment. Dis. 1953)

*Typical findings
BIBLIOGRAPHY:
1. Klippel, L. M. and Feil, A.: Anomalie de la collonne vertébrale par absence des vertébrales cervicales; cage thoracique remontant jusquà las base due crane, Bull. Soc. Anat. Paris, *14:*185, 1912.
2. Ford, F. R.: *Diseases of the Nervous System in Infancy, Childhood and Adolescent,* 3rd Ed., Springfield, Charles C Thomas, 1952, p. 308.
3. Walsh, F. B.: *Clinical Neuro-Ophthalmology,* 2nd Ed., Baltimore, The Williams & Wilkins Co., 1957, p. 421.
4. Gorlin, R. J. and Pindborg, J. J.: *Syndromes of the Head and Neck,* New York, McGraw-Hill Book Co. (Blakiston Division), 1964.

SYNDROME: Kloepfer
SYNONYMS:
GEN. INFORMATION:

Hereditary, autosomal recessive with 100% penetrance. The disease is very rare. The syndrome occurred in 4 males and 3 females among 22 members of 4 siblings descendant from a common ancestor (Kloepfer). Pathological findings: (based on one autopsy case by Dr. J. Moossy, quoted by Kloepfer) severe brain damage with loss of nerve cells in cerebral cortex, widespread ferrugination of capillaries in the cortex and within the putamen. Subcortical demyelination with astrogliosis. Alterations in dentate nucleus and gliosis in cerebellar white matter. Excessive accumulation of lipochrome probably representing pigmentary degeneration in nerve cells of medulla, pons, dentate nucleus and some areas of the cerebral cortex. Onset of manifestations at 2 months of age. Death occurs between 20 and 31 years of life.

OCULAR FINDINGS:

Orbit	
Lids	
Motility	
Lacr. App.	
Vision	Progressive loss of vision to complete blindness is associated with the progressive dementia.
Vis. Fields	
Intraoc. Ten.	
Ant. Segm. and Sclera	
Ocul. Media	
Retina and Choroid	
Optic Nerve	

OTHER CLINICAL FINDINGS:
1. Severe blistering in sunlight
2. No increase in weight and height after erythema subsides at 5 to 6 years of age
3. Mental age does not progress beyond the level of imbeciles
4. During or immediately after adolescence progressive degenerative dementia
5. Progressive deafness

BIBLIOGRAPHY:
1. Kloepfer, H. W.: Progress report on study of a type of progressive juvenile dementia with oligophrenia and erythema, *Proceedings of the 10th Internat. Conger. of Genetics,* Vol. II, Montreal, Aug. 20-27, 1958, Toronto, University of Toronto Press, 1958, p. 146.
2. McKusick, V. A.: *Medical Genetics 1958-1960,* St. Louis, C. V. Mosby Co., 1961, p. 42.

SYNDROME: Klüver-Bucy
SYNONYMS: Temporal lobectomy behavior syndrome
GEN. INFORMATION:
Original symptoms found experimentally in animals were present after temporal lobectomy in a human, carried out therapeutically for temporal lobe epilepsy.

OCULAR FINDINGS:

Orbit	
Lids	
Motility	
Lacr. App.	
Vision	'Psychic blindness' (Seelenblindheit) or visual agnosia
Vis. Fields	
Intraoc. Ten.	
Ant. Segm.	
and Sclera	
Ocul. Media	
Retina and	
Choroid	
Optic Nerve	

OTHER CLINICAL FINDINGS:
1. Changes in emotional behavior (possible rage reactions)
2. Hypersexuality
3. Bulimia (changes in dietary habits)
4. Loss of recognition of people
5. Strong oral tendencies (*i.e.* licking, biting, chewing)
6. Deficiency of memory

BIBLIOGRAPHY:
1. Klüver, H. and Bucy, P.: 'Psychic blindness' and other symptoms following bilateral temporal lobectomies in Rhesus monkeys, Am. J. Physio. *119:*352, 1937.
2. Klüver, H. and Bucy, P.: Preliminary analysis of functions of the temporal lobes in monkeys, Arch. Neurol. & Psychiat. *42:*979, 1939.
3. Terzian, H. and Ore, G.: Syndrome of Klüver and Bucy: Reproduced in man by bilateral removal of the temporal lobes, Neurology *5:*373, 1955.

SYNDROME: Koerber-Salus-Elschnig
SYNONYMS: Sylvian aqueduct syndrome, nystagmus retractorius syndrome
GEN. INFORMATION:
Lesion in region of the aqueduct, third and fourth ventricle, or corpora quadrigemina. Most frequent lesions are tumor or inflammation, but nystagmus retractorius has also been described with quadrigeminal hemorrhage and in a case with cysticercus (Elschnig). The symptoms can be explained as due to pressure upon the posterior longitudinal fasciculi and preponderance of tonus of the rectus muscles.

OCULAR FINDINGS:

Orbit	
Lids	Lid retraction may be associated with midbrain lesions above the posterior commissure
Motility	Paresis of vertical gaze. Tonic spasm of convergence on attempted upward gaze. Clonic convergence movements or convergence nystagmus. Vertical nystagmus on gaze up or down. Nystagmus retractorius with spasmodic retraction of the eyes when on attempt is made to move them in any direcion. Extraocular muscle paresis. (occasionally)
Lacr. App.	
Vision	
Vis. Fields	
Intraoc. Ten.	
Ant. Segm. and Sclera	Pupillary abnormalities
Ocul. Media	
Retina and Choroid	
Optic Nerve	

OTHER CLINICAL FINDINGS:
1. Headaches, dizziness
2. Hypertension
3. Positive Babinski sign
4. Possible hemiparesis
5. Ataxia
6. Hemitremor

BIBLIOGRAPHY:
1. Salus, R.: On acquired retraction movements of the eyes, Arch. Ophth. 42:34, 1913.
2. Elschnig, A.: Nystagmus retractorius, ein cerebrales Herdysmptom, Med. Klin. 9:8, 1913.
3. Collier, J.: Nuclear ophthalmoplegia, with especial reference to retraction of the lids and ptosis and to lesions of the posterior commissure, Brain 50:488, 1927.
4. Kestenbaum, A.: Clinical methods of neuro-ophthalmologic examination, New York, Grune & Stratton, 1946.
5. Smith, J. L.; Zieper, I.; Gay A. J. and Cogan, D. G.: Nystagmus Retractorius, Arch. Ophth. 62:864, 1959.
6. Waltman, S. R.: Ocular Signs in midbrain disease, in Gay, A. J. and Burde R. M. (eds.) Clinical concepts in neuro-ophthalmology, Internat. Ophth. Clinics, 7:807, 1967.

SYNDROME: Krause

SYNONYMS: Congenital encephalo-ophthalmic dysplasia, encephalo-ophthalmic syndrome.

GEN. INFORMATION:
Apparently no hereditary factors involved. No predilection for either sex. More frequently in premature infants. Death frequently from intercurrent infections. Brain and retina are affected but not the spinal cord. Cerebral dysplasia with hyperplasia, hypoplasia and aplasia of cerebrum and cerebellum. The hydrocephaly may arise from arachnoidal and cerebral dysplasia. Microcephaly may result from cerebral and cerebellar agenesis. The syndrome is not always complete. Ocular findings usually present several months after birth. Cerebral signs occur later with development of cerebral agenesis etc. Clinically only the brain or only the eye may appear to be affected, however at autopsy, signs of the disease are usually found in the other part. Ocular pathology may be unilateral.

OCULAR FINDINGS:

Orbit	Microphthalmos, enophthalmos
Lids	Ptosis
Motility	Strabismus
Lacr. App.	
Vison	Blindness
Vis. Fields	
Intrac. Ten.	Sec. glaucoma
Ant. Segm. and Sclera	Iris atrophy. Anterior and posterior synechiae. Scleral atrophy.
Ocul. Media	Persistant remnants of hyaloid artery. Intraocular hemorrhages and exudates. Cyclitic membranes. Cataracts.
Retina and Choroid	Retinal hypoplasia and hyperplasia; choroidal and retinal malformation; retinal glial membranes, cones and septums; retinal detachment. Choroidal atrophy. First mildest sign may be a small area of retinal atrophy.
Optic Nerve	Optic nerve malformation, colobomata.

OTHER CLINICAL FINDINGS:
1. Congenital cerebral dysplasia
2. Hydrocephalus or microcephaly
3. Mental retardation
4. Heterotopia

BIBLIOGRAPHY:

1. Wehrli, E.: Ueber die Mikro-und Makrogyrie der Gehirnsanlage, Entwicklungsstorungen der Retina mit Besprechung der Epithelrosetten und der Pathogenese der Glioma. Arch. f. Ophth. 60:302, 1905.
2. Gartner, S.: Congenital retinal folds and microcephaly, Arch. Ophth. 25:93., 1941.
3. Krause, A. C.: Congenital encephalo-ophthalmic dysplasia, Arch. Ophth. 36:387, 1946.

SYNDROME: Laurence-Moon-Bardet-Biedl

SYNONYMS: Bardet-Biedl syndrome, Retinitis pigmentosa-polydactyly-adiposogenital syndrome

GEN. INFORMATION:

Monogenic recessive (Rieger), one dominant-autosomal and one recessive sex-linked gene, (Macklin). Abiotrophy of the diencephalohypophyseal region and the retinal neuroepithelium. Male preponderance. Predominantly in Caucasians but also reported in Japanese and Egyptians (2 cases in Negro, Snell and Walsh). Onset in childhood. Prognosis good. No shortening of life expectancy. Electroretinography shows changes compatible with malfunction of rod vision. X-ray findings: Shortening of metacarpals and metatarsals.* Symmetrical hyperostosis of the frontal bones (reported in 1 case, Van Bogaert and Borremans).

OCULAR FINDINGS:

Orbit	
Lids	Ptosis, epicanthus
Motility	Nystagmus, strabismus (nonparalytic or paralytic) internal ophthalmoplegia (Walsh):** External ophthalmoplegia (Sussman)**
Lacr. App.	
Vision	Night blindness during school age, progressive visual loss. Myopia or hypermetropia (emmetropia is rare)
Vis. Fields	Ring scotoma
Intraoc. Ten.	
Ant. Segm. and Sclera	Iris coloboma
Ocul. Media	Cataract,* keratoconus** (Walsh)
Retina and Choroid	Retinitis pigmentosa "bone corpuscles" and general distribution of pigments (15% of the cases): Macular degeneration or pigmentary changes: Attenuation of retinal vessels: Choroidal atrophy (similar to choroideremia)
Optic Nerve	Atrophy, pale waxy disc*

OTHER CLINICAL FINDINGS:

1. Obesity (Fröhlich's type)
2. Hypogenitalism
3. Polydaktyly
4. Reduced intelligence and mental retardation
5. Turricephalia
6. Shortness of structure
7. Atresia ani
8. Genu valgum
9. Congenital heart disease
10. Choreiform movements (Marmor and Lambert)
11. Congenital malformations of the urinary tract*
12. Metabolic disturbances

*Less frequent
**Single reports

BIBLIOGRAPHY:

1. Laurence, J.Z. and Moon, R. C.: Four cases of 'retinitis pigmentosa' in the same family and accompanied by general imperfections of development, Ophth. Rev. 2:32, 1866.
2. Bardet, G.: Sur un syndrome d'obésité infantile avec polydactylie et rétinite pigmentaire, Thesis, Paris, 1920.
3. Biedl, A.: Geschwisterpaar mit adiposogenitaler Dystrophie, Dtsch. med. Wschr. 48:1630, 1922, Ibid: Med. Klin, 18:1041, 1922.
4. Rieger, H.: Über die Erbichkeisverhältnisse des Biedl-Bardetschen Syndromes, Arch. Rass. Biol. 32:298, 1931.
5. Macklin, M.; The Laurence-Moon-Biedls syndrome: a genetic study, J. Hered., 27:97, 1936.
6. Francois, J.: *Heredity in Ophthalmology,* St. Louis, C. V. Mosby Co., 1961
7. Saraux, H. et al.: Le syndrome de Bardet-Biedl, Ann. Oculist 19:864, 1964.

SYNDROME: Leber
SYNONYMS: Optic atrophy-amaurosis-pituitary syndrome
GEN. INFORMATION:

Male preponderance (sex linked recessive? cytoplasmic?); the disease has been described in females, too. Seedorf, 1968, was able to trace a family through 8 generations (116 persons)without finding non-carriers. This supports the assumption that *every* daughter of a carrier inherits the trait for optic neuritis. Most frequent onset in third decade of life but also described in other age groups. X-ray findings: distortion of the sella turcica.

OCULAR FINDINGS:

Orbit	
Lids	
Motility	
Lacr. App.	
Vision	Loss of vision, which is sudden and severe, usually reaches its maximum after 1 or 2 months. Complete blindness is rare, however central vision remains seriously impaired. Only occasionally considerable visual improvement
Vis. Fields	Central or paracentral field defects (15 ot 40 degrees) of varying intensity
Intraoc. Ten.	
Ant. Segm. and Sclera	
Ocul. Media	
Retina and Choroid	Hemorrhages, exudates, edema, (may occur): Sheathing of vessels
Optic Nerve	Optic neuritis of low grade often initially until bilateral optic atrophy (partial or complete) occurs. Swelling of the discs with hemorrhages and exudates might be present, though usually transitory

OTHER CLINICAL FINDINGS:
Headaches and vertigo

BIBLIOGRAPHY:
1. Leber, T.: Ueber hereditär und congenital-angelegte Sehnervenleiden, v. Graefes Arch. Ophthal. *17:*249, 1871.
2. Walsh, F. B.: *Clinical Neuro-Ophthalmology,* 2nd Ed., Baltimore, The Williams & Wilkins Co., 1957, p. 605.
3. Ballantyne, A. F. and Michaelson, I. C.: *The Fundus of the Eye,* Edinburgh, E. & S. Livingstone Ltd., 1962.
4. Seedorf, T.: Leber's disease, Acta Ophth. *46:*4, 1968; Ibid: *46:*985, 1968.

SYNDROME: Lenoble-Aubineau
SYNONYMS: Nystagmus-myoclonia syndrome
GEN. INFORMATION:
Hereditary familial. The pathogenesis is not known. Pathological findings: Diffuse nonspecific meningovascular and glial changes of chronic toxemia. Muscle fasciculations occur spontaneously or can be elicited by cold or mechanical stimuli.

OCULAR FINDINGS:

Orbit	
Lids	
Motility	Congenital nystagmus associated with fasciculations of muscles spontaneously elicited by cold or mechanical stimulation
Lacr. App.	
Vision	
Vis. Fields	
Intraoc. Ten.	
Ant. Segm.	
and Sclera	
Ocul. Media	
Retina and	
Choroid	
Optic Nerve	

OTHER CLINICAL FINDINGS:
1. Tremors of the head and limbs (occasionally)
3. Overactive reflexes (Wilson)

BIBLIOGRAPHY:
1. Lenoble, E. and Aubineau, E.: Nystagmus-myoclonia syndrome, Rev. méd., Paris, *26*:471, 1906.
2. David, N. J.: Neuro-Ophthalmology of occlusive disease in the vertebral-basilar arterial system; in Smith, J. L. (ed.) *Neuro-Ophthalmology,* Vol. 2, St. Louis, C. V. Mosby Co., 1965.

SYNDROME: Louis-Bar

SYNONYMS: Cephalooculocutaneous telangiectasis, Ataxia—telangiectasia syndrome

GEN. INFORMATION:

Transmitted as an autosomal recessive trait. Life expectancy usually not longer than 2 decades. A thymic abnormality leading to an immunologic deficiency has been suggested as the cause for this syndrome (Peterson *et al.*). while others believe it to be a specific dysgammaglobulinemia (Fireman *et al.*). (Lymphoreticular malignancies as the cause of death in this disease have also been reported (Harley *et al.,* Arch. Ophth., 1967); Histopathologic findings: diffuse cerebral degeneration, degeneration of pyramidal cells in frontal area, loss of pigment cells in substantia nigra, loss of Purkinje cells and of the basket cell and granular layers of cerebral cortex (Harley *et al.*).

OCULAR FINDINGS:

Orbit	
Lids	Rapid blinking in upward gaze
Motility	"Pseudoophthalmoplegia," fixational nystagmus (Roth-Bielschowsky phenomenon), halting intermittently mainly on lateral and upward gaze (80% of patients). On head turning, eyes are involuntarily directed to opposite side with slow returning to the primary position. Ocular motor apraxic movement, loss of optokinetic responses, poor convergence ability
Vis. Fields	
Intraoc. Ten.	
Ant. Segm. and Sclera	Telangiectasia.* Fine bright, symmetrical red streaks temporal and nasal conjunctiva (usually first seen at age 4 to 6 years). Prominent veins in the canthal regions of the conjunctiva, whereas superior and inferior conjunctiva are not involved
Ocul. Media	
Retina and Choroid	
Optic Nerve	

OTHER CLINICAL FINDINGS:

1. Progressive cerebellar ataxia*
2. Slow and scanning speech*
3. Mental retardation (80%)
4. Cutaneous telangiectasis and fine spots of pigmentation*
5. Recurrent sinopulmonary infections (70 to 80%)
6. Daysynergi and intention tremor
7. Diminished tendon reflexes, hypotonia (85%)
8. Diminished growth (about 65% of cases)

*In all patients

BIBLIOGRAPHY:

1. Louis-Bar, Mme.: Sur un syndrome progressif comprenant des têlangiectasies capillaires cutaneé et conjonctivales symétriques, à disposition naevoïde et des troubles cérèbelleux, Confinia neurol. *4:*32, 1941.
2. Peterson, R. D. A.; Kelly, W. D. and Good, R. A.: Ataxia-Teleangiectasia: Its association with a defective thymus, immunological-deficiency disease, and malignancy, Lancet, *1:*1189, 1964.
3. Fireman, P.; Boesman, M. and Gitlin, D.: Ataxia & teleangiectasia: A dysgammaglobulinemia with deficient γ_1 A (β_2A)-globulin, Lancet, *1:*1193, 1964.
4. Karpati, G.: Ataxia-telangiectasia, Amer. J. Dis. Child. *110:*51, 1965.
5. Peterson, R. D.; Cooper, M. D. and Good, R. A.: Lymphoid tissue abnormalities with ataxia-telangiectasia, Am. J. Med. *41:*342,1966

SYNDROME: Lowe
SYNONYMS: Oculo cerebro renal syndrome
GEN. INFORMATION:
The essential enzyme or protein abnormality is unknown. The syndrome seems to be caused by a pathological gene. Since all cases reported are males,it has been concluded that the defect is a sex linked recessive trait (Streiff, E. B.:Ophthalmologica *135*:632, 1958). The presence of lenticular opacities in the mothers of a number of cases suggested a possible expression of the carrier state (Wilson and Donnel: Arch Ophth. *70*:5, 1963)

OCULAR FINDINGS:

Orbit	
Lids	
Motility	Nystagmus
Lacr. App.	
Vision	
Vis. Fields	
Intraoc. Ten.	Congenital glaucoma, hydrophthalmos,
Ant. Segm. and Sclera	Miotic pupils, no pupillary reaction, ectropion uveii, malformation of the anterior chamber angle and the iris. Schlemm's canal may be absent with imperfect angle cleavage (Adams). Blue sclera
Ocul. Media	Cloudy cornea, cataracts (punctate cataracts may be found in the mother
Retina and Choroid	Reduced ganglion cells in the retina [single report and was associated with long standing glaucoma (See Ref. 5)]
Optic Nerve	

OTHER CLINICAL FINDINGS:
1. Mental, psychomotor and growth retardation
2. Systemic acidosis
3. Renal symptoms (aminoaciduria, oligoammoniuria,* albuminuria, intermittent glycosuria, renal tubular acidosis, low titratable acidity*)
4. Musculoskeletal abnormalities (rickets, osteomalacia, muscular hypotony, hyporeflexia)

*Variable

BIBLIOGRAPHY:
1. Lowe, C. U.; Terrey, M.; and MacLachlan, E. A.: Organic-aciduria, decreased renal ammonia production, hydrophthalmos and mental retardation, Amer. J. Dis. Child., *83*:164, 1952.
2. Schoen, E. J.; and Young, G.: "Lowe's Syndrome": Abnormalities in renal tubular function in combination with other ocular defects, Am. J. Med., *27*:781, 1959.
3. Adams, S. T.; Granten, W. M. and Smith, T. R.: Congenital glaucoma (possibly Lowe's syndrome), Arch. Ophth., *68*:191, 1962.
4. Chutorian, A.; and Rowland, L. P.: Lowe Syndrome, Neurology *16*:115 (11), 1966.
5. Fisher, N. F.; Hallet, J.; and Carpenter, G.: Oculocerebrorenal syndrome of Lowe, Arch. Ophth. *77*:642, 1967.

SYNDROME: Marchesani
SYNONYMS: Weil-Marchesani syndrome, inverted Marfan syndrome, brachymorphy with spherophakia, dystrophia mesodermalis congenita hyperplastica.
GEN. INFORMATION:
While the syndrome is undoubetdly hereditary, its precise mode of transmission has not yet been established. Some observations suggest dominant inheritance, while others suggest recessiveness. It has also been suggested that the skeletal changes represent the expression of the gene in the heterozygous condition (brachydactyly and brachymorphia frequently occur in the antecedants and collaterals without ocular pathology), whereas their combination with ocular findings represents homozygous manifestations (Marchesani; Kloepfer and Rosenthal: Am. J. Hum. Gen., 1955). Onset 9 months to 13 years of age. Prognosis depends on various conditions within this syndrome. Ocular-pathological findings: dysplasia of the ciliary body (Marchesani, 1939); Defective closure of the fetal fissure (Becker, 1935; Stellwag, 1953); Vasotrophic disturbances of the vascular capsule of the lens (Thums, 1937).

OCULAR FINDINGS:

Optic	
Lids	
Motility	
Lacr. App.	
Vision	Lenticular myopia. Complete blindness may occur
Vis. Fields	
Intraoc. Ten,	Secondary glaucoma (rare), due to luxation of the lens
Ant. Segm. and Sclera	Iriodonesis
Ocul. Media	Ectopia lentis, spherophakia, microphakia, microcornea. The lenticular changes can be regarded secondary to mesodermal changes in the anterior segment of the globe
Retina and Choroid	Chorioretinal changes (rare)—(Rahman). Retinal pigment degeneration (Rahman)
Optic Nerve	Optic atrophy (Rahman)

OTHER CLINICAL FINDINGS:
1. Brachydactyly
2. Reduced growth, symmetrical and athletic with abundant subcutaneous tissue
3. Short neck and large thorax
4. Short and clumsy hands and feet
5. Decreased joint flexibility(occasionally)
6. Hearing defects

BIBLIOGRAPHY:
1. Marchesani, O.: Brachydactylie und angeborene Kugellinse als Systemerkrankung, K. Mbl. Augenhk. *103:*392, 1939.
2. Zabriskie, J. and Reisman, M.: Marchesani syndrome, J. Pediat., *52:*158, 1958.
3. Francois, J.: *Heredity in Ophthalmology,* St. Louis, C. V. Mosby Co., 1961.
4. Jones, R. F.: The Syndrome of Marchesani, Brit. J. Ophth. *45:*377, 1961.
5. Rahman, M. and Rahman, S.: Marchesani's syndrome, Brit. J. Ophth., *47:*182, 1963.

132

SYNDROME: Marcus Gunn
SYNONYMS: Jaw-winking syndrome and inverse jaw-winking syndrome.
GEN. INFORMATION:
Familial occurrence rare. Irregular dominant inheritance seems to exist in a few reported cases (Ref. 2, 4). Abnormal connections between central mechanism innervating the external pterygoid muscle and that innervating the levator, and supranuclear or supranuclear-nuclear involvement have been suggested of causing the clinical picture.

OCULAR FINDINGS:

Orbit	
Lids	Unilateral congenital ptosis more than 90% of cases, with the rest showing spontaneous onset, usually in older persons. Lid elevates rapidly when mouth is opened or mandible is moved to one or the other side. The left eye seems to be more frequently affected than the right eye
Motility	Palsy of external muscles (Lutz). Other external ocular muscle palsies, only as occasional finding
Lacr. App.	
Vision	
Vis. Fields	
Intraoc. Ten.	
Ant. Segm. and Sclera	
Ocul. Media	
Retina and Choroid	
Optic Nerve	

OTHER CLINICAL FINDINGS:

BIBLIOGRAPHY:
1. Gunn, R. M.: Congenital ptosis with peculiar associated movements of the affected lid, Tr. Ophth. Soc. U. K., *3*:283, 1883.
2. Lutz, Z.: The jaw winking phenomenon and its explanation, Arch. Ophth. *48*:144, 1919.
3. Wartenberg, R.: Inverted Marcus Gunn phenomenon (so-called Marin-Amat syndrome), Arch. Neurol & Psychiat, *60*:584, 1948.
4. Falls, H. F.: Three cases of Marcus Gunn phenomenon in two generations, Am. J. Ophth. *32* (2):53, 1949.
5. Simpson, D. G.: Marcus Gunn phenomenon following squint and ptosis surgery. Definition and review, Arch. Ophth. *56*:743, 1956.
6. Schultz, R. O. and Burian, H. M.: Bilateral jaw winking. Reflex in association with multiple congenital anomalies, Arch. Ophth. *64*:946, 1960.

SYNDROME: Marfan
SYNONYMS: Dolichosternomelia, arachnodactyly, hyperchondroplasia, dystrophia mesodermalis congenita,
GEN. INFORMATION:
Hypoplastic form of dystrophia mesodermalis congenita. Autosomal dominant, often with incomplete expression. Sporadic cases occur. Few observations suggest recessive inheritance (Jequier, 1944). Prognosis good. Infantile mortality is high. Pathological findings: elongated metacarpia, metatarsia and basal phalanges. Endocardial lesions simulating rheumatic fever, aortic medial necrosis. Laboratory findings: Serum mucoprotein level may be below normal, urinary hydroxyproline concentration is high (this is also found in hyperthyroidism and Paget's disease)-(Dull and Henneman: N. Engl. J. Med., 1963)

OCULAR FINDINGS:

Orbit	
Lids	
Motility	Divergent squint, nystagmus, paralysis of accommodation
Lacr. App.	
Vision	Myopia** (axial or lenticular), pronounced hypermetropia, astigmatism (Kurz, 1934)
Vis. Fields	
Intraoc. Ten.	Glaucoma (less frequently and secondary to lens dislocation)
Ant. Segm. and Sclera	Iridodonesis, coloboma, miosis, persistent pupillary membrane. Blue sclerae
Ocul. Media	Spherophakia, lens dislocation** (50% and frequently superior nasally), cataract (less frequently), megalocornea (less frequently).
Retina and Choroid	Detachment (less frequently), pigmentary retinopathy. Uveal coloboma (less frequently), macular coloboma, choroidal sclerosis
Optic Nerve	Coloboma

OTHER CLINICAL FINDINGS:
1. Arachnodactyly**
2. Skeletal anomalies**
3. Spina bifida (less frequent)
4. Asymmetric thorax
5. Relaxed ligaments
6. General muscular underdevelopment
7. Dolichocephaly and high arched palate**
8. Decrease in subcutaneous fat
9. Prominent ears
10. Tendency to infantilism
11. Congenital heart disease
12. Aneurysma dissecans**

**Typical findings

BIBLIOGRAPHY:
1. Marfan, A. B.: Un cas de déformation congénitale des quatre membres plus prononcées aux extremités characterisée par l'allongement des os avec un certae degré d'amincissement, Bull. et mem. Soc. méd. d. hôp. de Paris, *13:* 220, 1896.
2. Schwarzweller, F.: Die konstitutionelle Bedingtheit der sogenannten Arachnodaktylie, Erbarzt, *4:*96, 1937.
3. Futcher, P. H.; and Southworth, H.: Arachnodactyly and its medical complications, Arch. Int. Med., *61:*693, 1938.
4. Lloyd, R. I.: Arachnodactyly (Marfan's syndrome), Trans. Am. Ophthal. Soc., *45:*342, 1947.

SYNDROME: Marinesco-Sjögren
SYNONYMS: Congenital spinocerebellar ataxia - congenital cataract - oligophrenia syndrome
GEN. INFORMATION:
The syndrome is rare and apparently inherited as an autosomal recessive trait. Parental consanguinity was observed in some patients (Sjögren).

OCULAR FINDINGS:

Orbit	
Lids	
Motility	
Lacr. App.	
Vision	
Vis. Fields	
Intraoc. Ten.	
Ant. Segm. and Sclera	Aniridia in brother and sister, instead of cataracts, was described by Gillespie
Ocul. Media	Congenital cataracts
Retina and Choroid	
Optic Nerve	

OTHER CLINICAL FINDINGS:
1. Cerebellar ataxia
2. Oligophrenia
3. Skeletal abnormalities (small stature, scoliosis, genu valgum, restricted extensibility of the knee, defects of fingers and toes)
4. Mental retardation (single report)

BIBLIOGRAPHY:
1. Marinesco, G.; Draganesco, G.; Vasiliu, O.: Nouvelle maladie familiale caractérésée par une cataracte congénitale et un arrêt du developpement somato-neuro-psychique, Encéphale 26:97, 1931.
2. Sjögren, T.: Hereditary congenital spinocerebellar ataxia combined with congenital cataracts and oligophrenia, Acta Psychiat. Neurol. Suppl. 46, Nils Antoni Anno Aetatis LX; Ibid: Confinia neurol. 10:293, 1950.
3. Gillespie, F. D.: Aniridia, cerebellar ataxia, and oligophrenia in siblings, Arch. Ophth. 73:338, 1965.

SYNDROME: Melkersson-Rosenthal
SYNONYMS: Melkersson, idiopathic fibroedema, Miescher's cheilitis granulomatosis
GEN. INFORMATION:
Occurance during childhood or youth. Disturbance of blood supply to the facial nerve. Etiology is unknown (viral?). Possible etiologic factors considered have been: Disturbance of parasympathetic cells in the geniculate ganglia of their central nuclei, allergic reactions, sarcoidosis, tuberculosis, etc. The facial palsy resembles that of Bell's palsy. There is no sex predominance or racial predilection. The lingua plicata is always congenital and sometimes familial.

OCULAR FINDINGS:

Orbit	Bilateral recurrent exophthalmos*
Lids	Lagophthalmos, lid edema, blepharochalasis*
Motility	Paralysis medial recti*
Lacr. App.	Lacrimation secondary to the 'crocodile tear' phenomenon from aberrant 7th nerve regeneration.
Vision	
Vis. Fields	
Intraoc. Ten.	
Ant. Segm.	Burning sensations
and Sclera	
Ocul. Media	Exposure keratitis and corneal ulcers, keratitis sicca,* corneal opacities
Retina and	
Choroid	
Optic Nerve	Retrobulbar neuritis*

OTHER CLINICAL FINDINGS:
1. Chronic edema face and lips
2. Peripheral facial palsy (may be bilateral) and may precede the edema by weeks to even years
3. Furrowed tongue
4. Granulomatous cheilitis, glossitis, parotitis*
5. Migraine

*In isolated case reports
BIBLIOGRAPHY:
1. Rosenthal, C.: Klinisch-erbbiologischer Beitrag zur Konstitutionspathologie: Gemeinsames Auftreten von (rezidivierender familiärer) Fazialislähmung, angioneurotischem Gesichtsödem und Lingua plicata in Arthritismus-Familien, Ztschr. ges. Neurol. & Psychiat. *131*:475, 1930.
2. Kettel, K.: Melkersson's Syndrome-report of five cases with special reference to the pothologic observations, Arch. Otolaryng. *46*:341, 1947.
3. Koch, H.: Augenveränderungen beim Melkersson-Rosenthal Syndrome, Heidelberg-Berichte 57, Kongress 1951.
4. Stevens H.: Melkersson's Syndrome, Neurology *15*:263, 1965.
5. Paton, D.: The Melkersson-Rosenthal Syndrome, Am. J. Ophth. suppl. 3, *59*:705, 1965.

SYNDROME: Ménière
SYNONYMS:
GEN. INFORMATION:
Etiology is unknown, but most likely virus infection. Lesion of the inner ear with hydrops and distentions of the endolymph canals of the labyrinth (Hallpick and Cairns). The prognosis is good. The disease is more common in males, mainly between age 40 and 60 years. Attacks come usually suddenly at irregular intervals and last from minutes to several hours or days. Unconsciousness occurs in somewhat less than 10% of patients. EEG has been found abnormal in 25% of patients (Barac *et al.* 1966). Differential diagnosis: cerebellopontine angle tumor. Lermoyez's syndrome.

OCULAR FINDINGS:

Orbit	
Lids	
Motility	Nystagmus (rapid component toward the normal side)-mainly during attacks
Lacr. App.	
Vision	Diplopia (during and after attacks possible)—(Dandy)
Vis. Fields	
Intraoc. Ten.	
Ant. Segm.	Loss of corneal reflex*
and Sclera	
Ocul. Media	
Retina and	
Choroid	
Optic Nerve	

OTHER CLINICAL FINDINGS:
1. Paroxysmal attacks of vertigo, tinnitus
2. Gradually progressing deafness, though not prerequisite for the diagnosis.
3. During attacks pallor, nausea, vomiting, fainting.

*Single observation
BIBLIOGRAPHY:
1. Ménière, P.: Mémoire sur des lésions de l'oreille interne, Gaz. méd., Paris, 1861.
2. Dandy, W. E.: Ménière's disease. Its diagnosis and treatment, South. Med. J. *30*:621, 1937.
3. Adler, F. H.; McNally, W. J.; Stuart, E. A.; and Alpers, B. J. : Symposium on vertigo, Tr. Am. Acad. Ophth., 1941, pp. 33-54.
4. Walsh, F.: *Clinical Neuro-Ophthalmology,* 2nd Ed., Baltimore, The Williams & Wilkins Co. 1957.

SYNDROME: Meyer-Schwickerath-Weyers
SYNONYMS: Microphthalmos syndrome, oculodentodigital dysplasia
GEN. INFORMATION:

None of the very rare findings of this syndrome seem to have given a clearly genetic mode of inheritance, though Berliner (Arch. Ophth. 1941). Described the clinical findings in two cousins of 1st degree. Meyer-Schwickerath *et al.* pointed to two types of hereditary microphthalmos syndromes: (1) Dysplasia oculo-dento-digitalis, and (2) Dyscranio-pygo-phalangie. Type I is characterized by microphthalmia with possible iris pathology and glaucoma. Oligodontia and brown pigmentation of teeth. Comptodactyly and possible absence of middle phalanges 2nd to 5th toes. Type II consists of severe microphthalmos to anophthalmos. Polydactyly. Developmental anomalies of nose and oral cavity. These authors suggested that both types derived from a similar teratogenetic principle, but where the symptoms and extent of malformation is less severe in Type I than in Type II which has in addition a number of other malformations of internal organs and is fatal.

OCULAR FINDINGS:

Orbit	Microphthalmos
Lids	Shortened lid aperture
Motility	
Lacr. App.	
Vision	Myopia (Meyer-Schwickerath), Hyperopia (Lohmann)
Vis Fields	
Intraoc. Ten.	Glaucoma
Ant. Segm. and Sclera	Iris anomalies (excentric located pupil, changes in normal iris texture, remnants of pupillary membrane along iris margins)
Ocul. Media	Microcornea
Retina and Choroid	
Optic Nerve	

OTHER CLINICAL FINDINGS:
1. Thin, small nose with anteverted nostrils and hypoplastic alae
2. Syndactyly
3. Camptodactyly (4th and 5th fingers)
4. Anomalies of middle phalanx of 5th finger and toes
5. Dental enamel hypoplasia
6. Sparse hair growth

BIBLIOGRAPHY:
1. Meyer-Schwickerath, G.; Grüterich, E. and Weyers, H.: Mikrophthalmus-syndrom, Klin. Mbl. Augenhk. *131:*18, 1957.
2. Weyers, H.: Zur Dyscephalie mit Cataracta congenita und Hypotrichose, Ztschr. Kinderhk., *74:*468, 1954.
3. Lohmann, W.: Mikrophthalmus in Kombination mit Kamptodaktylie, Arch Augenhk. *86:*136, 1920.

SYNDROME: Mikulicz-Radecki
SYNONYMS: Mikulicz syndrome, dacryosialoadenopathy, Mikulicz-Sjörgen syndrome.

GEN. INFORMATION:

The syndrome is not an individual disease but includes a number of clinical entities. Among those have been listed tuberculosis, leukemia, lymphosarcoma, sarcoidosis, Hodgkin's disease, or lymphoma of unknown etiology. Prognosis: chronic course with frequent recurrences. This syndrome also has been considered as a milder form of Sjören's syndrome (Bain). Associated findings may be extensive depending on the etiology of the syndrome and in particular when sarcoidosis is the underlying cause (See also Schaumann's syndrome).

OCULAR FINDINGS:

Orbit	
Lids	Bulging upper lid due to swelling of lacrimal gland
Motility	
Lacr. App.	Bilateral painless enlargement of lacrimal glands. Decreased or absent lacrimation
Vision	
Vis. Fields	
Intraoc. Ten.	
Ant. Segm.	
and Sclera	
Ocul. Media	
Retina and	
Choroid	
Optiv Nerve	

OTHER CLINICAL FINDINGS:

1. Symmetrical enlargement of salivary glands and parotis
2. Dryness of mouth and larynx
3. Neurological complications
4. X-ray finding: normal branching of the parotid duct system and complete evacuation of contrast medium during emptying phase.

BIBLIOGRAPHY:

1. Mikulicz-Radecki, J. von: Ueber eine eigenartige symmetrische Erkrankung der Thränen-und Mundspeicheldrüsen, in Beiträge zur Chirurgie. Festschr. gewid. T. Billroth., Stuttgart, 610-30, 1892.
2. Radding, J.: Mikulicz's syndrome in chronic leukemia, North-West Med., 49:772, 1950.
3. Morgan, W. C.: The probably systemic nature of Mikulicz's syndrome and its relation to Sjögren's syndrome, New England J. Med. 251:5, 1954.
4. Bain, G. O.: The pathology of Mikulicz-Sjögren disease in relation to disseminated lupus erythematosus, Canad. M. A. J. 82:143, 1960.

SYNDROME: Millard-Gubler
SYNONYMS: Abducens-facial hemiplegia alternans
GEN. INFORMATION:
Lesion in the base of the pons affecting the nuclei of the sixth and seventh nerves and fibers of the pyramidal tract (vascular, encephalitis, tumors).

OCULAR FINDINGS:

Orbit	
Lids	
Motility	Diplopia, internal strabismus, paralysis external rectus muscle (often bilateral). In cases where it is unilateral there is deviation of the eyes to the side opposite the lesion and inability to move them toward the side of the lesion. Abduction of the eye is prevented by the destruction of the 6th nerve nucleus. The opposite eye cannot be voluntarily adducted but can converge and can move in this position by rotatory and caloric stimulation (Walsh)
Lacr. App.	
Vision	
Vis. Fields	
Intraoc. Ten.	
Ant. Segm. and Sclera	
Ocul. Media	
Retina and Choroid	
Optic Nerve	

OTHER CLINICAL FINDINGS:
1. Paralysis of one side of the face
2. Contralateral hemiplegia of arm and leg from involvement of the pyramidal tract

BIBLIOGRAPHY:
1. Gubler, A.: De l'hémiplégie alterne envisagée comme signe de lésion de la protubérance annulaire et comme preuve de la décussation des nerfs faciaux, Gaz. hebd. Méd. Chir. *3:*749, 789; 811, 1856.
2. Walsh, F. B.: *Clinical Neuro-Ophthalmology,* 2nd Ed., Baltimore, The Williams & Wilkins Co., 1957, p. 262.

SYNDROME: Möbius

SYNONYMS: Congenital facial diplegia, congenital paralysis of the 6th and 7th nerves, congenital oculofacial paralysis, von Graefe's syndrome.

GEN. INFORMATION:
Rare congenital disturbance. Defective development of the 6th and 7th nerves. Pathological findings: Aplasia of the motor cerebral nuclei. Defective development of the medial longitudinal fasciculus. Poor development of the olives and pyramidal tract (Heubner). Since the development of the intracranial nuclei engaged in this syndrome reaches its height during the 4th and 5th weeks of the fetal life, the lesion of the fetus, caused by an unknown factor, may occur during this period (Ref. 3). Heredity has been excluded.

OCULAR FINDINGS:

Orbit	Proptosis (6%)
Lids	Ptosis
Motility	Weakness of abductor muscles. Normal convergence, limitation to internal rotation in lateral movements. Convergent squint (studied by electromyography-Merz-Wojtowicz)
Lacr. App.	
Vision	
Vis. Fields	
Intraoc. Ten.	
Ant. Segm. and Sclera	
Ocul. Media	
Retina and Choroid	
Optic Nerve	

OTHER CLINICAL FINDINGS:
1. Facial diplegia
2. Deafness
3. Loss of vestibular responses
4. Webbed fingers or toes
5. Supernumerary digits
6. Muscle defects of chest, neck and tongue
7. Club foot

BIBLIOGRAPHY:
1. Möbius, P. J.; Über angeborene doppelseitige Abducens-Facialislähmung, Münch. Med. Wschr., *35*:91, 1888.
2. Hicks, A. M.: Congenital paralysis of lateral rotators of eyes with paralysis of muscles of face, Arch. Ophth., *30*:38, 1943.
3. Merz, M; and Mojtowicz, S.: The Möbius syndrome, Am. J. Ophth. *63* (Part II): 837, 1967.

SYNDROME; Morgagni
SYNONYMS: Hyperostosis frontalis interna syndrome, intracranial exostosis, metabolic craniopathy
GEN. INFORMATION:
Dominant inheritance. Almost confined to females. Onset about middle age (45 years). X-ray findings: Bony protrusions into the optic canal (not a frequent finding in this syndrome). Hyperostosis of the tabula interna of the frontal bone. Either the squamous, the orbital, or both portions of the bone are involved. The tabula externa is never affected. The petrous bone is occasionally involved causing 7th and 8th crainal nerve symptoms.

OCULAR FINDINGS:

Orbit	
Lids	
Motility	
Lacr. App.	
Vision	
Vis. Fields	Field loss of various degree dure to optic nerve injury by bony protrusions in the optic canal.
Intraoc. Ten.	
Ant. Segm. and Sclera	
Ocul. Media	
Retina and Choroid	Circumscribed bilateral chorioretinitis (Rubino)
Optic Nerve	Optic nerve injury within the optic canal by bony protrusions with resulting blindness.

OTHER CLINICAL FINDINGS:
1. Hyperostosis frontalis interna
2. Obesity (mainly trunk and proximal portions of the limbs)
3. Mental incapacity (occasionally)
4. Hirsutism, menstrual disorders
5. Fatigue
6. Hypertension and arteriosclerosis
7. Headache
8. Somnolence and lethargy
9. Vertigo
10. Tinnitus

BIBLIOGRAPHY:
1. Morgagni, G. B.: De sedibus et causis morborum peranatomen indagatis libri quinque (2 vols.) Venetiis, typog. Remondiniana, 1761. Engl. Transl. by B. Alexander, 3 vols.,, London, 1769. (Selections in Med. Classics 4:640, 1940.)
2. Rubino, A.: Sindrome de Morgagni con emianopsia bitemporale a quadrant superiori associata a retinite pigmentosa circoscrita, Riv. Oto-Neuro-Oftal. 22:237,, 1947.
3. Falconer, M. A. and Pierard, B. E.: Failing vison caused by a bony spike compressing the optic nerve within the optic canal. Report of two cases associated with Morgagni's syndrome benefited by operation, Brit. J. Ophth., 34:265, 1950.

SYNDROME: Morquio-Brailsford
SYNONYMS: Brailsford-Morquio dystrophy, familial osseous dystrophy, keratosulfatoria, mucopolysaridosis (MPS)IV.
GEN. INFORMATION:
Hereditary dystrophy of cartilage and bone. Transmitted as a recessive character. Slight predilection for male. Familial influences common. Relative rare occurance. Becomes apparent between ages of 4 to 10 years. Etiology unknown. Spine most severely affected of skeletal system. (Differential diagnosis to exclude Hurler's syndrome and Leri's syndrome). With progression of the disease, there in increasing disability. Excess production of keratosulfate. (See also: Hurler, Hunter, Sanfillipo-Good and Scheie's Syndromes)

OCULAR FINDINGS:

Orbit	Enophthalmos*
Lids	Ptosis *
Motility	
Lacr. App.	Excessive tear secretion*
Vision	
Vis. Fields	
Intraoc. Ten.	Ocular hypotomy*
Ant. Segm.	Miosis*
and Sclera	
Ocul. Media	Occasionally hazy corneae
Retina and	Fundi and ERG response normal (Gills *et al.*)
Choroid	
Optic Nerve	

OTHER CLINICAL FINDINGS:
1. Dwarfism
2. Skeletal deformities (progressive)
3. Chest and spine deformities particularly severe
4. Delayed ossification of epiphyses
5. Decreased muscle tone
6. Joint crepitation
7. Intelligence usually normal
8. Normal skull

*Ocular finging correspond to Horner's syndrome and have been described as being caused by bilateral cervical sympathetic irritation in this syndrome (Giraud and Bert, 1934).

BIBLIOGRAPHY:
1. Morquio, L.:Sur une forme de dystrophie osseuse familiale, Bull. Soc. Pediat. Paris, *27:*145, 1929.
2. Braisford, J. E.: Chondro-osteo-dystrophy, Roentgenographic and clinical features of child with dislocation of vertebrae, Am J. Surg. 7:404, 1929.
3. Whiteside, J. D. and Cholmeley, J. A.: Morquio's disease-a review of the literature with a description of four cases, Arch. Dis. Childhood, *27:*487, 1952.
4. Gills, J. P.; Hobson, R.; Hanley, W. B., and Mckusick, V. A.: Electroretinography and fundus oculi findings in Hurler's syndrome and allied mucopolysaccharidoses, Arch. Ophth. *74:*596, 1965.
5. McKusick, V. A.: The Genetic Mucopolysaccharidoses, Medicine (See Ref. 4)

SYNDROME: Naegeli
SYNONYMS: Melanophoric nevus syndrome
GEN. INFORMATION:
Autosomal dominant inheritance. Both sexes equally affected (Franceschetti and Jadassohn). The syndrome was recognized as a separate entity from incontinentia pigmenti (Bloch-Sulzberger's syndrome) by Franceschetti and based on the mode of inheritance. Ocular findings are infrequent. The skin pigmentation appears usually during the second year of life. Inflammatory lesions of the skin and blisters as seen in incontinentia pigmenti are *not* present in Naegeli's syndrome.

OCULAR FINDINGS:

Orbit	
Lids	
Motility	Nystagmus, strabismus
Lacr. App.	
Vision	
Vis. Fields	
Intraoc. Ten.	
Ant. Segm.	
and Sclera	
Ocul. Media	
Retina and	Pseudoglioma
Choroid	
Optic Nerve	Papillitis, optic atrophy

OTHER CLINICAL FINDINGS:
1. Pigmentary skin changes in reticular fashion
2. Dental abnormalities with yellowish spots on buccal side of teeth
3. Lowered function of sweat glands (hipohydrosis) mainly palms and soles
4. Moderate keratosis palmaris and plantaris (absent in Bloch-Sulzberger's syndrome)

BIBLIOGRAPHY:
1. Naegeli, O.:Familiärer Chromatophorennaevus, Schweiz. med. Wschr. *8:*48, 1927.
2. Franceschetti, A. and Jadassohn, W.: A propos de 'l'incontinentia pigmenti', délimitation de deux syndromes différents figurant sous le même terme, Dermatologica, *108:*1, 1954.

SYNDROME: Naffziger
SYNONYMS: Scalenus anticus syndrome
GEN. INFORMATION:
Compression of brachial plexus and subclavian artery by the scalenus anticus muscle. The symptoms vary from mild to severe and show in the mild form remissions and exacerbations. The symptoms usually disappear with scalenectomy and removal of cervical rib if present (approx. 20% of cases). Differential diagnosis: Cervical rib, spinal chord tumor, Pancoast tumor, ruptured nucleus pulposus, spinal column tuberculosis, cervical spondylosis. (See also: Pancoast and Naffziger syndromes)

OCULAR FINDINGS:

Orbit	
Lids	Ptosis (unilateral)
Motility	
Lacr. App.	
Vision	
Vis. Fields	
Intraoc. Ten.	
Ant. Segm.	Small pupil, loss of ciliospinal reflex (same side as ptosis)
and Sclera	
Ocul. Media	
Retina and	
Choroid	
Optic Nerve	

OTHER CLINICAL FINDINGS:
1. Weakness ipsilateral hand grip
2. Reduced ipsilateral biceps reflex
3. Diminution of pulse volume on affected side
4. Numbness and coldness in hand and fingers

BIBLIOGRAPHY:
1. Naffziger, H. D., quoted in Ochsner, A.; Gage, M. and DeBakey, M.: Scalenus anticus (Naffziger) syndrome, Am. J. Surg. *28*:669, 1935.
2. Adson, A. W. and Coffey, J. R.: Cervical rib, Ann. Surg., *85*:839, 1927.
3. Collins, R. D.: *Neurologic Diagnosis,* Philadelphia, J. B. Lippincott Co., 1962.

SYNDROME: Niemann-Pick
SYNONYMS: Essential lipoid histiocytosis
GEN. INFORMATION:

Phosphatide lipidosis with degeneration of the ganglion cells of the central nervous system and lipid storage involving the entire reticuloendothelial system and parenchymatous tissue.

Recessive mode of inheritance with onset of the clinical signs during the first months of life. Smiliar to Tay Sach's syndrome there is a predisposition for the disease among Jews. Prognosis is poor with death usually within first 2 years of life, but may in some chronic cases last to late childhood. Pathological findings: Accumulation of mainly lecithin and sphingomyelin in reticuloendothelial cells of liver, spleen, marrow and lymphnodes. CNS and vascular endothelium are affected less extensively.

OCULAR FINDINGS:

Orbit Lids Motility Lacr. App. Vision Vis. Fields Intraoc. Ten. Ant. Segm. 　and Sclera Ocul. Media	Vision may be reduced but usually no complete blindness
Retina and Choroid	Red spot of the macula similar to that of Tay-Sachs syndrome, though retinal pathology is not as frequent in Niemann-Pick syndrome. Histopathological changes are seen in ganglion cells with vacuolization and swelling and cells of the nuclear layers may be affected
Optic Nerve	Progressive optic atrophy may be present concomitant with the retinal pathology

OTHER CLINICAL FINDINGS:
1. Mental retardation, idiocy
2. Extensive hepatosplenomegaly
3. Epileptic seizures
4. Progressive physical deterioration
5. Skin pigmentation
6. Deafness

BIBLIOGRAPHY:
1. Niemann, A.: Ein unbekanntes Krankheitsbild; Jahrb. f. Kinderheilk. *29:*1, 1914.
2. Pick, L.: Niemann-Pick's disease and other forms of so-called xanthomatoses, Amer. J. Med. Sc. *185:*601, 1933.
3. Crocker, A. C.:The cerebral defect in Tay-Sachs disease and Niemann-Pick disease, J. Neurochem. *7:*69, 1961
4. Duke-Elder, Sir Stewart: *System of Ophthalmology,* Vol. X, St. Louis, C. V. Mosby Co., 1967.

SYNDROME: Noonan
SYNONYMS:
GEN. INFORMATION:
This syndrome is recognized as a new one with many of the features similar to Turner's syndrome, however, with normal chromosomal analysis. It is assumed that it is a familial disease with an X-linked dominant inheritance or a multifactorial inheritance. Males and females are equally affected. The severity of the pulmonary stenosis is not clearly to ascertain from physical signs, EKG or x-ray examination, but rather requires cardiac catheterization

OCULAR FINDINGS:

Orbit	Hypertelorism, exophthalmos
Lids	Ptosis (unilateral or bilateral), antimongoloid slanting palpebral fissures
Motility	
Lacr. App.	
Vision	
Vis. Fields	
Intraoc. Ten.	
Ant. Segm.	
and Sclera	
Ocul. Media	
Retina and	
Choroid	
Optic Nerve	

OTHER CLINICAL FINDINGS:

1. Valvular pulmonary stenosis
2. Short stature
3. Webbed neck
4. Low hairline in the back
5. Cubitus valgus
6. Mental retardation (not a constant feature)
7. Deformed chestwall
8. Micrognathia
9. Low set ears
10. Dystrophic nails
11. Short 5th finger
12. Abnormal dermatoglyphic pattern

BIBLIOGRAPHY:

1. Noonan, J. A.: Hypertelorism with Turner phenotype: A new syndrome with associated congenital heart disease, Am. J. Dis. Child. *116*:373, 1968.
2. Nora, J. J. and Sinha, A. K.: Direct familial transmission of the Turner phenotype, Am. J. Dis. Child. *116*:343, 1968.
3. Calermajer, J. M.; Bowdler, J. D. and Cohen, D. H.: Pulmonary stenosis in patients with the Turner phenotype in male, Am. J. Dis. Child. *116*:351, 1968.
4. Kaplan, M. S., Opitz, J. M. and Gosset, R. S.: Noonan's syndrome, Am. J. Dis. Child. *116*:359, 1968.
5. Wright, N. L.; Summitt, E. L. and Ainger, L. E.: Noonan's syndrome and Ebstein's malformation of the tricuspid valve, Am. J. Dis. Child. *116*:367, 1968.

SYNDROME: Nothnagel
SYNONYMS: Ophthalmoplegia-cerebellar ataxia syndrome
GEN. INFORMATION:
Lesion of the superior cerebellar peduncle, red nucleus and emerging oculo-motor fibers. Pathological findings: Pineal tumor, tumor or vascular disturbance in the corpora quadrigemina and in the vermis cerebelli. Midbrain lesion with involvement of the area of the third nerve nucleus and brachium conjunctivum.

OCULAR FINDINGS:

Orbit	
Lids	
Motility	Oculomotor paresis. Gaze paralysis most frequent upward combined with evidence of some degree of internal or external ophthalmoplegia
Lacr. App.	
Vision	
Vis. Fields	
Intraoc. Ten.	
Ant. Segm. and Sclera	
Ocul. Media	
Retina and Choroid	
Optic Nerve	

OTHER CLINICAL FINDINGS:
Cerebellar ataxia
BIBLIOGRAPHY:
1. Nothnagel, C. W. H.:*Topische Diagnostik der Gehirnkrankheiten,* Berlin, A Hirschwarld, 1879, p. 220.
2. Hiller, F.: The vascular syndromes of the basilar and vertebral arteries and their branches, J. Nerv. & Ment. Dis., *116:*988, 1952.

SYNDROME: Oculocerebellar-tegmental
SYNONYMS:
GEN. INFORMATION:
Vascular lesion of the mesencephalon with softening in the peduncular tegmentum.

OCULAR FINDINGS:

Orbit	
Lids	
Motility	Paralysis of associated ocular movements (internuclear anterior ophthalmoplegia)
Lacr. App.	
Vision	
Vis. Fields	
Intraoc. Ten.	
Ant. Segm. and Sclera	
Ocul. Media	
Retina and Choroid	
Optic Nerve	

OTHER CLINICAL FINDINGS:
1. Sudden onset of hemiplegia with rapid recovery
2. Bilateral cerebellar syndrome

BIBLIOGRAPHY:
Rodriquez, B.; Rodriquez, B. R. and Oreggia, A.: A new type of peduncular syndrome. Internulear ophthalmoplegia and bilateral cerebellar syndrome from a tegmental lesion, Arch. Urug. de Med., *10:*353, 1945 (Abstract, A. J. O., *29:*511, 1946).

11

SYNDROME: Oculo-oro-genital
SYNONYMS:
GEN. INFORMATION:
Vitamin B$_1$ deficiency and possible vitamin A deficiency. Prognosis good with adequate diet. All symptoms improved after normal diet was resumed. This is in contrast to central nervous system deficiency syndrome in which visual loss and neurological symptoms remained after re-establishemnt of adequate diet.

OCULAR FINDINGS:

Orbit	
Lids	
Motility	
Lacr. App.	
Vision	Loss of vision according to severeness of optic atrophy
Vis. Fields	
Intraoc. Ten.	
Ant. Segm. and Sclera	Conjunctivitis, varying from mild to severe (93%)
Ocul. Media	Keratitis
Retina and Choroid	
Optic Nerve	Optic atrophy (attributed to B$_1$ and A deficiency)

OTHER CLINICAL FINDINGS:
1. Stomatitis, glossitis
2. Dermatitis of the scrotum developing through several phases: pruritus, erythema, exfoliation, ulceration: Subjectively with burning and itching
3. Erythema of the pharynx and soft palate
4. Small sensitive ulcers of buccal membranes
5. Diarrhea
6. Fatigue, muscular weakness
7. Mental depression, dizziness
8. Painful feet

BIBLIOGRAPHY:
1. Bloom, S. M.; Merg, E. H. and Taylor, W. W.: Nutritional amblyopia in American prisoners, Am. J. Ophth. *29:*1248, 1946.
2. Denny-Brown, D.: Neurological conditions resulting from prolonged and severe dietary restrictions, Medicine, *26:*41, 1947.
3. Jacobs, E. C.: Oculo-oro-genital syndrome: A deficiency disease, Ann. Int. Med., *35:*1049, 1951.
4. MacBryde, C. M.: Weight loss and undernutrition, in MacBryde, C. M. (ed.): *Signs and Symptoms,* 4th ed., Philadelphia, J. B. Lippincott Co., 1964, p. 817

SYNDROME: Ophthalmoplegic-migraine
SYNONYMS:
GEN. INFORMATION:
Anatomical, clinical, pathological and experimental evidence exists that unilateral increase in cerebral volume can produce ipsilateral herniation of the hippocampal gyrus of the temporal lobe through the incisura tentorii, resulting in all the symptoms of this syndrome. The herniation depends on anatomical variations correlated with unilateral cerebral edema due to vascular origin, vasomotor phenomena, intracranial aneurysm or tumor. The clinical findings are often transitory but with recurrence leading in certain cases to permanent manifestations.

OCULAR FINDINGS:

Orbit	Severe unilateral supraorbital pain
Lids	Ptosis
Motility..	Transitory partial or complete homolateral oculomotor paralysis. Sixth nerve is occasionally involved, rarely the fourth
Lacr. App.	
Vision	
Vis. Fields	
Intraoc. Ten.	
Ant. Segm. and Sclera	Anisocoria (occasional finding), normal pupil reactions
Ocul. Media	
Retina and Choroid	Retinal hemorrhages
Optic Nerve	Papilledema (may be bilateral)

OTHER CLINICAL FINDINGS:
1. Migraine headache, not present in all instances
2. Dizziness
3. Diminution in sense of smell
4. Hypalgesia contralateral side of face

BIBLIOGRAPHY:
1. Adie, W. J.: Permanent hemianopia in migraine and subarachnoid hemorrhage, Lancet, 2:237, 1930.
2. Alpers, B. F. and Yaskin, H. E. Pathogenesis of ophthalmoplegic migraine, Arch. Ophth. 45:555, 1951.
3. Harrington, D. O. and Flocks, M.: Ophthalmoplegic migraine. Pathogenesis; Report of pathological findings in case of recurrent oculomotor paralysis, Arch. Ophth., 49:643, 1953.

SYNDROME: Ophthalmoplegic-retinal degeneration
SYNONYMS: Barnard-Scholz syndrome, Kearns-Sayre syndrome
GEN. INFORMATION:
The association of ophthalmoplegia with retinal degeneration to be more than merely coincidental was first suggested by Barnard and Scholz (1944). The etiology for the ophthalmoplegia has been various, including possible nuclear ophthalmoplegia and ocular myopathy (Kiloh-Nevin). Kearns and Sayre (1958) reported this syndrome associated with heart block in two patients as a possible new syndrome.

OCULAR FINDINGS:

Orbit	
Lids	Slowly progressive weakness of muscles of the eyelids (may be first sign), until after years severe ptosis. Müller's muscle seems not to be involved
Motility	Ocular myopathy of external ocular muscles without evidence of CNS involvement with final complete external ophthalmoplegia. Usually slight divergent strabismus. Muscular involvement can be unilateral or bilateral (possibly assymetric in degree)
Lacr. App.	
Vision	
Vis. Fields	
Intraoc. Ten.	
Ant. Segm. and Sclera	Pupils unaffected
Ocul. Media	
Retina and Choroid	Retinitis pigmentosa
Optic Nerve	

OTHER CLINICAL FINDINGS:
1. Facial, neck and shoulder muscles occasionally also involved
2. Heart block*
3. Possible association with progressive muscular dystrophy

*See: Gen. Information above

BIBLIOGRAPHY:
1. Barnard, R. I. and Scholz, R. O.: Ophthalmoplegia and Retinal Degeneration, Am. J. Ophth. 27:621, 1944.
2. Erdbrink, W. L.: Ocular Myopathy Associated with Retinitis Pigmentosa, Arch. Ophth. 57:335, 1957.
3. Kearns, T. P. and Sayre, G. P.: Retinitis Pigmentosa, External Ophthalmoplegia and Complete Heart Block, Arch. Ophth. 60:280, 1958.
4. Kiloh, L. G. and Nevin, S.: Progressive dystrophy of the external ocular muscles (Ocular myopathy), Brain, 74:115, 1951.
5. Drachman, D. A.: Progressive external ophthalmoplegia-a finding associated with neurodegenerative disorders, in Smith, J. L.: Neuro-Ophthalmology, Vol. IV, St. Louis, C. V. Mosby Co., 1968, p. 124

SYNDROME: Page
SYNONYMS: Hypertensive diencephalic syndrome
GEN. INFORMATION:
Irritation of the parasympathetic and sympathetic centers in the diencephalon.
Intradermal histamine 0.25 mg reproduces the syndrome (Schroeder and Gold-
men). The prognosis is unpredictable. The syndrome is more frequently seen in
women. Onset at ages 18 to 30 years with attacks arising spontaneously at times,
but usually under excitement. The symptoms last usually for few minutes but
may occur several times in a day. Phenomena also occur in these patients which
suggests regression to more archiac emotional patterns, possibly having their
origin in the thalamus and hypothalamus (Page).

OCULAR FINDINGS:

Orbit	
Lids	
Motility	
Lacr. App.	Excessive lacrimation
Vision	
Vis. Fields	
Intraoc. Ten.	
Ant. Segm.	
and Sclera	
Ocul. Media	
Retina and	Arteriosclerotic and hypertensive fundus changes
Optic Nerve	

OTHER CLINICAL FINDINGS:
1. Vasomotor blush over face, neck and trunk followed by perspiration
2. Tachycardia, palpipation
3. Elevated blood pressure with additional 20 to 30mm Hg rise during attacks
4. Respiration is reduced and may become labored
5. Increased bowel sounds
6. Salivation
7. Sexual frigidity
8. Tremor of hands and general trembling
9. Slight enlargement of thyroid gland
10. Tightness of scalp

BIBLIOGRAPHY:
1. Page, I. H.: A syndrome simulating diencephalic stimulation occurring in
patients with essential hypertension, Amer. J. Med. Sc., *190:*9, 1935.
2. Page, I. H.: Acetyl ß-methyl cholin (mecholin). Observations concerning
its action on the blood pressure, skin temperature and the heart as exhibited
by the electrocardiograms of hypertensive patients, Amer. J. Med. Sc. *189:*
55, 1935.
3. Schroeder H. A. and Goldman, M. L.: Test for the presence of the 'hypertensive diencephalic syndrome' using histamine, Am. J. Med. 6:162, 1949.

SYNDROME: Pancoast
SYNONYMS: Hare syndrome, superior pulmonary sulcus syndrome
GEN. INFORMATION:
Tumor in the pulmonary apex. Erosion of the first 3 ribs is frequent. Vertebral changes may occur later on. Primary bronchogenic carcinoma most frequent cause (50%) but any other tumor in this location may produce the syndrome. Prognosis is poor, with death usually within a year. Symptomatology in earlier stages is similar to that present in lower radicular syndrome (Déjerine-Klumpke) and scalenus anticus syndrome (Naffziger). X-ray findings include homogeneous opacity in the apex of the lung and possibly bony destruction of upper thoracic vertebrae.

OCULAR FINDINGS:

Orbit	Mild enophthalmos*
Lids	Ptosis* Narrowing of the palpebral fissure*
Motility	
Lacr. App.	
Vision	
Vis. Fields	
Intraoc. Ten.	
Ant. Segm.	Miosis*
and Sclera	
Ocul. Media	
Retina and	
Choroid	
Optic Nerve	

OTHER CLINICAL FINDINGS:
1. Pulmonary apical tumor
2. Severe shoulder pain
3. Paresthesia, pain and paresis of the homolateral arm with atrophy of arm and hand muscles

*Horner's syndrome caused by involvement of the sympathetic
BIBLIOGRAPHY:

1. Pancoast, H.: Importance of careful roetgen-ray investigation of apical chest tumor, J. A. M. A., *83:*1407, 1924.
2. Pancoast, H.: Superior pulmonary sulcus tumor: tumor characterized by pain, Horner's syndrome, destruction of bone and atrophy of hand muscle, J. A. M. A., *99:*1391, 1932.
3. Jaffe, N. S.: Localization of lesions causing Horner's syndrome, Arch. Ophth. *44:*710, 1950.
4. Walsh, F. B.: *Clinical Neuro-Ophthalmology*, Baltimore, The Williams & Wilkins Co., 1957.

SYNDROME: Parinaud
SYNONYMS: Divergence paralyis, subthalamus syndrome, paralysis of vertical movements.
GEN. INFORMATION:
Pineal tumor, supranuclear lesions, vascular lesions, inflammation, hemorrhages, midbrain lesions, lesion of the posterior white commissure of the pons, the red nucleus, the superior cerebellar peduncle, etc. The supranuclear lesions which cause the paralysis of voluntary vertical movements are situated closely to the afferent pupillomotor pathways and therefore cause early pupillary signs. Differential diagnosis: myasthenia gravis, Wernicke's syndrome.

OCULAR FINDINGS:

Orbit	
Lids	Ptosis or wide separation of the lids may be present dependent on the location of the lesion. (Retraction of the lids with lesion in the mesencephalic gray matter and ptosis with lesions more anteriorly)
Motility	Paralysis of conjugate upward movement of the eye without paralysis of convergence; Occasionally paralysis of upward and downward movement. Diplopia is often present since nuclear involvement is common as well as supranuclear. Retraction nystagmus (occasional finding)
Vision	
Vis. Fields	Contralateral hemianopsia occurs when the lateral geniculate body becomes involved in case of infiltrating tumor
Intraoc. Ten.	
Ant. Segm. and Sclera	Wide pupils which fail to react to light but sometimes react during accommodation (Holmes)
Ocul. Media	
Retina and Choroid	
Optic Nerve	Papilledema (usually severe)

OTHER CLINICAL FINDINGS:
1. Vertigo
2. Contralateral cerebellar ataxia and chorioathetoid movements if the lesion involves the superior cerebellar peduncle after its decussation

BIBLIOGRAPHY:
1. Parinaud, H.: *Le Strabisme et Son Traitement,* Paris, G. Doin & Co., 1899.
2. Holmes, G.: Palsies of the conjugate ocular movements, Brit. J. Ophth. *5:*241, 1921.
3. Bielschowsky, A.: Lectures on motor anomalies of eyes, paralysis of conjugate movements of eyes, Arch. Ophth., *13:*569, 1935.
4. Waltman, S. R.: Ocular signs in midbrain disease, in Gay, A. J. and Burde, R. M. (eds). *Clinical Concepts of Neuro-Ophthalmology,* Internat. Ophth. Clinics *,7:*807, 1967.

SYNDROME: Parinaud's oculoglandular
SYNONYMS: Parinaud's conjunctiva-adenitis syndrome, cat-scartch-oculoglandular syndrome.
GEN. INFORMATION:
Most frequently seen in children but may occur in adults as well. Infection: transmission from patient to patient does not seem to occur. Incubation time about 7 to 10 days. (Tularemia, leptothrix, sporotrichosis, lymphogranuloma venerum, etc. have been suspected as the cause for the syndrome with leptothrix the most likely cause. (Verhoeff modifications of the Gram stain most suited to demonstrate these organisms.) The prognosis is good, spontaneous recovery in weeks or months (usually 3 to 5 weeks). Laboratory findings: leukocytosis with shift to left in the beginning.

OCULAR FINDINGS:

Orbit	
Lids	
Motility	
Lacr. App.	
Vision	
Vis. Fields	
Intraoc. Ten.	
Ant. Segm. and Sclera	Conjunctivitis, retrotarsal conjunctival granulations. Formation of granuloma about 3 mm high and 2 to 6 mm in diameter. Nodules consist of inflammatory exudate, mainly lymphocytes and plasma cells surrounding small zones of macrophages. Early necrosis. Inferior fornix usually affected and ulcertation is common
Ocul. Media	
Retina and Choroid	
Optic Nerve	

OTHER CLINICAL FINDINGS:
1. Tender, red papule at the site of a cat scratch
2. Regional preauricular and cervical lymphadenitis (often only one gland involved)
3. Irregular fever for 4 to 5 days and malaise

BIBLIOGRAPHY:
1. Parinaud, H. and Galezowski, X.: Conjonctivite infectieuse transmise par les animaux, Ann. Oculist. (Brux.) *101*:252, 1889.
2. Debre, R. *et al.*: La maladie des griffes de chat, Semain hôp. Paris, *26*:1895, 1950.
3. Cassady, J. and Culbertson, C. : Cat-scratch disease and Parinaud's oculoglandular syndrome, Arch Ophth., *50*:68, 1953.
4. Daniels, W. and MacMurray, F.: Cat scratch disease: report of 160 cases, J. A. M. A. *154*:1247, 1954.
5. Hogan, M. J. and Zimmerman, L. E.: *Ophthamlic Pathology, 2nd* Ed., Philadelphia, W. B. Saunders Co., 1962.

SYNDROME: Parkinson
SYNONYMS: Paralysis agitans, 'shaking palsy'
GEN. INFORMATION:
Late stages of epidemic encephalitis, present in association with arteriosclerosis, manganese and carbon monoxide poisoning. Widerspread destruction of the pigmented cells in the substantia nigra. Prognosis is poor.

OCULAR FINDINGS:

Orbit	
Lids	Fluttering of the eyelids. Blepharospasm or less frequent blepharoplegia, ptosis (often bilateral)
Motility	Nystagmus, paralysis of convergence, diplopia, paralysis external rectus muscle
Lacr. App.	
Vision	Weakness of accommodation
Vis. Fields	
Intraoc. Ten.	
Ant. Segm. and Sclera	Absent or sluggish pupillary reactions to light or convergence, mydriasis or anisocoria
Ocul. Media	
Retina and Choroid	
Optic Nerve	Optic neuritis (occasionally), papilledema (rare)

OTHER CLINICAL FINDINGS:
1. Slowness of movements
2. Loss of facial expression
3. "Cog wheel" rigidity of the arms
4. Rhythmical tremors

BIBLIOGRAPHY:
1. Parkinson, J.: An essay on the shaking palsy. London, Sherwood, Nesly and Jones, 1817.
2. Holden, W. A.: The ocular manifestations of epidemic encephalitis, Arch. Ophth., *50:*101, 1921.
3. Libby, G. F.: Epidemic encephalitis from the standpoint of the ophthalmologist, Tr. Am. Ophth Soc., *20:*181, 1922.
4. Hoyt, W. F.: Neurology of the orbicularis oculi, in Smith, J. L. (ed) *Neuro-Ophthalmology,* Vol. 2, St. Louis, C. V. Mosby Co., 1965, p. 167.

SYNDROME: Pelizaeus-Merzbacher
SYNONYMS: Aplasia axialis extracorticalis congenita
GEN. INFORMATION:
Rare disease with poor prognosis. Represents a subdivision of diffuse cerebral sclerosis predominantly involving the white matter of CNS. Brain stem involvement. Onset of symptoms in infancy or childhood with rapid or protracted course. Death usually from intercurrent complications. The pathogenesis is still controversial-(faulty inherent myelination; myelin destruction and removal; normal myelination with subsequent degeneration [leukodystrophy]; arrest of myelin at an early age.) Most often inherited as x-linked recessive, male members affected through normal-appearing carrier mothers. Female cases reported have at least two implications: (1) erroneous diagnosis; (2) autosomal recessive transmission. Affected feniales with milder phenotypic expression can be explained also by Lyon hypothesis (Ref. 6).

OCULAR FINDINGS:

Orbit	
Lids	
Motility	Incomitant lateral, rotary or vertical nystagmus or non-rhythmic wandering eye movements
Lacr. App.	
Vision	Visual impairment in advanced stage from occipital lobe involvement and still later from optic nerve changes. Final stages: expressionless staring without fixation
Vis. Fields	
Intraoc. Ten.	
Ant. Segm. and Sclera	Normal pupillary responses
Ocul. Media	
Retina and Choroid	Tapetoretinal degeneration characteristic of retinitis pigmentosa (Böhringer and Bischoff). Foveal reflex absent. Attenuated arterioles. (Path: Retinal ganglion cells reduced, nerve fiber layer thinned; most likely due to retrograde degeneration of optic nerve fibers without trans-synaptic degeneration
Optic Nerve	Pallor optic disc, optic atrophy, papilledema. (Path: demyelination of optic nerve and loss of optic nerve axon cylinders)

OTHER CLINICAL FINDINGS:
1. Retarded development (physical, mental, motor)
2. Gait instability, ataxia
3. Intention tremor and athetosis
4. Abnormal reflex responses (Babinski, abdominal reflex absent, patellar reflex increased).
5. Hearing and speech disturbances
6. Trophic disturbances
7. Spastic paralysis (advanced stage)
8. Dementia, epileptiform seizures (terminal)

BIBLIOGRAPHY:
1. Pelizaeus, F.: Über eine eigentümliche Form spastischer Lähmung mit Zerebralerscheinungen auf hereditärer Grundlage (multiple sclerose), Arch. Psych. Nervenkr. *16:*698, 1885.
2. Merzbacher, L.: Eine eigenartige familiär-hereditäre Erkrankungsform (aplasia axialis extracorticalis congenita), Zstchr. Ges. Neurol. Psychiat. *3:*1, 1910.
3. Bohringer, H. R. and Bischoff, A.: Über ein familiäres Syndrom mit degenerativer diffuser Sklerose (Typus Pelizaeus-Merzbacher), tapetoretinaler Degenration und Zwergwuchs, Ophthalmologica *137:*147, 1959.
4. Zeman, W.; Demyer, W. and Falls, H. F.: Pelizaeus-Merzbacher disease: A study in nosology, J. Neuropath, Exp. Neurol. *23:*334, 1964.
5. Rahn, E. K., Yanoff, M.; and Tucker, S.: Neuro-Ocular considerations in the Pelizaeus-Merzbacher syndrome, Am. J. Ophth. *66:*1143, 1968.
6. Thompson, J. S.; and Thompson, M. W.: The Lyon hopothesis of gene action on the X chromosome (p. 127) in Ibid: *Genetics in Medicine.* Philadelphia, W. B. Saunders Co., 1966.

SYNDROME: Pierre Robin
SYNONYMS: Robin's syndrome, micrognathia-glossoptosis syndrome
GEN. INFORMATION:
Etiology is unknown. Apparently no genetic pattern. Manifestations present at birth. A history of intrauterine disturbance during early pregnancy was reported in about 25% of cases and the syndrome was more frequently in the offspring of elderly mothers (Ref. 5). A pathogenesis for this syndrome based on arrested development seems most likely. Supportive therapy is of importance in early life to prevent secondary complications due to the difficulites in swallowing.

OCULAR FINDINGS:

Orbit	Microphthalmos (occasional finding), proptosis
Lids	Ptosis
Motility	Esotropia (occasional)
Lacr. App.	
Vision	High myopia, reduced vision
Vis. Fields	
Intraoc. Ten.	Congenital glaucoma
Ant. Segm. and Sclera	Conjunctivitis
Ocul. Media	Congenital cataract (rare)
Retina and Choroid	Retinal disinsertion, choroidal coloboma (single observation, Ref. 5)
Optic Nerve	

OTHER CLINICAL FINDINGS:
1. Micrognathia* 4. Acute dyspnea 7. Mental retardation (approx. 20%)
2. Cleft palate* 5. Cyanosis 8. Hearing defects
3. Glossoptosis* 6. Difficulties in 9. Skeletal deformations
   swallowing
The facial expression is bird like with flat base of the nose and high arched deformed palate with or without cleft. Swallowing will usually improve up to 6 years of age at which time it may be normal.

*Characteristic for the syndrome
BIBLIOGRAPHY:

1. Robin, P.: La chute de la base de la langue considérée comme une nouvelle cause de gêne dans la respiration naso-pharyngienne, Bull. Acad. méd. (Paris), *88*:37, 1923.
2. Robin, P.: Glossoptosis due to atresia and hypotrophy of the mandible, Am. J. Dis. Child., *48*:541, 1934.
3. MacKenzie, J.: The first arch syndrome, Arch. Dis. Child., *33*:477, 1958.
4. Smith, J. L.; Cavanaugh, J. J. A. and Stowe, F. C.: Ocular manifestations of the Pierre Robin syndrome, Arch. Ophth., *63*:984, 1960.
5. Smith, J. L. and Stowe, F.: The Pierre Robin syndrome (Glossoptosis, Micrognathia, Cleft Palate): A review of 39 cases with emphasis on associated ocular lesions, Pediatrics, *27*:128, 1961.

159

SYNDROME: Posner-Schlossman
SYNONYMS: Glaucomatocyclitic crisis
GEN. INFORMATION:
Episodes of high intraocular tension last from hours to several weeks (usually 2 weeks) and recur at varying frequency. Etiology is not known. Allergic factor has been suggested. Posner and Schlossman thought it possibly to be due to a central disturbance in the hypothalamus in the presence of an unstable peripheral autonomic nervous system. Woods believed it to be a low grade, intermittent, nongranulomatous inflammation confined to the ciliary body and due to the same etiologic factor as other nongranulomatous lesions of the uvea.

OCULAR FINDINGS:

Orbit	
Lids	
Motility	
Lacr. App.	
Vision	Slight blurring of vision, colored halos during episodes of high intraocular tension. No permanent visual loss
Vis. Fields	No field losses
Intraoc. Ten.	High intraocular pressure (unilateral), no pain
Ant. Segm. and Sclera	Glaucomatocyclitic crisis (benign and usually unilateral). Enlarged pupil anisocoria; absence of ciliary or conjunctival injection; only trace of aqueous flare. No posterior synehciae. Chamber angle open
Ocul. Media	Keratic precipitates may be present
Retina and Choroid	
Optic Nerve	

OTHER CLINICAL FINDINGS:
Allergy
BIBLIOGRAPHY:
1. Posner, A. and Schlossman, A.: Syndrome of unilateral recurrent attacks of glaucoma with cyclitic symptoms, Arch. Ophth. *39:*517, 1948.
2. Theodore, F. H.: Observations on glaucomatocyclitic crisis (Posner-Schlossman syndrome), Brit. J. Ophth. *36:*207, 1952.
3. Theodore, F. H. and Schlossman, A.: *Ocular Allergy,* Baltimore, The Williams & Wilkins Co., 1958, p. 353.
4. Woods, A. C.: Endogenous inflammations of the uveal tract. Baltimore, The Williams & Wilkins Co., 1961, p. 174.
5. Billet, E.: Syndrome of glaucomato-cyclitic crisis, Am. J. Ophth. *35:*214, 1952.

SYNDROME: Pseudo-Graefe
SYNONYMS: Fuchs' sign
GEN. INFORMATION:

Misdirection of regenerating oculomotor nerve fibers after injury of the 3rd nerve to the other muscles they are designated for, will lead to a variety of malfunctionings of the globe and upper lid upon muscle activation from stimuli received by the misdirected fibres. Most frequent cause is trauma, however aneurysm and tumor have been described as having produced the symptoms of Pseudo-Graefe's sign. Though the 'Pseudo Graefe' sign can be explained entirely on misdirected regeneration of oculomotor nerve fibers, it also has been thought possible as being produced by a short circuit of impulses from one cranial nucleus into another. The condition may occur beside the ones mentioned in exophthalmic goiter, tabes, anterior poliomyelitis, or vascular lesions of the brain stem.

OCULAR FINDINGS:

Orbit	
Lids	Elevation of the upper lid in downward gaze. *Not* the failure of the upper lid to descend on downward gaze but rather its elevation is called the Pseudo-Graefe sign. (Lagging in upper lid movement on downward gaze is referred to as Graefe's sign)
Motility	
Lacr. App.	
Vision	
Vis. Fields	
Intraoc. Ten.	
Ant. Segm. and Sclera	
Ocul. Media	
Retina and Choroid	
Optic Nerve	

OTHER CLINICAL FINDINGS:
BIBLIOGRAPHY:

1. Bender, M. B.: The nerve supply to the orbicularis muscle and the physiology of movements of the upper lid, with particular reference to the Pseudo-Graefe phenomenon, Arch. Ophth., *15*:21, 1936.
2. Bender, M. B. and Fulton, J. F.: Factors in functional recovery following section of the oculomotor nerve in monkeys, J. Neurol. & Psychol. *2*:285, 1939.
3. Walsh, F. B. and King, A. B.: Ocular signs of intracranial saccular aneurysms. Experimental work on collateral circulation through the ophthalmic artery, Arch. Ophth. *23*:1169, 1942.

SYNDROME: Pseudo hypoparathyroidism

SYNONYMS: Chronic renal tubular insufficiency syndrome, Seabright-bantam syndrome.

GEN INFORMATION:
Etiology is unknown. Higher frequency in females (2:1). Manifestations may be present from birth. The parathyroid glands are normally functioning but kidney and skeleton fail to respond to the parathormone. If patients receive parathyroid extract, their kidneys fail to respond with phosphate diuresis. Laboratory findings: Depressed serum calcium, elevated serum phosphorus, normal alkaline phosphatase. Prognosis is good under proper treatment. Attention: Pseudo-pseudohypoparathyroidism syndrome has normal Ca-PO$_4$ serum levels and no ocular changes. More recently it has been suggested that Pseudo-Pseudohypoparathyroidism represents the same syndrome as Pseudo-parathyroidism. Symptoms of the nervous system are caused by hypocalcemia. X-ray: Demineralization of bones may exist, similar to osteitis fibrosa cystica.

OCULAR FINDINGS:

Orbit	
Lids	
Motility	Strabismus
Lacr. App.	
Vision	
Vis. Fields	
Intraoc. Ten.	
Ant. Seam. and Sclera	Blue sclera
Ocul. Media	Punctate-cataracts, white opacities and ploychromatic cortex. (possibly due to the hyperphosphatemia)
Retina and Choroid	
Optic Nerve	Papilledema (rare)

OTHER CLINICAL FINDINGS:
1. Short stature and short metacarpals and metatarsals (esp. 4th digit)
2. Short limbs in relation to trunk
3. Metastatic ossification in subcutaneous tissue and exostoses. (This finding is very rare in idiopathic hypoparathyroidism)
4. Round face with short neck
5. Decalcification of teeth
6. Obesity, fat stubby hands
7. Tetany with positive Chvostek and Trousseau signs
8. Mental retardation
9. Absence of moniliasis is of differential diagnostic help

BIBLIOGRAPHY:
1. Albright, F.; Burnett, C. H.; Smith, P. H.; and Parson, W.: Pseudo-hypoparathyroidism-An example of 'Seabright-bantam syndrome', Endocrinology, *30:*922, 1942.
2. Alexander, S. B. and Tucker, H. St. G., Jr.: Pseudohypoparathyroidism: Report of a case with late manifestations, J. Clin. Endocrin., *9:*862, 1949.
3. Albright, F.; Forbes, A. P. and Henneman, P. H.: Pseudo-Psuedohypoparathyroidism, Tr. Am. A. Physicians, *65:*337, 1952
4. Klein, R.: Hypoparathyroidism; in: Gardner, L. I.: *Endocrine and Genetic Diseases of Childhood.* Philadelphia, W. B. Saunders Co. 1969, p. 373.

SYNDROME: Raeder

SYNONYMS: Paratrigeminal paralysis, Horton's Headache, histamine cephalalgia

GEN. INFORMATION:
Interruption of sympathetic fibers about the carotid artery and involvement of the fifth nerve. Meningioma and aneurysm of the internal carotid artery most frequent causes. Pachymeningitis occasional etiologic factor. Prognosis is poor. The majority of patients never show an organic lesion. Raeder's syndrome has been divided into 2 groups (Boniuk and Schlezinger) both presenting neuralgia but with or without parasellar cranial nerve involvement. The former requiring extensive studies to determine the intracranial lesion. The syndrome has almost exclusively been reported in the male (only 1 female case in a total of 27).

OCULAR FINDINGS:

Orbit	Mild enophthalmos
Lids	Mild ptosis (unilateral)
Motility	Diplopia possible
Lacr. App.	Epiphora
Vision	
Vis. Fields	Scotoma possible
Intraoc. Ten.	Hypotonia
Ant. Segm. and Sclera	Unilateral miosis
Ocul. Media	
Retina and Choroid	
Optic Nerve	

OTHER CLINICAL FINDINGS:
1. Facial pain
2. Occasionally weakness of the jaw muscles
3. Headaches (V, region)
4. Hypertension
5. Associated inflammatory processes are not infrequent (30%)

BIBLIOGRAPHY:
1. Raeder, J. G.: "Paratrigeminal" paralysis of oculo-pupillary sympathetic, Brain, *47:*149, 1924.
2. Bedrossian, E.: Raeder's syndrome, Arch. Ophth. *48:*620, 1952.
3. Boniuk, M.; and Schlezinger, N. S.: Raeder's paratrigeminal syndrome, Am. J. Ophth., *54:*1074, 1962.
4. Minton, L. R.; and Bounds, G. W., Jr.: Raeder's paratrigeminal syndrome, Am. J. Ophth *58:*271, 1964.

SYNDROME: Raymond

SYNONYMS: Raymond-Cestan syndrome, Cestan syndrome, pontine syndrome, dissociation of lateral gaze syndrome

GEN. INFORMATION:

The syndrome is caused by lesion involving the pyramidal tracts as they traverse the pons. The posterior longitudinal bundle and the medial lemniscus may also be involved. Most frequently lesion of small branches of the basilar artery although tumor and vascular thrombosis has to be considered.

OCULAR FINDINGS:

Orbit	
Lids	
Motility	Ipsilateral abducens palsy, paralysis of lateral conjugate gaze
Lacr. App.	
Vision	
Vis. Fields	
Intraoc. Ten.	
Ant. Segm. and Sclera	
Ocul. Media	
Retina and Choroid	
Optic Nerve	

OTHER CLINICAL FINDINGS:

1. Contralateral hemiplegia
2. Anesthesia of the face, limbs and trunk

BIBLIOGRAPHY:

1. Behr, C.: Zur topischen Diagnose der Abduzenslähmung, Ztschr. Augenhk. *55*:293, 1925.
2. Hiller, F.: The vascular syndromes of the basilar and vertebral arteries and their branches, J. Nerv. & Ment. Dis. *116*:988, 1952.
2. David, N. J.: Neuro ophthalmology of occlusive disease in the vertebral-basilar arterial system; in Smith, J. L. (Ed.) *Neuro-Ophthalmology,* Vol. 2, St. Louis, C. V. Mosby Co., 1965, p. 206.

SYNDROME: Refsum

SYNONYMS: Heredopathia atactica polyneuritiformis syndrome

GEN. INFORMATION:

Recessive hereditary disease. A disorder of lipid metabolism (failure to oxidize phytol with resulting accummulation of phytanic acid in serum and tissues*). Interstitial hypertrophic polyneuropathy has been suggested, based on pathological findings. Delamination of myelin sheaths has been given as another etiological factor. Course is slowly progressive with death after few years. Laboratory findings: Increase of protein in cerebrospinal fluid without increase of cells.* EEG shows slowing of brain waves. Neuropathological findings revealed thickening of connective tissue surrounding peripheral nerves, lipid granules in neurons, astrocytes, meninges, perivascular macrophages and in hepatic and renal cells.

OCULAR FINDINGS:

Orbit	
Lids	
Motility	Progressive external ophthalmoplegia (occasionally)
Lacr. App.	
Vision	Night blindness
Vis .Fields	General constriction
Intraoc. Ten.	
Ant. Segm. and Sclera	Pupillary abnormalities
Ocul. Media	Corneal opacities (Baum et al., A. J. O. 60: 699, 1965)-(single observation.)
Retina and Choroid	Retinal degeneration beginning in macula (atypical)* or retinitis pigmentosa
Optic Nerve	

OTHER CLINICAL FINDINGS:

1. Spinocerebellar ataxia*
2. Deafness(progressive)
3. Polyneuritis-like affection of limbs*
4. CNS degeneration
5. Ichthyosis
6. Sensory changes
7. Wasting of extremities
8. Complete heart block

*Main features of the syndrome

BIBLIOGRAPHY:

1. Refsum, S.: Heredo-ataxia hemeralopica polyneruitiformis familial syndrome. Acta Psychiat. Scand. Suppl. 38:1, 1946.
2. Jager, B. V.; Fred, Herbert L.; Butler, Ronald B.: and Carnes, William H.: Occurrence of retinal pigmentation, ophthalmoplegia, ataxia, deafness and heart block, A. J. Med. 29:888, 1960.
3. Jampel, R. S.; Okazaki, H.; and Bernstein, H.: Ophthalmoplegia and retinal degeneration associated with spinocerebellar ataxia, Arch Ophth. 66:247, 1961.
4. Nordhagen, E.; and Grøndahl, J.: Heredopathy atactica polyneuritiformis (Refsum's disease), Acta Ophth. 42:629, 1964
5. Drachman, D. A. ; Progressive external ophthalmoplegia- a finding associated with neurodegenerative disorders. in Smith, J. L.: Neuro-Ophthamology, Vol. IV, St. Louis, C. V. Mosby Co., 1968.

12

SYNDROME: Reiter

SYNONYMS: Fiessinger-Leroy syndrome, conjunctivo-urethro-synovial syndrome, idiopathic blenorrheal arthritis, polyarthritis enterica

GEN. INFORMATION:
Etiology is unknown: (virus infection has been suggested). Disease is not frequent mainly in males. Onset within the age of 16 to 42 years. Prognosis is good. Duration of symptoms dependent on administered therapy. Laboratory findings: show leukocytosis, increased sedimentation rate, albuminuria, mild anemia. Destructive arthropathy may occur if treatment is not employed. Laboratory finding: Mild to moderate leukocytosis, increased blood sedimentation rate, pyuria. Pathology: Epithelial parakeratosis and acanthosis with infiltration of polymorphonuclear leukocytes, and intraepithelial microabscesses. Lymphocytic infiltration of connective tissue below epithelium. Hyperemia, edema and acute or chronic inflammation of synovial tissues.

OCULAR FINDINGS:

Orbit	
Lids	
Motility	
Lacr. App.	
Vision	
Vis. Fields	
Intraoc. Ten.	
Ant. Seam. and Sclera	Sterile mucopurulent conjunctivitis, usually bilateral. Occasionally conjunctivitis can be so mild that it is easily overlooked. Duration about 1 to 4 weeks, rarely up to several months. Photophobia and epiphora may precede the symptoms of conjunctivitis. Iritis (occasionally)
Ocul. Media	Keratitis (occasionally)
Retina and Choroid	
Optic Nerve	

OTHER CLINICAL FINDINGS:
1. Skin erythema (occasionally)
2. Genital ulcerations
3. Urethritis with discharge (may be mucoid or purulent)from meatus (subsides spontaneously within 1 to 4 weeks)
4. Cystitis with dysuria, abacterial pyuria and hematuria (occasionally)
5. Oral ulceration (occasionally)
6. Arthritis with pain, swelling, heat and effusion
7. Peripheraly lymphadenopathy
8. Anorexia
9. Nausea and vomiting
10. Cough
11. Pleuritis
12. Fever (occasionally)

BIBLIOGRAPHY:
1. Reiter, H.: Über eine bisher unbekannte Spirochätenerkrankung (Spirochaetosis arthritica), Dtsch. med. Wschr., *42:*1535, 1916.
2. Paronen, I.: Reiter's Disease. A study of 344 cases observed in Finland. Acta med. Scand., Suppl. 212:1-114, 1948.
3. Hall, W. H.; and Fingold, S. A.; A study of 23 cases of Reiter's syndrome, Ann. Int. Med., *38:*533, 1953.
4. Foxworthy, D.: Adrenocorticotropin and cortisone in treatment of severe Reiter's syndrome, Ann. Int. Med. *44:*52, 1956.

SYNDROME: Retino-hypophysary
SYNONYMS:
GEN. INFORMATION:
So called "benign" syndrome is not absolutely benign with regard to vision since permanent impairment of vision is associated with this syndrome. X-ray findings: alterations of the bony structure of the sella turcica with decalcifications and osteolysis of the posterior clinoid process.

OCULAR FINDINGS:

Orbit	
Lids	
Motility	
Lacr. App.	
Vision	Reduced central vision
Vis. Fields	Atypical alterations
Intraoc. Ten.	
Ant. Segm. and Sclera	
Ocul. Media	
Retina and Choroid	Narrowing of retinal vessels
Optic Nerve	Optic neuritis, optic atrophy

OTHER CLINICAL FINDINGS:
1. Glycosuria
2. Headache
3. Vertigo
4. Psychic disturbances

BIBLIOGRAPHY:
Lijó Pavia, J.: Retino-hypophysary syndrome. Treatment with gonadotropine. Four new cases. Rev. oto-neuro-oftal., *22:*5, 1947 (Abstract, Am. J. Ophth. *31:* 382, 1948); Ibid: Abstract, Am, J. Ophth. *33:*1007. 1950

SYNDROME: Riegers

SYNONYMS: Dysgenesis mesodermalis corneae et irides, dysgenesis mesostromalis

GEN. INFORMATION:

The syndrome is inherited by an autosomal dominant mode. The developmental defect has been suggested to occur at the 5th to 6th week of fetal life. Busch *et al.* observed this condition through 5 generations of one family with both males and females equally affected. Others have found only males, or only females belonging to one family with this syndrome.

OCULAR FINDINGS:

Orbit	Microphthalmia (occasional finding)
Lids	
Mitlity	
Lacr. App.	
Vision	
Vis. Fields	
Intraoc. Ten.	Congenital glaucoma with chamber angle anomalies (see under Ocul. media below)
Ant. Segm.	
and Sclera	Hypoplasia of the iris, deformed and acentric pupil, anterior synechiae, aniridia not infrequent
Ocul. Media	Microcornea, corneal opacities in Descemet's membrane parallel to the limbus with remaining strands to the atrophic iris, dislocated lens
Retina and	
Choroid	
Optic Nerve	Optic atrophy

OTHER CLINICAL FINDINGS:

1. The face often appears unusually wide
2. Hypodontia and underdeveloped maxilla (may be causing the appearance of feature listed under(1)
3. Suppression of dentation
4. Masculinization in females (quoted in Gorlin and Pindborg)
5. Myotonic dystrophy (Busch *et al.*) of different degree or intensity

BIBLIOGRAPHY:

1. Rieger, H.: Beiträge zur Kenntnis seltener Missbildungen der Iris, Graefes Arch. f. Ophth. *133:*602, 1935.
2. Unger, L.: Hereditäre Irisatrophie mit Sekundärglaukom, Klin. Mbl. Augenhk., *126:*362, 1955.
3. Wilson, J. P.: A case of partial anondontia, Brit. Dent J. *99:*199, 1955
4. Busch, G.; Weiskopf, J. and Busch, K. Th.: Dysgenesis mesodermalis et ectodermalis Rieger oder Riegersche Krankheit, Klin. Mbl. Augnehk. *136:*512, 1960.
5. Gorlin, R. J. and Pindborg, J. J. *Syndromes of the Head and Neck,* New York, McGraw-Hill Book Co. (Blakiston Division), 1964.

SYNDROME: Riley-Day
SYNONYMS: Congenital familial dysautonomia
GEN. INFORMATION:
Inherited in autosomal recessive manner. Occurs in Jewish children. Exact mechanism of production of symptoms not fully known. Most affected functions are under autonomic control, but tendon reflexes and pain response are not. Lab findings: Abnormal EEG possible. Adrenal hypofunction and liver dysfunction possible.

OCULAR FINDINGS:

Orbit	
Lids	
Motility	
Lacr. App.	Congenital failure of tear production
Vision	
Vis. Fields	
Intraco. Ten.	
Ant. Segm. and Sclera	Absence of pupil dilater muscle fibers (Howard)
Ocul. Media	Corneal anesthesia, neuro paralytic keratitis, keratitis sicca, corneal ulcers
Retina and Choroid	
Optic Nerve	

OTHER CLINICAL FINDINGS:

1. Excessive salivation
2. Failure to thrive
3. Recurrent respiratory infections
4. Diarrhea
5. Emotional instability
6. Insensitivity to pain
7. Skin blotching
8. Hyporeflexia
9. Spontan. fractures
10. Lability of blood pressure*
11. Epilepsy*
12. Ureteric malformations

*Less frequent

BIBLIOGRAPHY:
1. Riley, C. M.; Day, R. L.; Greeley, D. M.; and Langford, W. S.: Central autonomic dysfunction with defective lacrimation; report of 6 cases, Pediatrics, *3*:468, 1949.
2. Yatsu, F.; and Zussman, W.: Familial dysautonomia (Riley-Day syndrome): Case report with postmortem findings of a patient at age 31, Arch. Neurol. *10*:459, 1964.
3. Keith, C. G.: Riley-Day Syndrome, Brit. J. Ophth. *49*:667, 1965.
4. Howard, R. O.: Familial dysautonomia (Riley-Day syndrome), Am. J. Ophth. *64*:392, 1967.

SYNDROME: Rochon-Duvigneaud
SYNONYMS: Superior orbital fissure syndrome
GEN. INFORMATION:
Etiology may be inflammatory, traumatic, tumor or vascular. Meningioma of the sphenoid and carotid aneurysm have ahigh incidence in the cause of the syndrome. Arachnoiditis seems to represent the most frequent inflammatory etiology, though syphilis and tuberculosis have been reported in association with it. X-ray findings are characteristic for the various lesions involved. The symptomatology is similar as in orbital opex syndrome (Rollet) and spheno cavernous syndrome.

OCULAR FINDINGS:

Orbit	Mild exophthalmos may be present, sometimes with sudden onset
Lids	Lid edema, caused by disturbance of veinous drainage of the ophthalmic vein
Motility	Partial or complete ophthalmoplegia (III, IV and VI)
Lacr. Aoo.	
Vision	Visual loss with possible blindness depending on the extent of optic nerve involvement
Vis. Fields	
Intraoc. Ten.	
Ant. Segm. and Sclera	Decreased corneal sensitivity
Ocul. Media	
Retina and Choroid	
Ootuc Nerve	Papilledema and optic atrophy may develop particularly with tumor etiology

OTHER CLINICAL FINDINGS:
1. Decreased sensitivity in area of nasociliary, lacrimal, frontal and ophthalmic nerve distribution

BIBLIOGRAPHY:
1. Rochon-Duvigneaud, A.: Quelques cas de paralysie de tous les nerfs orbitaires (ophtalmoplégie totale avec amaurose et anesthésie dans le domaine de l'ophtalmique d'origine syphilitique), Arch. d'opht. *16:*746, 1896
2. Holt, H. and de Rötth, A.:Orbital apex and sphenoid fissure syndrome, Arch. Ophth. *24:*731, 1940.
3. Walsh, F. B.: *Clinical Neuro- Ophthalmology,* Baltimore, The Williams & Wilkins Co., 1957.
4. Hartmann, E. and Gilles, E.:*Roentgenologic Diagnosis in Ophthalmology,* Philadelphia, J. B. Lippincott Co., 1959.

SYNDROME: Rollet
SYNONYMS: Orbital apex-sphenoidal syndrome
GEN. INFORMATION:

Lesion in the apex of the orbit (neoplastic, hemorrhagic, or inflammatory) involving the 3rd, 4th and 6th cranial nerves, the ophthalmic branch of the 5th, sympathetic fibers when they pass through the sphenoidal fissure and the optic nerve. The clinical manifestations and symptoms vary greatly with the extent of the lesion. Pain is a frequent and early sign. The symptomatology of the superior orbital fissure syndrome and spheno-cavernous syndrome are very similar to the orbital apex syndrome. Rollet first described actually syphilitic periostoses of the sphenoidal fissure, whereas Rochon-Duvigneaud first pointed to the sphenoidal syndrome. Déjean classified the orbital apex syndrome in 4 groups. -1) complete form involving II, III, IV, V, VI and sympathetic; -2) lesions limited to the fissure (II is spared); -3) only III, IV, VI involved; -4) lesions of isolated nerves.

Orbit	Varying degree of exophthalmos
Lids	Ptosis, hyperesthesia or anesthesia of the upper lid
Motility	Ophthalmoplegia (partial or complete) depending on degree of nerve involvement
Lacr. App.	
Vision	Impairment of vision of varying degrees
Vis. Fields	Defects according to optic nerve involvement
Intraoc. Ten.	
Ant. Segm. and Sclera	Usually wide pupil with loss of reaction on accommodation
Ocul. Media	Neuralgic pain in the region of the ophthalmic branch V. Anesthesia of the cornea
Retina and Choroid	
Optic Nerve	Papilledema, optic neuritis, otpic atrophy

OTHER CLINICAL FINDINGS:
1. Hyperesthesia or anesthesia of the forehead
2. Vasomotor disturbances

BIBLIOGRAPHY:
1. Rollet, J.: Dict. de De schambres, Syphilis, p. 344, 1865.
2. Rollet, J: Dict Traité des maladies véneriennes, 15:993, Paris, V. Masson & fils, 1865.
3. Rochon-Duvigneaud, A.:Quelques cas de paralysie de tous les nerfs orbitaires (ophtalmoplégie totale avec amaurose et anesthésie dans le domaine de l'ophtalmique d'origine syphilitique), Arch. d'opht,. 16:746, 1896.
4. Déjean, C.: Le syndrome paralytique du sommet de l'orbite, Arch. d'opht. 44:657, 1927.
5. Holt, H. and de Rötth, A.: Orbital apex and sphenoid fissure syndrome Arch. Ophth., 24:731, 1940

SYNDROME: Romberg
SYNONYMS: Parry-Romberg syndrome, progressive hemifacial atrophy, progressive facial hemiatrophy
GEN. INFORMATION:
It appears that the syndrome may be transmitted autosomal dominant with little penetrance of the gene. The condition has been suggested as a heredodegeneration caused by irritation in the peripheral trophic sympathetic system (Ref. 4.) Onset of the syndrome after trauma was described by Crikelair *et al.* 1962. A relationship between this syndrome and scleroderma has also been pointed out (Ref. 4, a. o.). Onset of the symptoms usually during 2nd decade, slowly progressing over several years and then becoming stationary for lifetime.

OCULAR FINDINGS:

Orbit	Enophthalmos due to lack of intraorbital fat. Outer canthus may be lowered caused by loss of underlying bone. Absence of nasal portion of eyebrow
Lids	Ptosis,
Motility	Paresis of ocular muscles
Lacr. App.	
Vision	
Vis. Fields	
Intraoc. Ten.	
Ant. Segm. and Sclera	Mydriasm, absent pupil reflex to light, iritis, iridocyclitis, heterochromia iridis
Ocul. Media	Keratitis elagophthalmos, neuroparalytic keratitis, cataracts
Retina and Choroid	Choroiditis
Optic Nerve	

OTHER CLINICAL FINDINGS:
1. Atrophy of soft tissue one side of the face including tongue (slowly progressive)
2. Trigeminal neuralgia and /or paresthesia (early findings)
3. Epilepsy (usually contralateral side and late appearing)
4. Vitiligo (occasionally)
5. Alopecia and poliosis not uncommon and may precede atrophic skin changes
6. Migraine

BIBLIOGRAPHY:

1. Romberg, M. H.:*Trophoneurosen, Klin, Ergebn.,* Berlin, A. Förster, 1846.
2. Parry, C. H.: Collections from unpublished papers, London, Underwood, Vol. l, 1825.
3. Walsh, F. B.: Facial hemiatrophy, Am. J. Ophth. *22:*1, 1939.
4. Wartenberg, R.: Progressive facial hemiatrophy, Arch. Neurol & Psychiat. *54:*75, 1945.
5. Archambault, L. and Fromm, N. K.: Progressive faciacl hemiatrophy, Arch. Neurol. & Psychiat, *27:*529, 1932.

SYNDROME: Rothmund
SYNONYMS: Rothmund-Thomson, telangiectasia-pigmentation-cataract syndrome, ectodermal syndrome, congenital poikiloderma with juvenile cataract
GEN. INFORMATION:
The syndrome is most likely transmitted as an autosomal recessive trait. However, the observation in mother and son (Hallmann and Patiala:Acta derm. vener.: 1951) points to possible other modes of transmission. Parental consanguinity has been present in some instances. Females are more frequently affected, about 2:1 (Taylor: Arch. Derm., 1957). Werner's syndrome in adults has certain similarities with this syndrome, its mode of inheritance, however, is more likely that of an autosomal recessive trait and it develops somewhat more frequent in males.—The skin changes in Rothmund-Thomson syndrome (see below: Other Clin. Find.) pass from an inflammatory phase, in which exposed skin areas are more severely affected, into a period in which atrophy and telangiectasia are predominant. Reticular or macular pigmentation follow. Sensitivity to sunlight exist in about one third of patients.

OCULAR FINDINGS:

Orbit	Eyebrows may be sparse or absent
Lids	Cilia are sometimes diminished or absent
Motility	
Lacr. App.	
Vision	
Vis. Fields	
Intraoc. Ten.	
Ant. Segm. and Sclera	
Ocul. Media	Bilateral cataracts (anterior subcapsular, posterior stellate or perinuclear type), approx. in 50% of patients. Appearance most frequently during period of 4th to 7th year of life. Corneal lesions occasionally
Retina and Choroid	
Optic Nerve	

OTHER CLINICAL FINDINGS:
1. Poikiloderma (onset between 3rd to 6th months of life)-see also above: Gen. inf.
2. Hypogonadism (about in 25% of patients); hypomenorrhea
3. Head deformity (enlarged with depressed nasal bridge as well as microcephaly have been described; (Tomson)
4. Small stature, with short or malformed distal phalanges,-acrocyanosis may be pronounced.
5. Alopecia
6. Ungula dystrophy
7. Dental disorders

BIBLIOGRAPHY:
1. Rothmund, A.: Über Katarakte in Verbindung mit einer eigntümlichen Hautdegeneration, v. Graefes Arch. f. Ophth., *14*:159, 1868.
2. Thomson, M. S.: A hitherto undescribed familial disease, Brit. J. Dermat. *35*:455, 1923.
3. Thomson, M. S.: Poikiloderma congenitale, Brit. J. Dermat. *48*:221, 1936.
4. Thannhauser, S. J.: Werner's syndrome (Progeria of the adult) and Rothmund's syndrome. Ann. Int. Med., *23*:559, 1945.
5. Franceschetti, A. and Maeder, G.: Cataracte et affections cutanées du type poikilodermie (syndrome de Rothmund) et du type sclerodermie (syndrome de Werner), Schw. Med Wschr. *79*:657, 1949.
6. Lepard, C. W.:Poikiloderma congenitale (Rothmund's syndrome), Tr. Am. Ophth. Soc., *54*:301, 1956.
7. Silver, H. K.: Rothumnd-Thomson syndrome: An oculocutaneous disorder, Am. J. Dis. Child. 111:182, 1966.

SYNDROME: Rubella
SYNONYMS: Congenital rubella syndrome
GEN. INFORMATION:
Rubella infection of the mother during first trimester of pregnancy. Exposure to rubella may be sufficient without that the mother has presented erythema. The virus is demonstrable in the newborn though it may be very difficult to grow *in vitro*. Unusual dermatoglyphic findings, such as distal axial triradii, radial loops on digits other than the second, and simian creases were reported (Achs *et al.*, 1966). Rubella virus, as environmental teratogen, might affect the development of dermal patterns (Ushida and Soltan, 1969)

OCULAR FINDINGS:

Orbit	
Lids	
Motility	Nystagmus (occasionally)
Lacr. App.	
Vision	Visual disturbances and diplopia (less common)
Vis. Fields	
Inttraoc. Ten.	Glaucoma (also without cataracts)
Ant. Segm. and Sclera	Iris cysts and mottled appearance, vascular distortion in anterior chamber angle
Ocul. Media	Corneal haziness and/or opacities clear usually spontaneously. von Hippels posterior corneal ulcer (central absence of Descemet's membrance and endothelium). Cataracts (pygnotic nuclei extending into nucleus of lens)
Retina and Choroid	Retinal pigmentary changes-the appearance and central distribution of lesions are quite distinguishable from retinitis pigmentosa. The retinopathy is not progressive and has little, if any effect on vision
Optic Nerve	Waxy atrophy of optic disc

OTHER CLINICAL FINDINGS:

1. Low birth weight
2. Diarrhea
3. Pneumonia
4. Urinary infection
5. Hearing loss
6. Heart disease
7. Fever
8. Convulsions
9. Reflex changes
10. Ataxia
11. Involuntary movements

BIBLIOGRAPHY:
1. Selzer, G.: Virus isolation, inclusion bodies and chromosomes in rubella inflicted human embryo, Lancet, *2:*336, 1963.
2. Hampton, Roy F., Fuste, F., Hiatt, R. L.; Deutsch, A. R.; and Korones, S. B.: Congenital rubella syndrome, Am. J. Ophth. *62:*222, 1966.
3. Roy, F. H.: Pupillary dilatation in the congenital rubella syndrome, EENT Digest, *29:*51, Oct. 1967.
4. Krill, A. E.: The retinal disease of rubella, Arch. Ophth. *77:*445, 1967.

SYNDROME: Rubinstein-Taybi
SYNONYMS:
GEN. INFORMATION:
Possibly genetically determined. Inheritance may be polygenic or multifactorial (Ref. 1), *i.e.* only if the required genes are present at the necessary locations, the infant will present the typical features of the syndrome.

OCULAR FINDINGS:

Orbit	Enophthalmos*
Lids	Antimongoloid slant of lid fissure (89% Ref. 3), epicanthus (58% Ref. 3.), long eye lashes and highly arched brows Blepharoptosis*
Motility	Strabismus (72% Ref. 3.) Exotropia more common than esotropia
Lacr. App.	Obstruction of nasolacrimal ducts*
Vision	Refractive error(55% Ref. 3) either myopic or hyperopic
Vis. Fields	
Intraoc. Ten.	
Ant. Segm. and Sclera	Coloboma*
Ocul. Media	Cataract*
Retina and Choroid	
Optic Nerve	Optic atrophy*

OTHER CLINICAL FINDINGS:

1. Motor and mental retardation
2. Broad thumbs and toes
3. Highly arched palate
4. Abnormalities of face and limbs
5. Neonatal feeding problems
6. Allergies
7. Urinary infections
8. Heart murmurs

*less frequent

BIBLIOGRAPHY:
1. Rubinstein, J. H. and Taybi, H.: Broad thumbs and toes and facial abnormalities, Am. J. Dis. Child, *105*:588, 1963.
2. Taybi, H.; and Rubinstein, J. H.: Broad thumbs and toes and unusual facial features, Am J. Roentgen. *93*:362, 1965
3. Coffin, G. S.: Brachydactyly, peculiar facies and mental retardation, Am. J. Dis. Child. *108*:351, 1964
4. Roy, F. H.; Summit, R. L;. Hiatt, R. L.; and Hughes, J. G.: Ocular Manifestations of the Rubinstein-Taybi Syndrome, Arch. Ophth. *79*:272, 1968.

SYNDROME: Sabin-Feldman
SYNONYMS:
GEN. INFORMATION:
Etiology is unknown. The syndrome is very similar to toxoplasmosis. Toxoplasma dye and complement fixation tests are negative. Chorioretinopathy associated with *positive* tests showed 90% incidence (of 23 cases) of cerebral calcifications, while in infants with chorioretinopathy and *negative* tests, cerebral calcifications were present only in 5% (of 20 cases). Defective development rather than destructive lesions of necrosis seems to be the basis of this syndrome (Ref. 1). Microscopic findings are similar to those found in toxoplasmosis (Ref. 2).

OCULAR FINDINGS:

Orbit	Microphthalmia*
Lids	
Motility	Strabismus*
Lacr. App.	
Vision	
Vis. Fields	
Intraoc. Ten.	
Ant. Segm. and Sclera	Fixed pupils*
Ocul. Media	Posterior lenticonus*, microcornea*
Retina and Choroid	Chorioretinitis or atrophic degenerative chorioretinal changes
Optic Nerve	Optic atrophy*

OTHER CLINICAL FINDINGS:
1. Cerebral calcifications, infrequent but can be present. (See above: Gen. Information)
2. Convulsions (frequent)
3. Retarded development*
4. Hydrocephalus*
5. Microcephaly

*Occasional findings

BIBLIOGRAPHY:
1. Sabin, A. B. and Feldman, H. A.: Chorioretinopathy associated with other evidence of cerebral damage in childhood: A syndrome of unknown etiology separable from congenital toxoplasmosis, J. Pediat. *35:*296, 1949.
2. Hogan, M. J.; and Zimmerman, L.E.: *Ophthalmic Pathology*, 2nd Ed., Philadelphia, W. B. Saunders Co., 1962, p. 488.

SYNDROME: Sanfillipo-Good
SYNONYMS: Heparitinuria, Mucopolysaccharidosis type (MPS)III
GEN. INFORMATION:
Autosomal recessive inheritance. Excess urinary excretion of heparitin sulfate
(See also: Hurler, Hunter, Morquio-Brailsford and Scheie's syndrome)

OCULAR FINDINGS:

Orbit	
Lids ·	
Motility	
Larcr. App.	
Vision	Nightblindness may exist
Vis. Fields	
Intraoc. Ten.	
Ant. Segm.	
and Sclera	
Ocul. Media	Usually no macroscopic corneal opacifications as seen in MPS 1
Retina and	Slight narrowing of retinal vessels, pigment deposits in the
Choriod	fundi and markedly subnormal ERG with or without scotopic responses (Gills *et al.*)
Optic Nerve	

OTHER CLINICAL FINDINGS:
1. Mental deficiency progressing to severe degrees within a few years
2. Seizures
3. Gargoyl features very mild

BIBLIOGRAPHY:
1. Sanfillipo, S. J.; and Good, R. A.: A laboratory study of the Hurler's syndrome, Am. J. Dis. Child. *102:*766, 1961.
2. Sanfillipo, S. J.; and Good, R. A.: Urinary acid mucopolysaccharides (AMP) in the Hurler syndrome and Morquio's Disease, J. Pediat. *614:*296, 1962.
3. McKusick, V. A.: The Genetic Mucopolysaccharidoses, Medicine (see Ref. 4)
4. Gills, J. P.; Hobson, R.; Hanley, W. B.; and McKusick, V. A.: Electroretinography and fundus oculi findings in Hurler's disease and allied mucopolysaccharidoses, Arch. Ophth. *74:*596, 1965.

SYNDROME: Schaumann
SYNONYMS: Besnier-Boeck-Schaumann syndrome, Boeck's sarcoid, sarcoidosis
GEN. INFORMATION:
Etiology is unknown. Predominantly Negroes in the United States are involved. Onset mainly in the third and fourth decade of life. Chronic course with spontaneous remissions and clinical recovery. Laboratory findings: reversed A/G ratio. Enlarged hilar nodes. Schaumann bodies and asteroid bodies are frequently found in this disease.

OCULAR FINDINGS:

Orbit	
Lids	
Motility	
Lacr. App.	
Vision	
Vis. Fields	
Intraoc. Ten.	
Ant. Segm. and Sclera	Granulomatous uveitis with iris nodules, cells and flare in the anterior chamber
Ocul. Media	Vitreous floaters and increased cellular activity in the vitreous. Bandshaped keratitis
Retina and Choroid	Inflammatory retinal exudates
Optic Nerve	

OTHER CLINICAL FINDINGS:
1. Lymphadenopathy
2. Hilar nodes
3. Lack of energy and fatigue
4. O. T. test negative

BIBLIOGRAPHY:
1. Schaumann, J.: Benign lymphogranuloma and its cutaneous manifestations, Brit. J. Derm. *36:*615 1924.
2. Ozazewski, J. C. and Bennett, V.: Ocular Sarcoidosis, A. J. O. *35:*547, 1952.
3. Geeraets, W. J.; McNeer, K.; Maxey, E. E. and Guerry, D.: Retinopathy in sarcoidosis, Acta Ophthalmologica, *40:*492, 1962.
4. Motohashi, A.: Ocular sarcoidosis complicated by central nerve palsy, Ophthalmology *8:*287, 1966.

SYNDROME: Scheie
SYNONYMS: Mucopolysaccharidosis type (MPS) V
GEN. INFORMATION:
Autosomal recessive inheritance. Only chondroitin sulfate B is excreted in excess in the urine. Usual clinical picture of Hurler's syndrome is absent or minimal. (Histopath: Vacuolation secondary to presence of MPS within cells.) The syndrome should be recognized to avoid diagnosis of congenital glaucoma. (See also: Hurler, Hunter, Sanfillipo-Good, Morquio-Braislford syndromes)

OCULAR FINDINGS:

Orbit	
Lids	
Motility	
Lacr. App.	
Vision	Nightblindness may exist
Vis. Fields	Fields may show general constriction, ring scotomata
Intraoc. Ten.	
Ant. Segm. and Sclear	
Ocul. Media	Diffuse corneal haze to marked corneal clouding (progressive) and interfering with vision in second decade. Appa rently
Ocul. Media	poor response to keratoplasty
Retina and Coroid	Fundi may be normal and normal ERG response may be present, particularly in young patients. But also severe diminishing of ERG response and absence of scotopic ERG responses can be present with advanced age (Gills *et al.*)
Optic Nerve	

OTHER CLINICAL FINDINGS:
1. Normal intelligence
2. Broad facies
3. Limitaion of motion
4. Thickened joints
5. Aortic valvular disease

BIBLIOGRAPHY:
1. Scheie, M. C.; Hambrick, G. W., Jr.; and Barness, L. A.; A newly recognized form fruste of Hurler's disease (Gargoylism), Am. J. Ophth. *53*:753, 1962.
2. McKusick, V. A.: The Genetic Mucopolysaccharidoses. Medicine (See Ref. 3)
3. Gills, J. P.; Hobson, R.; Hanley, W. B. and McKusick, V. A.: Electroretinography and fundus oculi findings in Hurler's syndrome and allied mucopolysaccharidoses. Arch. Ophth. *74*:596, 1965.

179

SYNDROME: Schilder
SYNONYMS: Encephalitis periaxialis diffusa
GEN. INFORMATION:
Lesions most frequently situated in the subcortical white matter. More frequent in males. Occurs at any age. Sometimes slight increase in spinal fluid pressure. Mild pleocytosis, with almost all lymphocytes. Absence of leukocytes. Demyelinization of the hemispheres of the brain and the cerebellum. The prognosis is poor, lethal in about 1 year.

OCULAR FINDINGS:

Orbit	
Lids	
Motility	Nystagmus, extraocular palsy may occur either nuclear or supranuclear in origin
Lacr. App.	
Vision	Progressive loss of vision, loss of spatial orientation
Vis. Fields	Hemianopsia (in occipital lobe involvement)
Intraoc. Ten.	
Ant. Segm. and Sclera	
Ocul. Media	
Retina and Choroid	
Optic Nerve	Optic nerve, chiasm and tract involvement might lead to blindness. Papilledema due to increased intracranial pressure present in 15 to 20%

OTHER CLINICAL FINDINGS:
1. Progressive spastic paralysis
2. Progressive mental deterioration
3. Irritability and peevishness
4. Deafness if the temporal lobe becomes involved
5. Tremor
6. Scanning speech

BIBLIOGRAPHY:
1. Schilder, P.: Zur Kenntnis der sogenannten diffusen Sklerose (ueber encephalitis periaxialis diffusa) Z. Ges. Neurol. Psychiat. *10:* 1, 1912.
2. Symonds, C. P.: A contribution to the clinical study of Schilder's encephalitis, Brain. *51:*24, 1928.
3. Meyer, A. and Tennent, T.: Familiar Schilder's disease, Brain, *59:*100,1936.

SYNDROME: Siegrist
SYNONYMS: Pigmented choroidal vessels
GEN. INFORMATION:
The disease is rare. More frequently seen in females (2:1). Malignant hypertension is the most frequent cause for the symptomatology.

OCULAR FINDINGS:

Orbit	Exophthalmos
Lids	
Motility	
Lacr. App.	
Vision	Decreasing vision with poor prognosis
Vis. Fields	
Intraoc. Ten.	
Ant. Segm. and Sclera	
Ocul. Media	
Retina and Choroid	Granular pigmented spots in the choroid, fairly uniform, following the course of larger choroidal vessels with extension radially toward the periphery. These changes are related to arteriosclerotic choroidal changes and may be seen following chorioretinitis of pregnancy and albuminuric choroiditis
Optic Nerve	

OTHER CLINICAL FINDINGS:
1. Hypertension
2. Albuminuria

BIBLIOGRAPHY:
1. Siegrist: Report at 9th Internat. Congress, Utrecht, 36, 1899 quoted in Duke-Elder, Sir Stewart: *Textbook of Ophthalmology,* Vol. III, St. Louis, C. V. Mosby Co., 1941.
2. Elschnig, A.: Die diagnostische und prognostische Bedeutung der Netzhauterkrankung bei Nephritis, Wien. med. Wschr. *54:*494, 1904.
3. Ballantyne, A. J. and Michaelson, I. C.: *The Fundus of the Eye.* Edinburgh, E. & S. Livingstone Ltd., 1962.

SYNDROME: Sjögren
SYNONYMS: Gougerot-Sjögren syndrome, secreto-inhibitor syndrome
GEN. INFORMATION:
The etiology is unknown, possible disturbances in endocrine function, congenital or familial, autosomal recessive. The syndrome occurs almost exclusively in women, above 40, frequently at the time of menopause. Symptoms are caused by failure of the lacrimal and conjunctival glands to maintain adequate secretion. The clinical picture of the syndrome is inconstant. Similarities exist with Mikulicz' syndrome and the latter has been suggested to be a less highly developed variant of Sjögren's syndrome (Bain, 1960). Laboratory findings: Frequently found increase in plasma globulin fraction. Plasma electrophoresis has revealed elevation of gamma globulin. Microcytic, hypochromic anemia may exist. Sedimentation rate is usually increased.

OCULAR FINDINGS:

Orbit	
Lids	Blepharoconjunctivitis
Motility	
Lacr. App.	Deficient lacrimal secretion. Positive Schirmer test. Electrophoresis of tears shows no lysozyme. Glandular tissue is replaced by dense aggregates of small lymphocytes sticking to blood vessel walls and hyaline connective tissue
Vision	Slightly blurred vision
Vis. Fields	
Intraoc. Ten.	
Ant. Segm. and Sclera	Dryness, burning sensation, photophobia, stringy discharge. Conjunctival scraping reveals keratinization of the epithelium, mucous in absence of leukocytes
Ocul. Media	Keratoconjunctivitis sicca (positive stains with fluoresceine). The corneal epithelium is thinner than normal. Superficial corneal ulcers. Marked ulceration on the conjunctiva and cornea is rare, even in severe cases
Retina and Choroid	
Optic Nerve	

OTHER CLINICAL FINDINGS:
1. Dryness of mouth and other mucous membranes
2. Enlarged salivary glands
3. Dysphagia
4. Scleroderma-like skin changes
5. Painless swelling of joints
6. Polyarthritis (the frequency of this systemic finding has been given as high as 40 to 60% (Bloch *et al.* 1960, and Heaton, 1959), whereas Henderson (1950) regarded it as an incidental finding.)
7. Muscle weakness
8. Areflexia
9. Alopecia
10. Purpura

BIBLIOGRAPHY:
1. Sjögren, H.: Zur Kenntnis der Keratoconjunctivitis sicca, Acta Ophth., Suppl. 2, Stockholm, 1933.
2. Gougerot, M.: Insuffisance progressive et atrophie des glandes salivares et muqueuses de la bouche des conjunctives (et parfois des muqueuses nasale, laryngée, vulvaire), Bull. Soc. franc. dermat. et syph., *32:*376, 1925.
3. Henderson, J.: Keratoconjunctivitis sicca, review with survey of 121 additional cases, A. J. O., *33:*197, 1950.
4. Bain, G. O.: The pathology of Mikulicz-Sjögren disease in relation to disseminated lupus erythematosus. Canad. M. A. J., *82:*143, 1960.

SYNDROME: Sjögren-Larsson
SYNONYMS: Oligophrenia-ichthyosis-spastic diplegia syndrome
GEN. INFORMATION:

The syndrome of oligophrenia, congenital ichthyosis, spastic disorders and ocular involvement is very rare. Autosomal recessive mode of inheritance. Prepared chromosmal karyotypes were normal (Selmanowitz and Porter, 1967). Prognosis poor with life expectancy half that of normal. Consanguinity seems to play major factor. X-ray findings: Pneumoencephalography may reveal cortical atrophy and enlargement of the entire ventricular system as a result of shrinkage of gray matter. Path: Loss of neurones and gliosis throughout gray matter, (Baar *et al.* 1965).

OCULAR FINDINGS:

Orbit	Hypertelorism (mild, if present)
Lids	Ichthiosis of lid skin may occur
Motility	Variable small angle intermittent esotropia (Ref. 3)
Lacr. App.	
Vision	Reduced visual acuity related to retinal pathologic condition. Visual testing often impossible because of mental status
Vis. Fields	
Intraoc. Ten.	
Ant. Segm. and Sclera	
Ocul. Media	
Retina and Choroid **Optic Nerve**	Chorioretinitis with macular and perimacular pigment degeneration or bright, glistening intraretinal dots. Atypical retinitis pigmentosa, but ERG responses usually normal. Fluoresceineangiography demonstrates leaks in arterial and venous phase at the site of the lesion. However, macular lesions sharplyborderlined and symmetrical in both eyes without dye leakage into the retina itself were reported (Gilbert *et al.:* 1968)
Choroid **Optic Nerve**	Fundus changes occur in 20 to 30% of affected individuals

OTHER CLINICAL FINDINGS:

1. Oligophrenia-idiocy
2. Ichthyosis (congenital)
3. Spastic disorders
4. Epilepsy
5. Osseous and dental dysplasia
6. Slow hand tremor
7. Speech defect
8. Atrophy to leg muscles
9. Generalyzed hyperreflexia

BIBLIOGRAPHY:

1. Sjögren, T. and Larsson, T.: Oligophrenia in combination with congenital ichthyosis and spastic disorders; a clinical and genetic study, Acta Psych. et Neurol. Scan. Suppl. 113, 1957.
2. Selmanowitz, Victor J. and Porter, Michael J.: The Sjögren-Larsson Syndrome, A. J. Med. *42:*412, 1967.
3. Gilbert, W. R.; Smith, J. L. and Nyhan, W. L.: The Sjögren-Larsson Syndrome. in Smith, J. L.: *Neuro-Ophthalmology,* Vol. IV, St. Louis, C. V. Mosby Co., 1968.

SYNDROME: Sphenocavernous
SYNONYMS:
GEN. INFORMATION:
Lesion in the cavernous sinus. Since structures may be involved which continue to go through the superior orbital fissure, localization of the lesion is often difficult. Symptoms may be similar to the superior orbital fissure syndrome (Rochon-Duvigneaud) and to the orbital apex syndrome in the absence of marked exophthalmos.

OCULAR FINDINGS:

Orbit	Proptosis
Lids	Edema
Motility	Paresis of III, IV and VI. The paralysis of the abducens nerve precedes the paralysis of the oculomotor nerve since the abducens is situated between the internal carotid artery and the cavernous sinus wall, whereas in the fissure it is more lateral of the two nerves and therefore further away from the superior and inferior walls
Lacr. App.	
Vision	Diplopia
Vis. Fields	
Intraoc. Ten.	
Ant. Segm. and Sclera	Conjunctival edema
Ocul. media	
Retina and Choroid	
Optic Nerve	

OTHER CLINICAL FINDINGS:
Paresis of first, sometimes second and third division of the Vth nerve
BIBLIOGRAPHY:
1. Lereboullet. J. and Pluvinage, R.: Le syndrome sphéno-cáverneux, sa nosologié, son étiologie ses frontiéres, Rev. Oto.-Neuro-Ophthal., *22:*644, 1950; Ibid: Bull. et mém. Soc. méd. hôp. Paris, 1940.
2. Jefferson, G.: Concerning injuries, aneurysms and tumours involving the cavernous sinus, Tr. Ophth. Soc. U. Kingdom, *73:*117, 1953.
3. Hartmann, E. and Gilles, E.: *Roentgenologic Diagnosis in Ophthalmology,* Philadelphia, J. B. Lippincott Co., 1959.
4. Daves, M. L. and Loechel, W. E.: *The Interpretation of Tomograms of the Head,* Springfield, Charles C Thomas 1962.

SYNDROME: Stevens-Johnson

SYNONYMS: Dermatostomatitis, erythema multiforme exudativum, syndroma muco-cutaneooculare, Baader's dermatostomatitis syndrome, mucosal-respiratory syndrome, (Fuchs (2) syndrome)

GEN. INFORMATION:

Etiology is unknown (bacterial? virus? allergy?) Many cases, however, seem to be idiopathic. An electronmicroscopic study of one case (Newman. Oral Surg. 1956) demonstrated, however, presence of virus-type bodies. Differential diagnosis: Reiter's syndrome. Occurs in young adults (males), rarely in other age groups. Complete recovery may occur. Recovery usually within months. Recurrences may occur but is unpredictable. Very severe cases may be fatal. None of the ocular manifestations have been regarded pathognomonic for this syndrome, though many lesions may develop.

OCULAR FINDINGS:

Orbit	
Lids	
Motility	
Lacr. App.	
Vision	In severe cases partial or total blindness may occur
Vis. Fields	
Intraoc. Ten.	
Ant. Segm. and Sclera	The conjunctival lesions have been grouped in fibromembraneous and papulovesicular types. This shows clinically as conjunctivitis with vesicular and bullous lesions and ulcerations and chemosis. Hypopyon, iritis (less frequent)
Ocul. Media	Keratitis, corneal ulcers (less frequent), keratoconjunctivitis sicca (occasionally)
Retina and Choroid	
Optic Nerve	

OTHER CLINICAL FINDINGS:

1. General malaise, headaches, chills and fever
2. Acute respiratory infection
3. Severe skin and mucous membrane eruptions(erythema multiforme), dorsum of hands and feet are most frequently affected. The lesions may be maculopapular to vesiculobullous eruptions and occasionally nodular in appearance
4. Rhinitis, balanitis, vulvovaginitis, urethritis (non specific), cystitis
5. Involvement of internal organs with ulceration of gastrointestinal tract and nephritis (Short: Lancet, 1957)

BIBLIOGRAPHY:

1. Stevens, A. M. and Johnson, C. F.: A new eruptive fever associated with stomatitis and ophthalmia, Am. J. Dis. Child. 24:526, 1922.
2. Fuchs, E.: Herpes iris conjunctivae. Kl. Mbl. Augenhk. 14:333, 1876.
3. Baader, E.: Dermatostomatitis, Arch. Derm. & Syph. 149:261, 1925.
4. Robinson, H. M. and McCrumb, F. R.: Comparative analysis of the mucocutaneous-ocular syndromes, Arch. Dermat. & Syph., 61:539 1950.
5. Walsh, F. B.: Clinical Neuro-Ophthalmology, 2nd Ed., Baltimore, The Williams & Wilkins Co., 1957, p. 468.
6. Gorlin, R. J. And Pindborg, J. J.: Syndromes of the Head and Neck, New York, McGraw-Hill Book Co. (Blakiston Division), 1964.

SYNDROME: Sturge-Weber

SYNONYMS: Meningocutaneous syndrome, vascular encephalotrigeminal syndrome, neurooculocutaneous angiomatosis, encephalofacial angiomatosis.

GEN. INFORMATION:

Inheritance still debated. (47 chromosomes with trisomy for number 22 has been suggested. Later, partial trisomy was described. (Patau: Am. J. Human Genet., 1961) Variations: Jahnke's syndrome without glaucoma; Schirmer's syndrome with early glaucoma; Lawford's syndrome with late glaucoma and no increase in volume of globe; Mille's syndrome with choroidal angioma but no glaucoma. X-ray findings: Calcified angiomata and localized double-contoured linear calcification outlining the cerebral convolutions (pathognomonic for this syndrome). Similar angiomas have been described in many other organs (Givner). The nevus flammeous of the face is often located along the course of the trigeminal nerve and ipsilateral to the cerebral angiomatosis. Histopathology: Cerebral calcification in cortical gray matter also in areas unrelated to blood vessels. Venous angiomatas of the pial vessels.

OCULAR FINDINGS:

Orbit	
Lids	
Motility	
Lacr. App.	
Vision	
Vis. Fields	
Intraoc. Ten.	Unilateral hydrophthalmos (about 20%), or secondary glaucoma (late) in about 10% of cases (Ref. 4)
Ant. Segm. and Sclera	Conjunctival angioma (telangiectases), iris decoloration, nevoid marks or vascular dilation of the episclera
Ocul. Media	
Retina and Choroid	Glioma, detachment, choroidal angiomata, vessel proliferation most frequently unilateral
Optic Nerve	

OTHER CLINICAL FINDINGS:

1. Vascular-'portwine nevus'-(face, scalp, limbs, trunk, leptomeninges)
2. Contralateral paresis
3. Hemiatrophy
4. Mental retardation
5. Jacksonian epilepsy
6. Acromegaly
7. Adipositas
8. Facial hemihypertrophy

Depending on location of intracranial angiomas

BIBLIOGRAPHY:

1. Sturge, W. A.: A case of partial epilpesy, apparently due to a lesion of one of the vasomotor centers of the brain, Tr. Clin. Soc. London, *12:*1962, 1879.
2. Weber, F. P.: A note on the association of extensive haemangiomatous naevus of the skin with cerebral (meningeal) haemangioma, Proc. roy. Soc. Med. *22:*25, 1929.
3. Anderson, J. R.: Hydrophthalmia or congenital glaucoma, its causes, treatment and outlook, London, Cambridge University Press, 1939, p. 180.
4. Alexander, G. L. and Norman R. M.: *The Sturge-Weber Syndrome,* Bristol, John Wright & Sons, Ltd., 1960.
5. Ballantyne, A. F. and Michaelson, I. C.:*The Fundus of the Eye,* Edinburgh, E & S livingston, Ltd., 1962.
6. Francois, J. and Matton-Van Leuven, M. T.: Chromosome abnormalities and ophthalmology, J. Ped. Ophth., *1:*5, 1964.

SYNDROME: Symonds
SYNONYMS: Otitic hydrocephalus syndrome, serous meningitis syndrome
GEN. INFORMATION:
Occurs in children and adolescents. Good prognosis, frequently with protracted course over weeks or months with occasionally spontaneous recovery. The condition with increased cerebrospinal fluid, but without increase in protein or cells and often associated with otitis media had been called 'serous meningitis' (Quincke: Dtsch. Ztschr. Nervenheilk.; 1897). Since signs of meningeal inflammation are apparently absent, Symonds introduced the designation of 'otitic hydrophthalmos' which at the same time eliminates the classification of 'internal' or 'external' since there is a general increase in cerebrospinal fluid. Between attacks the patient feels well which is of differential diagnostic value against aseptic meningitis and brain abscess.

OCULAR FINDINGS:

Orbit	
Lids	
Motility	Sixth nerve palsy ipsilateral side with otitis media. Diplopia
Lacr. App.	
Vison	Impaired vision depending on optic nerve involvement
Vis. Fields	
Intraoc. Ten.	
Ant. Segm. and Sclera	
Ocul. Media	
Retina and Choroid	Hemorrhages and exudates
Optic Nerve	Moderate to marked papilledema followed by secondary optic atrophy

OTHER CLINICAL FINDINGS:
1. Greatly increased pressure of spinal fluid often >300 mm without increased cells or protein
2. Intermittent headaches
3. Drowsiness, nausea, vomiting (inconstant)
4. Otitis media
5. Mastoiditis
6. Meningitis ⎫ may produce similar symptoms, but do not be-
7. Brain abscess ⎬ long to the syndrome
8. Lateral sinus thrombosis ⎭

BIBLIOGRAPHY:
1. Symonds, C. P.: Otitic hydrocephalus, Brain, *54:*55, 1931.
2. Symonds, C. P.: Otitic hydrocephalus: report of 3 cases, Brit. M. J., *1:*53, 1932.
3. Ford, F. R.: *Diseases of the Nervous System in Infancy, Childhood and Adolescence,* Springfield, Charles C Thomas, 1952, p.505-512.
4. Walsh, F. B.: *Clinical Neuro-Ophthalmology,* Baltimore, The Williams & Wilkins Co., 1957, P. 486.

SYNDROME: Takayasu
SYNONYMS: Matoluell syndrome, aortic arch syndrome, pulseless disease, reversed coaractation syndrome.
GEN: INFORMATION:
No evidence of heredity. Two types of the disease have been described: (1) caused by occlusive inflammatory lesion, appearing as a nonspecific arteritis with histologic evidence of disorganization of the elastic membrane, adventitia and media, and presence of giant cells. This type is usually seen in young women (more frequent in Japanese). (2) Occlusive vascular disease without inflammation. Often associated with atherosclerose and syphilis (Ross and McKusick, Arch. Int. Med., 1953). This type has usually its onset within the fifth and sixth decades of life and both sexes are equally affected.

OCULAR FINDINGS:

Orbit	
Lids	
Motility	
Lacr. App.	
Vision	Transient blindness or blurring of vision (Dowling and Smith)
Vis. Fields	
Intraoc. Ten.	
Ant. Segm.	
and Sclera	Iris atrophy (Ref. 2)
Ocul. Media	Cataracts (Histol: coagulation necrosis)
Retina and	Retinal microaneurysms, 'sausage' shaped veinous dilatations.
Chorodi	Central retinal artery pressure reduced. (Histol: decreased number of ganglion cells in ganglion cell layer (Ref. 3)
Optic Nerve	Optic atrophy with demyelination

OTHER CLINICAL FINDINGS:
1. Diminished or absent pulsation of arteries (head, neck, upper limbs)
2. Orthostatic syncope, vertigo
3. Facial atrophy
4. Epileptiform seizures
5. Perforated nasal septum with atrophic mucosa.
6. Hemiplegia (transient)
7. Weakness, fatigue
8. Intermittent claudication
9. Loss of teeth and oral ulceration in more advanced cases.

BIBLIOGRAPHY:
1. Takayasu, S.:A case with unusual changes in the central vessels of the retina, Acta Soc. Ophth. Jap., *12:*554, 1908.
2. Matorell, F. and Fabre, J.:The syndrome of obliteration of the supra-aortic branches, Angiology, *5:*39, 1954.
3. Dowling J. L., Jr. and Smith, T. R.: An ocular study of pulseless disease, Arch. Ophth. *64:*236, 1960
4. Hirose, K.:A study of fundus changes in the early stages of Takayasu-Ohnishi (Pulseless)disease, Am J. Ophth. *55:*295, 1963.

SYNDROME: Tapetal-like Reflex
SYNONYMS:
GEN. INFORMATION:
The syndrome is very rare. A family in which females presented tapetal-like reflex and males showed typical retinitis pigmentosa was described by Falls and Cotterman. A sex linked gene may be responsible for both anomalies (Mann). The name 'tapetal-like reflex' stems from the clinical appearance of the ocular fundus but should not suggest any anatomical similarity to the tapetum lucidum in the choroid of certain animals. The bright reflex has been suggested as being due to pathological changes in Bruch's membrane, causing a roughening of its surface with increased light reflection (Mann). Evidence of degenerative changes in the retinal pigment epithlium in addition to those in Bruch's membrane was given by Cicarrelli.

OCULAR FINDINGS:

Orbit	
Lids	
Motility	
Lacr. App.	
Vision	
Vis. Fields	Ring scotoma possible (Cicarelli)
Intraoc. Ten.	
Ant. Segm. and Sclera	
Ocul. Media	Discrete bright yellow spots in posterior polar region apparently located deep to the retinal vessels (Mann). Tapetal-like reflex and retinitis pigmentosa may be present in members of the same family (see above: Gen. Inf.)
Retina and Choroid	
Optic Nerve	

OTHER CLINICAL FINDINGS:
BIBLIOGRAPHY:
1. Niccol, W.:A family with bilateral developmental defects at the macula, Trans. Ophth. Soc. U. K., *58:*763, 1938.
2. Falls, H. F. and Cotterman, C. W.: Choroidal degeneration, Arch. Ophth., *40:*685, 1948.
3. Klien, B.: The heredodegeneration of the macula lutea, A. J. O., *33:*371, 1950.
4. Mann, J.:*Developmental Abnormalities of the Eye.* 2nd Ed., Philadelphia, J. B. Lippincott Co., 1957.
5. Ciccarelli, E. C.:A new syndrome of tapetal-like fundic reflexes with ring scotoma, Arch. Ophth., *67:*316, 1962.

SYNDROME: Tay-Sachs
SYNONYMS: Familial amaurotic idiocy (infantile type)
GEN. INFORMATION:
Similar to Spielmeyer-Vogt syndrome as the juvenile type of familial amaurotic idiocy. The syndrome is most often transmitted by an autosomal recessive gene and only occasionally by dominant inheritance. It occurs almost exclusively in Jewish infants and is more frequently seen in females. Death occurs usually during first 2 years of life. Histopathological findings: Ganglion cells of the retina and brain are filled with amorphous granular material and swelling of the cells. In late stages neuronal loss with extensive gliosis and diffuse demyelination. The stored material is recognized as ganglioside.

OCULAR FINDINGS:

Orbit	
Lids	
Motility	Nystagmus and strabismus have been described and are mainly related to the retinal and optic nerve pathologic conditions
Lacr. App.	
Vision	Blindness with progressing disease
Vis. Fields	
Intraoc. Ten.	
Ant. Segm. and Sclera	
Ocul. Media	
Retina and Choroid	Whitish-gray macular area with cherry red spot in the center, retinal pigmentary changes with involvement of the macula may occasinonally be seen instead of the typical red spot. The grayish coloration of the macula is due to the swollen ganglion cells accumulated in the perifovedal macular region. The retinal vessels become progressively narrowed.
Optic Nerve	Progressive ascending optic atrophy

OTHER CLINICAL FINDINGS:
1. Hyperacusis most often initial sign
2. Mental retardation
3. Convulsions
4. Muscles are at the beginning often flaccid but become spastic with progression of the disease.
5. Evidence of increasing visual loss at age 3 to 5 months.

BIBLIOGRAPHY:
1. Tay, W.:Symmetrical changes in the yellow spot in each eye of an infant, Trans. Ophth. Soc. U. K., *1:*55, 1881.
2. Sachs, B.:An arrested cerebral development with special reference to its cortical pathology, J. Nerv. & Ment. Dis. *14:*541, 1887.
3. Duke, J. R. and Clark, D. B.: Infantile amaurotic familial idiocy (Tay-Sachs Disease) in the Negro Race, Am. J. Ophth. *53:*800 1962.
4. Aronson, S. M.: Epidemiology; in B. W. Volk:*Tay-Sachs disease,* New York, Grune & Stratton, 1964, p. 118.
5. Carakushansky, G.:The Lipidoses; in Gardner, L. l.: *Endocrine and Genetic Diseases of Childhood,* Philadelphia, W. B. Saunders Co., 1969, p. 966.
6. Cogan, D. G.: Heredodegeneration of the retina, in Smith, J. L. (Ed.): *Neuro-ophthalmology,* Vol. ll, St. Louis, C. V. Mosby Co., 1965, p. 44.

SYNDROME: Temporal arteritis
SYNONYMS: Cranial arteritis syndrome, giant cell arteritis
GEN. INFORMATION:
Etiology is unknown. Apparently more frequent in females. Occurrence in Caucasians at 55 to 80 years of age. All three coats of the temporal artery show inflammatory thickening. Thrombosis of the vessel may occur. Histological changes are usually segmental. The narrowing or occlusion of the vessel lumen accounts for ischaemic lesions which in the brain may result in death and in the eye to optic atrophy with visual loss. The severe visual impairment is due to arteritis of the vessels supplying the optic nerve itself rather than to central retinal artery occlusion. The prognosis is good if treatment is started early but depends on the degree of involvement. Mortality is listed as 12.5% (Ballentine and Michaelson 1962). Self-limited course over weeks to several months. Ocular involvement in about 40%.

OCULAR FINDINGS:

Orbit	
Lids	Transient ptosis may occur if vascular changes involve the motorsystem of the eye
Motility	Diplopia
Lacr. App.	
Vision	Partial or complete loss of vision on the affected side. Occasionally bilateral
Vis. Fields	Temporal blurring and coloured scotomata may precede the sudden loss of irrecoverable vision
Intraoc. Ten.	
Ant. Segm. and Sclera	Photophobia
Ocul. Media	
Retina and Choroid	Detachment exudates and hemorrhages. Narrowing of retinal vessels and obstruction of the central retinal artery (10%): On occasion retinal artery branch obstruction (Johnson *et al.* 1943) (See above: Gen. Inf.)
Optuc Nerve	Optic atrophy. Usually slight or moderate edema of the disc with occasionally hemorrhages on or around the disc

OTHER CLINICAL FINDINGS:
1. Thorbbing headache
2. Hyperalgesia of the scalp
3. Malaise anorexia weakness
4. Weight loss
5. Fever
6. Unilateral painful temporal arteritis caused by the adventitial inflammation. More recent concepts have favored an antigen-antibody reaction involving primarily the elastic tissures of the artery (Ref. 6)

BIBLIOGRAPHY:

1. Hutchinson J.: On a peculiar form of thrombotic arteritis of the aged which is sometimes productive of gangrene, Arch. Surg. Lond, *1*:323, 1889-1890.
2. Johnson, R. H.; Robinson, D. H.; and Horton, B. T.: Arteritis of the temporal vessels associated with loss of vision, Am. J. Ophth. *26*:147, 1943.
3. Kilbourne, E.; and Wolff, H.: Cranical arteritis, Ann. Int. Med., *24*:1, 1946.
4. Anderson, B.; Nicholson, W. M.; and Iverson, L.: Temporal arteritis with associated optic atrophy, South. Med. J., *41*:426, 1948.
5. Cullen, J. F.: Occult temporal arteritis: Brit. J. Ophth. *51*:513, 1967.
6. Meadows, S. P.: Temporal or giant cell arteritis—ophthalmic aspects. in Smith, J. L. (edit.)(*Neuro-Ophthalmology*, Vol. IV, St. Louis, C. V. Mosby Co., 1968, p. 148.

SYNDROME: Tolosa-Hunt
SYNONYMS: Painful ophthalmoplegia
GEN. INFORMATION:
The clinical entity is not to be confused with 'ophthalmoplegic migraine' which is based on a vascular etiology. Symptoms last from days to weeks. Spontaneous remission possible, sometimes with residual neurologic deficit. Attacks recur at intervals of months or years. No sturctures outside the cavernous sinus are apparently involved. Inflammatoy lesion of cavernous sinus most likely etiology. Differential diagnosis include diabetic ophthalmoplegia, intracavernous carotid aneurysm and nasopharyngeal tumor.

OCULAR FINDINGS*

Orbit	Steady 'growing' retroorbital pain (may precede the ophthalmo-plegia for several days or might be absent)
Lids	Ptosis
Motility	Involvement of III, IV, VI and lst division of V cranial nerves
Lacr. App.	Scintillating scotomata, blurred vision to complete blindness
Vision	(depending on optic nerve involvement)
Vis. Fields	
Intraoc. Ten.	
Ant. Segm. and Sclera	Sluggish pupil reaction to light, fixed pupil
Ocul. Media	Corneal sensitivity may be diminished
Retina and Choroid	
Optic Nerve	Optic nerve may be involved

OTHER CLINICAL FINDINGS:
Usually no systemic reactions

*Ocular findings occur to various extent, depending on nerve involvement.
BIBLIOGRAPHY:
1. Tolosa, E.: Periarteritic lesions of carotid siphon with clinical features of carotid infraclinoidal aneurysm, J. Neurol., Neurosurg. & Psychiat. *17:*300, 1954.
2. Hunt, W. E.; Meaçher, J. N.; Le Fever, H. E.; and Zeman, W.: Painful Ophthalmoplegia, Neurology, *11:*56, 1961.
3. Smith, J. L.; and Taxdal, D. S. R.: Painful Ophthalmoplegia: The Tolosa-Hunt Syndrome, Am. J. Ophth. *61:*1466, 1966.
4. Berg, E.; and Gay, A. J.: Tolosa-Hunt Syndrome, E. E. N. T. Digest, *29:*51, April 1967.
5. Other, A.: Painful ophthalmoplegia, Acta Ophth. *45:*371, 1967.

SYNDROME: Trisomy-D$_1$
SYNONYMS: Trisomy 13–15, Patua's syndrome
GEN. INFORMATION:
Specific chromosome anomaly. Extra chromosome in the D-group. At present the exact chromosome cannot be distinguished. Fatal in first few months of life. Frequency about 1/10,000. A typical case of the syndrome was described by McEnery and Brenneman, 1937. Laboratory findings: Unusual nuclear projection of neutrophils.** Unusual persistence of fetal hemoglobin. Path.: Single umbilical artery.

OCULAR FINDINGS:

Orbit	Anophthalmia, microphthalmia** hyperteleorism, small orbitae, shallow supraorbital ridges, absent eye brows, intraocular cartilage (Ref. 4)
Lids	Slanting palpebral fissures
Motility	
Lacr. App.	
Vision	
Vis. Fields	
Intraoc. Ten.	
Ant. Segm. and Sclera	Iris coloboma**
Ocul. Media	Cataracts, vascularized membrane on the posterior lens capsule, corneal opacities
Retina and Choroid	Retinal dysplasia
Optic Nerve	Coloboma,* optic atrophy

OTHER CLINICAL FINDINGS:

1. Apneic spells** (death within 3 months)
2. Developmental deficiency of nervous system**
3. Seizures (minor motor)*
4. Deafness**
5. Cleft lip and palate*
6. Polydactyly
7. Hemangiomata* (capillary type)
8. Horizontal hand palm creases**
9. Hyperconvex fingernails**
10. Flexion of fingers and hands
11. Spina bifida
12. Interventricular septal defects*
13. Dextrocardia
14. Renal abnormalities,* cryptorchidism, abnormal scrotum**

*50% or more

**Patients presenting all the signs and symptoms identified by ** have been proved to have partial or complete D$_1$ trisomy (Smith, 1969)

BIBLIOGRAPHY:
1. McEnery, E. T.; and Brenneman, J.: Multiple facial anomalies, J. Pediat. *11*:468, 1937.
2. Smith, D. W.; et al.: Autosomal trisomy syndromes, Lancet, 2:211, 1961.
3. Atkins, L.; and Rosenthal, M. K.: Multiple congenital abnormalities associated with chromosomal trisomy, New. Engl. J. Med., 265:314, 1961.
4. Cogan, D. G.; and Kuwabara, T.:Ocular Pathology of the 13–15 Trisomy syndrome, Arch. Ophth. 72:246, 1964.
5. Francosi, J.; and Matton-Van Leuwen, M. T.: Chormosomal abnormalities and ophthalmology, J. Ped. Ophth., *1*:5, 1964.
6. Smith, D. W.: The 18 Trisomy and D$_1$ Trisomy Syndromes, in Gardner, L.I.: *Endocrine and Genetic Diseases of Childhood,* Philadelphia, W. B. Saunders Co., 1969.

SYNDROME: Trisomy-18
SYNONYMS: E-syndrome
GEN. INFORMATION:
Karyotype of 47 chromosomes with chromosome number 18 existent in triplicate. The number 18 chromosome has been identified as the extra autosome by both structural analysis (Patau *et al.,* 1961) and DNA replication studies (Yunis *et al.,* 1964). Female-male ratio 3:1. Age of the mother at time of conception often over 40 years. Though due to non-disjunction in almost all cases, the syndrome (like trisomy 21 or Down's syndrome)may rarely be caused by a parental translocation (Brodie and Dallaire, 1962). Combination of this syndrome with the XXX syndrome was described (Uchida, 1. A. and Bowman, J. M.: Lancet, *2:*1094, 1961). There is a multitude of inconsistant malformations affecting every organ system.

OCULAR FINDINGS:

Orbit	
Lids	Unilateral ptosis (Crawford, 1961), inner epicanthic folds, small palpebral fissures
Motility	
Lacr. App.	
Vision	Amaurosis*
Vis. Fields	
Intraoc. Ten.	Congenital glaucoma*
Ant. Segm. and Sclera	
Ocul. Media	Corneal opacities, lens opacities
Retina and Choroid	
Optic Nerve	Optic atrophy*

OTHER CLINICAL FINDINGS:
1. Mental retardation
2. Facial manifestations** (Low set ears, small mouth, micrognathic mandible, high palate arch, ao.)
3. Prominent occiput**
4. Flexion of fingers (2nd overlapping 3rd)
5. Hypertonicity
6. Male: cryptorchism**
7. Failure to thrive**
8. Meckel's diverticulum
9. Heart, vessel and renal anomalies, Ventricular septum defect**
10. Occasionally umbillical hernia
11. Hypertrichosis
12. Webbed neck

*(Townes *et al.,* 1962)
**50% or more

BIBLIOGRAPHY:
1. Townes, P. L.; Manning, J. A.; and DeHart, G. K., Jr.: Trisomy-18 (16–18) associated with congenital glaucoma and optic atrophy, J. Pediat. *61:*755, 1962.
2. Gardner, L. I.: Symposium on genetics, Ped. Clin. N. A. *10:* 2, 1963.
3. Francois, J.; and Matton-Van Leuwen, M. T.: Chromosomal abnormalities and ophthalmology, J. Ped. Ophth., *1:*5, 1964.
4. Smith, D. W. The 18 Trisomy and D₁ Trisomy Syndromes, in Gardner, L. I.: *Endocrine and Genetic Diseases of Childhood,* Philadelphia W. B. Saunders Co., 1969.

SYNDROME: Trisomy-22
SYNONYMS:
GEN. INFORMATION:
Forty seven chromosomes were found at chromosome analysis. Karyotypes showed trisomy for chromosome 21/22, which on satellite distribution appeared to be 22 (Turner and Jennings). Trisomy-22 was reported having been present in 2 patients with Sturge-Weber syndrome (Hayward and Bower). This finding has not been confirmed for other patients with Sturge-Weber syndrome, which instead showed the normal 46 chromosomes (Gustavson and Höök: Lancet, 1961; Lehman and Forssmann: Lancet, 1961; Hall: Lancet. 1961). The clinical findings are sparse in comparison with those of Down's syndrome (Trisomy 21), though it has been suggested more recently that chromome 22 may play a role in Down's syndrome (Ref. 4)—(See also Down's syndrome). From the discrepancies and controversies of the various reported findings, the true clinical expression of a Trisomy-22 becomes somewhat dubious and the question arises if the cases attributed to a Trisomy-22 may not have been very mild forms of Down's syndrome in spite of absence of the classical symptoms associated with that disease.

OCULAR FINDINGS:

Orbit	
Lids	
Motility	
Lacr. App.	
Vision	High myopia
Vis. Fields	
Intraoc. Ten.	
Ant. Segm. and Sclera	
Ocul. Media	
Retina and Choriod	
Optic Nerve	

OTHER CLINICAL FINDINGS:
1. Schizophrenia
2. Micrognatia
3. Large nostrils
4. Flat occiput
5. Overextension of elbows

BIBLIOGRAPHY:
1. Hayward, M. D. and Bower, B. D.: Chromosomal trisomy associated with the Sturge-Weber syndrome, Lancet, 2:844, 1960.
2. Turner, B. and Jennings, A. N.: Trisomy for chromosome 22, Lancet 2:49, 1961.
3. François, J.:*Heredity in Ophthalmology,* St. Louis, C. V. Mosby Co., 1961.
4. Neu, R. L. and Kajii, T.: Other autosomal abnormalities; in Gardner, L. I.: *Endocrine and Genetic Diseases of Childhood,* Philadelphia, W. B. Saunders Co., 1969.

SYNDROME: Turner
SYNONYMS: Turner Albright syndrome, gonadal dysgenesis, genital dwarfism syndrome.
GEN. INFORMATION:
Ovarian or gonadal agenesis. Negative nuclear sex chromatin pattern. In a majority of patients karyotypic analysis reveals 45 chromosomes with an XO sex chromosome constitution. Remaining 20% present a number of different forms of sex chromosome mosaicism. This suggests that sex chromosome abnormalities relate etiologically to the appearance of this syndrome (Ref. 4). Females are generally involved (very rarely in males). Laboratory findings: diminution of 17-ketosteroid excretion. Marked increase in follicle stimulating hormone in the urine, Path: Rudimentary or streak gonads seen as narrow white ridges of connective tissue parallel to the fallopian tubes in the broad ligaments. The streaks consist of dense stroma, similar to that found in normal ovaries, occasional rete tubules, mesonephric remnants, small clumps of Leydig cells, but no germ cells or seminiferous tubules.

OCULAR FINDINGS:

Orbit	Mild exophthalmos, hypertelorism
Lids	Ptosis, epicanthal folds (occasionally)
Motility	Squint (rare), either nonparalytic esotropia or exotropia, abducens palsy*
Lacr. App.	
Vision	Color blindness*
Vis. Fields	
Intraoc. Ten.	Primary open angle glaucoma*
Ant. Segm. and Sclera	Blue sclera
Ocul. Media	Oval corneae (Wilkins), corneal nebulae, cataracts
Retina and Choroid	Deficiency in retinal pigment
Optic Nerve	

OTHER CLINICAL FINDINGS:
1. Webbed neck (pterygium colli)
2. Diminished growth
3. Mandibulofacial disproportion pigmented nevi
4. Cubitus valgus
5. Masculine chest and trunk
6. Late appearance of pubic and axillary hair
7. Congenital deafness
8. Mental retardation
9. Failure in development in sex organs
10. Coarctation of aorta (25%-Rainier- Pope, 1964) and only in those with pterygium colli.
11. Idiopathic hypertension
12. Renal abnormalities

* Single observations

BIBLIOGRAPHY:
1. Turner, H. H.: Syndrome of infantilism, congenital webbed neck and cubitus valgus, Endocrinology, *23*:566, 1938.
2. Wilkins, L.: *The Diagnosis and Treatment of Endocrine Disorders in Childhood and Adolescence,* Springfield, Charles C Thomas, 1950.
3. Vaharu, T. V. *et al.*: XX/XO mosaicism in a girl, J. Ped., *61*:751. 1962
4. Lessell, S.: and Forbes, A. P.: Eye Signs in Turner's syndrome, Arch. Ophth. *76*:211, 1966.
5. Khodadoust, A. and Paton, D.: Turner's syndrome in a male, Arch. Ophth. *77*:309, 1967
6. Stempfel, R. S., Jr.: Abnormalities of sexual differentiation (p. 500) in Gardner, L. I.: *Endocrine and Genetic Diseases of Childhood,* Philadelphia, W. B. Saunders Co., 1969.

SYNDROME: Unverrichts
SYNONYMS: Familial myoclonia syndrome
GEN. INFORMATION:
Fatal hereditary form of diffuse neuronal disease, transmitted as an autosomal recessive trait. Begins in late childhood. If associated with basophilic deposits in CNS, retina and other organs as well, the syndrome is sometimes known as Lafora's disease. (Lafora and Glüch: Z. Ges. Neurol. Psychiat, 6:1, 1911)

OCULAR FINDINGS:

Orbit	
Lids	
Motility	
Lacr. App.	
Vision	Amaurosis
Vis. Fields	
Intraoc. Ten.	
Ant. Segm. and Sclera	
Ocul. Media	
Retina and Choroid	Laminated Lafora bodies in ganglion cell and inner nuclear layers of the retina, either intra-or extracellular. May also be present in inner plexiform and nerve fiber layers and the optic nerve (Ref. 2)
Optic Nerve	

OTHER CLINICAL FINDINGS:
1. Major epilepsy
2. Widespread myoclonus
3. Dementia
4. Tetraplegia
5. Pseudobulbar palsy

BIBLIOGRAPHY:

1. Unverricht, H.: Die Myoklonie, Leibzig, 128 (1891)
2. Yanoff, M. and Schwarz, G. A.: The retinal pathology of Lafora's disease: A form of glycoprotein-acid mucopolysaccharide dystrophy, Trans. Am. Ac. Ophth. 69:701, 1965.
3. Schwarz, G. A. and Yanoff, M.: Lafora's disease: Distinct clinico-pathologic form of Unverrichts syndrome, Arch. Neurol. 12:172, 1965.
4. Duke-Elder, Sir Stewart and Dobree, J. H.: Diseases of the retina in Duke-Elder, *System of Ophthalmology,* Vol. X; St. Louis, C. V. Mosby Co., 1967, p. 450.

SYNDROME: Usher
SYNONYMS: Hereditary retinitis pigmentosa-deafness syndrome
GEN. INFORMATION:
Retinitis pigmentosa associated with deaf mutism was described first by von Graefe. Usher pointed first to heredity as the leading factor of this combination. The frequency with which retinitis pigmentosa occurs in deaf-mutism varies greatly in literature reports (from 1.5%, Cernea-1956, to 19.4% Lindenow-1945). Deafness is usually dominantly inherited and rarely recessive or sex linked. (See also: Hallgren's syndrome)

OCULAR FINDINGS:

Orbit	
Lids	
Motility	
Lacr. App.	
Vision	Concentric contraction but no ring scotomata (Hardy)
Vis. Fields	
Intraoc. Ten.	
Ant. Segm. and Sclera	
Ocul. Media	
Retina and Choroid	Retinitis pigmentosa with dotted, fine pigmentation in mid-periphery and bone-corpuscle configurated pigment deposits mainly along the vessels toward the periphery. Yellow-white dots in outer retina and choroid (Hardy)
Optic Nerve	

OTHER CLINICAL FINDINGS:
Deaf-mutism, however deafness is not always complete
BIBLIOGRAPHY:
1. Usher, C. H.: On the inheritance of retinitis pigmentosa with notes of cases, Roy. Lond. Ophth. Hosp. Rep. *19*:130, 1913/1914.
2. Usher, C. H.: On a few hereditary eye affections, Tr. Ophth. Soc. U. K. *55*:164, 1935.
3. Bossu, A. and Luypaert, R.: Le syndrome d' Usher, Ann. Oculist. *191*:529, 1958.
4. Hardy, G.: Deafness and retinitis pigmentosa, Am. J. Ophth. *23*:315,1940.
5. Graefe, A. von: Exceptionales Verhalten des Gesichtsfeldes bei Pigmentierung der Netzhaut, Graefes Arch. Ophth. II *4*:250, 1858.

SYNDROME: Uveitis-rheumatoid arthritis
SYNONYMS:
GEN. INFORMATION:
General collagen disorder? Most frequently in children, but occurs also in adults. Prognosis is often poor. Though the co-existence of rheumatoid manifestations and uveitis is well recognized, the two entities are not to be regarded as cause and effect but as parallel symptoms of the same process. Laboratory findings: The so-called rheumatoid factor (an abnormal globulin) found in patients with rheumatoid disease is present in approx. 20% of patients with uveitis (Rheins *et al.*: A. J. O., 1965)

OCULAR FINDINGS:

Orbit	
Lids	
Motility	
Lacr. App.	
Vision	
Vis Fields	
Intraoc. Ten.	
Ant. Segm. and Sclera	In general, rheumatoid iridocyclitis occurs in two distinct types—acute recurrent and chronic. The acute form shows manifestations from mild to severe and unilateral occurrence followed by the other eye within a period of a year. Severeness of uveitis and arthritis are unrelated. In acute rheumatoid conditions uveitis is rare. In chronic forms anterior uveitis is found rather than posterior. In chronic polyarthritis in children (Still's disease) or in chronic progressive ankylosing spondylitis of adults iridocyclitis is common. Scleritis (less frequently), scleromalacia perforance (occasionally in adults).
Ocul. Media	Band-shaped keratopathy and keratic precipitates (fine to macular). Fine vitreous opacities.
Retina and Choroid	Choroidal inflammation, macular edema
Optic Nerve	Papillitis

OTHER CLINICAL FINDINGS:
1. Rheumatoid arthritis
2. Hepatosplenomegaly (occasional)

BIBLIOGRAPHY:
1. Davis, M.: Endogenous uveitis in children: Associated band-shaped keratopathy and rheumatoid arthritis, Arch. Ophth., *50:*443, 1953.
2. Theodore, F. M. and Schlossman, A.: *Ocular Allergy,* Baltimore, The Williams & Wilkins Co., 1958.
3. Woods, A. C.: *Endogenous Inflammations of the Uveal Tract,* Baltimore, The Williams & Wilkins Co., 1961.
4. Epstein, W. V.: New information on the structure of γ-globulin in relation to studies of rheumatoid arthritis, in: Maumenee, A. E. and Silverstein, A. M. (eds.): *Immunopathology of Uveitis,* Baltimore, The Williams & Wilkins Co., 1964.
5. Duke-Elder, Sir Stewart: *System of Ophthalmology,* Vol. IX, St. Louis, C. V. Mosby Co., 1966.

SYNDROME: Uyemura
SYNONYMS: Fundus albipunctatus with hemeralopia and xerosis
GEN. INFORMATION:
This syndrome is very rare and has been observed mainly in the far east. It closely resembles retinitis punctata albescens with nightblindness, decreased vision, visual field restriction, optic nerve atrophy, a disease which progresses with age. Even more closely to Uyemura's syndrome is the clinical picture of fundus albi punctatus and nightblindness. The latter can be related to congenital idiopathic nightblindness or Oguchi's disease and remains usually stationary through life. Uyemura's syndrome however is based on A-avitaminosis and responds fully to vitamin A treatment with disappearance of all symptoms provided the xerosis has not affected the cornea with scar formation.

OCULAR FINDINGS:

Orbit	
Lids	
Motility	
Lacr. App.	
Vision	Nightblindness (transient), decreased dark adaptation
Vis. Fields	
Intraoc. Ten.	
Ant. Segm. and Sclera	Conjunctival xerosis. Bitot's spots
Ocul. Media	
Retina and Choroid	White spots of the fundus
Optic Nerve	

OTHER CLINICAL FINDINGS:
BIBLIOGRAPHY:

1. Uyemura, M.: Über eine merkwürdige Augenhintergrundsveränderung bei zwei Fällen von idiopathischer Hemeralopie, Klin. Mbl. Augenhk. *81:*471, 1928.
2. Franceschetti, A.; and Chomé-Bercioux, N.: Fundus albipunctatus cum hemeralopia, Ophthalmologica, *121:*185, 1951.
3. Fuchs, A.: White spots of the fundus combined with nightblindness and xerosis (Uyemura's syndrome), Am. J. Ophth *.48:*101, 1959.

SYNDROME: van der Hoeve

SYNONYMS: Osteogenesis imperfecta, osteopsathyrosis, Ekman syndrome, Lobstein syndrome, Spurway syndrome.

GEN. INFORMATION:

The syndrome is considered to be inherited as an autosomal dominant trait, although only one third of the patients give a family history of the syndrome. Progressive from birth on, with osteosclerosis starting about age 20 years, but patients mostly live to advanced age. Laboratory findings: Serum calcium, phosphorus and phosphatase usually normal. Urinary excretion of amino acids may be increased (Chowers *et al.*: J. A. M. A., 1962)

OCULAR FINDINGS:

Orbit	
Lids	
Motility	
Lacr. App.	
Vision	Hyperopia*
Vis. Fields	
Intraoc. Ten.	Glaucoma*
Ant. Segm. and Sclera	Blue sclera** (most constant finding) the degree of blueness varies among cases. The blue color is either due to thinned sclera and/or greater translucency of the fibrous coat, increase in mucopolysaccharide content, or deficiency in collagen fibers (Ref. 5)
Ocul. Media	Cornea may be thinned leading to megalocornea and keratoconus.* Cataract (rare)
Retina and Choroid	
Optic Nerve	

OTHER CLINICAL FINDINGS:

1. Brittle bones**
2. Deafness (60%)** (bilateral and progressive)
3. Hyperflexibility of ligaments**
4. Dental defects**
5. Unusual fineness of the hair
6. Disproportioned skull with temporal bulge and large occiput.
7. Micromelia (short limbs)
8. Multiple fractures (frequent)

* Occasional findings (Ref. 7)   ** Characteristic for this syndrome

BIBLIOGRAPHY:
1. Ekman, O. J.: Dissertatio Medica Descriptionen et Casus Aliquot Osteomalaciae Sistens, Uppsala, J. Erdman, 1788.
2. Lobstein, J. B.: Traité de l' Anatomie Pathologique, Vol. II, Paris, F. G. Lerrault, 1833, p. 204.
3. Spurway, J.: Hereditary tendency to fracture, Brit. Med. J., 2:844, 1896.
4. Van der Hoeve, J., and Keyn, A.: Blaue Sklera, Knochenbrüchigkeit und Schwerhörigkeit, Arch. f. Ophth., 95:81, 1918.
5. Ruedemann, A. D.: Osteogenesis imperfecta congenita and blue sclerotics, Arch. Ophthal., 49:6, 1953,
6. Engfeldt, B.: Engstrom, A., and Zetterström, R.: Biophysical studies of the bone tissue in osteogenesis imperfecta, J. Bone & Joint Surg. 36:654, 1954.
7. Mckusick, V. A.: *Heritable Disorders of Connective Tissue,* St. Louis, C. V. Mosby Co., 1966.

SYNDROME: Vermis
SYNONYMS:
GEN. INFORMATION:
Mainly medulloblastomas arising primarily in the posterior vermis but invade the fourth ventricle secondarily and compress the bulb. The symptomatology is practically the same than that of ependymonas of the fourth ventricle. In late stages symptoms of bulbar compression may develop with possible sudden death. The condition is apparently more frequent in children (Bailey). Ventriculography aids in localizing the tumor.

OCULAR FINDINGS:

Orbit	
Lids	
Motility	Nystagmus (non-characteristic)
Lacr. App.	
Vision	
Vis. Fields	
Intraoc. Ten.	
Ant. Segm. and Sclera	
Ocul. Media	
Retina and Choroid	
Optic Nerve	Papilledema

OTHER CLINICAL FINDINGS:
1. Enlargement of the head
2. Vomiting (early sign)—direct pressure upon bulbar centers
3. Stiffness and pain of the neck and shoulders
4. Equilibratory disturbances
5. Incoordination of the limbs (only little)
6. Absence of definite laterality of cerebellar signs
7. Severe headache (more pronounced in adults than in children)

BILBIOGRAPHY:
1. Bogaert, van L. and Martin, P.: Les tumeurs du IV. vent. et le syndrome cérébelleux de la ligne médiane, Rev. neurol., 2:431, 1928.
2. Martin, P.: Rapport sur les tumeurs du IV eventricule au point de vue clinique oto-neuro-ophatlmologique et neurochirurgical, J. belge de neurol. et de psychiat., 30:255, 1930.
3. Bailey, P.; Buchanan, D. and Bucy, P. O.: *Intracranial Tumors of Infancy and Childhood,* Chicago, University of Chicago Press, 1939, p. 37.

SYNDROME: Vogt-Koyanagi-Harada
SYNONYMS: Harada's disease, Uveitis-vitiligo-alopecia-poliosis syndrome
GEN. INFORMATION:

Virus infection? (Injection of aqueous humor of affected individuals into the cerebrum of mice did not cause any symptoms.*) Italians and Japanese more commonly affected than other groups. Occurs usually in young adults. The disease is chronic over many months with often considerable loss of vision and hearing. Tendency toward recovery of visual function (frequently incomplete). Laboratory findings: Increased number of lymphocytes in spinal fluid with slightly increased pressure. EEG demonstrated diffuse cerebral involvement (Cowper). Originally the disease described by Harada and the Vogt-Koyanagi syndrome were regarded as separate entities. Bruno and McPherson suggested, however, that both are manifestations of the same condition, the varying symptoms differing only in their intensity and distribution, a concept now generally wide accepted.

OCULAR FINDINGS:

Orbit	
Lids	White lashes*
Motility	
Lacr. App.	
Vision	Strongly reduced vision during acute disease, but sometimes with subsequent remarkable improvement*
Vis. Fields	
Intraoc. Ten.	Secondary glaucoma
Ant. Segm. and Sclera	Bilateral uveitis,* sympathetic ophthalmitis, exudative iridocyclitis.
Ocul. Media	Steamy cornea, profuse vitreous opacities.
Retina and Choroid	Bilateral serous retinal detachment and edema with spontaneous reattachment after weeks. Depigmentation and patches of scattered pigment later on. Bilateral acute diffuse exudative choroiditis.* Occasionally retinal hemorrhages
Optic Nerve	Papilledema

OTHER CLINICAL FINDINGS:

1. Alopecia
2. Poliosis (90%)
3. Vitiligo* } (approx. 50%)
4. Hearing defect* }
5. Headaches*
6. Vomiting*
7. Meningeal irritation*
8. Tinnitus

* Particularly pronounced in 'Harada's disease'

BIBLIOGRAPHY:

1. Vogt, A.: Frühzeitiges Ergrauen der Zilien und Bemerkungen über den sogenannten plötzlichen Eintritt dieser Erscheinung, Kl. Mbl. Augenhk. *44:*228, 1906.
2. Harada, E.: Acta. Soc. Ophthal. Jap. *30:*356. 1926.
3. Koyanaga, Y.: Dysacusis, Alopecia, und Poliosis bei schwerer Uveitis nicht traumatischen Ursprungs, Kl. Mbl. Augenhk. *82:*194, 1929.
4. Bruno, M. G.; and McPherson, S. D., Jr.: Harada's disease, Am. J. Ophth. *32:*513, 1949.
5. Cowper, A. R.: Harada's disease and Vogt-Koyanagi syndrome, Uveoencephalitis, Arch. Ophth *45:*367, 1951.
6. Swartz, E.: Vogt-Koyanagi syndrome precipitated by lens extraction, report of a case, A. J. O., *39:*488, 1955.
7. Kamel, S.: The Vogt-Koyanagi syndrome, Bull. Ophth. Soc. Egypt, *50:*103, 1957.
8. Duke-Elder, Sir Stewart: *System of Ophthalmology,* Vol. IX, St. Louis, C. V. Mosby Co., 1966.

SYNDROME: von Herrenschwand
SYNONYMS: Sympathetic heterochromia
GEN. INFORMATION:
The syndrome is considered a congenital anomaly and the frequent association of heterochromia with Horner's syndrome and its association with vasomotor disturbances is at least suggestive of it. Others consider the heterochromia also in this syndrome as being caused by infection. Depigmentation of one iris due to sympathectomy has well been documented experimentally as after trauma or surgical intervention in man. (Angelucci: Arch. Ottal., 1893; Bistis: Z. Augenheilk., 1934) a. o. Both the sympathetic paralysis and the heterochromia may be transmitted as irregular autosomal dominant traits (Calhoun, Am. J. Ophth., 1919; and Durham, 1958). Sympathetic palsy from cervical ribs, tumor of the thyroid gland, enlarged cervical lymph nodes, scars following tuberculosis or syringomyelia in apex of the pleura, may cause this syndrome.

OCULAR FINDINGS:

Orbit	Enophthalmos
Lids	Ptosis
Motility	
Lacr. App.	
Vision	
Vis. Fields	
Intraoc. Ten.	
Ant. Segm. and Sclera	Heterochromia (unilateral iris) contrary to Fuchs' heterochromia the typical architecture and trabeculae of the deeper iris layers remain clearly outlined. Miosis may be present as part of Horner's trias.
Ocul. Media	
Retina and Choroid	
Optic Nerve	

OTHER CLINICAL FINDINGS:
Decrease of sweating ipsilateral side of face as part of the sympathetic paralysis.
BIBLIOGRAPHY:
1. Herrenschwand, F. von: Zur Sympathicusheterochromie, Klin. Wschr. 2:1059, 1923.
2. Davenport, C. B.: Heredity of eye-color in man, Science. N. S., 26:589, 1907.
3. Mann, I.: Developmental Abnormalities of the Eye, London, Cambridge University Press, 1937.
4. Durham, D. G.: Congenital heredity in Horner's syndrome. Arch. Ophth. 60:939, 1958.
5. Duke Elder, Sir Stewart: System of Ophthalmology, Vol. IX, St. Louis, C. V. Mosby Co., 1966.

SYNDROME: von Hippel-Lindau
SYNONYMS: Retinocerebral angiomatosis, angiomatosis retinae
GEN. INFORMATION:
Familial disease in at least 20% of the patients. Dominantly transmitted. Penetrance not always complete. Power of expression variable. Angiomata most frequently in the cerebellum and the walls of the fourth ventricle, more rare in brain stem and spinal cord. Visceral cysts in the kidneys (François) and less frequently in adrenals, ovaries, liver and spleen. Both eyes are affected in about 50% of cases. Onset usually in young adults, but may occur in small children (Appelmans, 1947). The initial pathology of the eye was thought to be a cluster of endothelial cells (angioblasts) which persist in an embryonic state and proliferate and invade the wall of the retinal vessels. Retinal cyst formation, glial overgrowth, hyaline changes and general retinal degeneration develop secondary as a result of the initial pathology (Ref. 5). Laboratory findings: Chromosome studies showed chromosomal aberrations with chromatid breakage, aneuploidy and polyploidy in 2 patients (Kobaysashi and Shimado), whereas Melmon and Rosen, 1964, reported that the karyotype was normal.

OCULAR FINDINGS:

Orbit	
Lids	
Motility	
Lacr. App.	
Vision	
Vis. Fields	
Intraoc. Ten.	Secondary glaucoma
Ant. Segm. and Sclera	Angiomatosis of the iris (François)
Ocul. Media	Vitreous hemorrhages and vascular proliferation
Retina nad Choroid	Angiomatosis, tortuosity of dilated retinal artery and vein (feeder vessels), exudates and hemorrhages, retinitis proliferans (less frequent). Changes are more frequently in the periphery. The choroid is usually not invaded. Severe hemorrhages and finally retinal detachment are late sequelae.
Optic Nerve	Occasionally involved along with retinal pathologic condition

OTHER CLINICAL FINDINGS:
1. Cerebellar angiomatosis (25% of patients with angiomatosis retinae (Lindau). This figure is considerably higher than that found on the North American continent (Ref. 5)
2. Epilepsy   3. Psychic disturbances to dementia

BIBLIOGRAPHY:
1. Hippel, F. von,: Vorstellung eines Patienten mit einem sehr ungewöhnlichen Netzhaut-bezw. Aderhautleiden, Ber. ophthal. Ges. *24:*269, 1895.
2. _____ ,: Die anatomische Grundlage der von mir beschriebenen sehr seltenen Erkrankung der Netzhaut, v. Graefes Arch. Ophth. *79:*350, 1911.
3. Lindau, A.: Zur Frage der Anglomatosis retinae und ihrer Hirnkomplikationen, Acta Ophth. *4:*193, 1927.
4. François, J.: *Heredity in Ophthalmology,* St. Louis, C. V. Mosby Co., 1961.
5. Kobaysashi, M.; and Shimado, K.: Chromosomal aberrations in Hippel-Lindau's disease, Jap. J. Ophth. *10:*38, 1966.

SYNDROME: von Recklinghausen
SYNONYMS: Neurofibromatosis, Neurinomatosis
GEN. INFORMATION:
Simple dominant (Etiology for unilateral exophthalmos within this syndrome: neurovascular theory; mechanical theory; coordination theory). Generally no sex linkage,—male likeage in isolated or familial cases in which it might be inherited as a recessive (Cockayne). Although present at birth usually not recognized until early childhood. The entire process becomes often activated at puberty, during pregnancy and menopause. Prognosis depending on severeness of ocular involvement. X-ray findings: Box-like widening of the sella turcica, enlarged orbit, especially roof, as congenital defect or erosion by tumor, periostal thickening, subperiosteal cysts, scoliosis.

OCULAR FINDINGS:

Obrit	Proptosis, displacement of the globe, pulsation of the globe synchronous with pulse but no bruit, enlargement of the optic foramen
Lids	Ptosis, elephantiasis, pigment spots
Motility	Muscle palsies
Lacr. App.	
Vision	
Vis. Fields	
Intraoc. Ten.	Unilateral hydrophthalmos. Glaucoma may be produced by dense abnormal tissue in the chamber angle obstructing aqueous outflow (Ref. 8)
Ant. Segm. and Sclea	Conjunctival nodules, iris nodules. Persistence of embryonal tissue in anterior chamber angle, defects of Schlemm's canal, peripheral anterior synechiae. Nodular swelling of ciliary nerves.
Ocul. Media	Nodular swelling of corneal nerves, cataract (rare)
Retina and Choroid	Diffuse and nodular involvement with thickening consisting of neurofibroma, fibroblasts, spindle cells containing pigment, ovoid corpuscles of convoluted nerve fibers
Optic Nerve	Primary optic atrophy due to tumor pressure, secondary atrophy due to papilledema, neurofibroma of the disc (Stallard)

OTHER CLINICAL FINDINGS:
1. Café-au-lâit skin pigmentations
2. Fibroma molluscum, lipoma and sebaceous adenoma, Schwannoma
3. Growth abnormalities
4. Spontaneous fractures
5. Facial hemihypertrophy

BIBLIOGRAPHY:
1. Recklinghausen, F. D. von: Ueber die multiplen Fibrome der Haut und ihre Beziehung zu den multiplen Neuromen. VI, 11:138, Berlin, Festschrift Path. Inst. Berlin, 1882. A. Hirschwald.
2. Stallard, H. B.: A case of intra-ocular neuroma of the left optic nerve head, Brit. J. Ophth., 22:11, 1938.
3. Davis, A. D.: Plexiform neurofibromatosis of the orbit and globe, Arch. Ophth., 22:761, 1939.
4. François, J.: The ocular manifestations of Recklinghausen's disease, Bull. roy. Med. belg., 9:365, 1947.
5. Kreibig, W.: Über Neurofibromatose des Auges, Klin. Mbl. Augenhk., 115:428, 1949.
6. Reese, A. B.: *Tumors of the Eye,* New York, Paul B. Hoeber, Inc., 1951.
7. Lieb, W. A.; Wirth, W. A.; and Geeraets, W. J.: Hydrophthalmos and neurofibromatosis, Confina Neurologica, 19:230, 1958.
8. Grant, W. M. and Walton, D. S.: Distinctive gonioscopic findings in glaucoma due to neurofibromatosis, Arch. Ophth., 79:127, 1968.

SYNDROME: von Sallmann-Paton-Witkop
SYNONYMS: Hereditary benign intraepithelial dyskeratosis
GEN. INFORMATION:
The syndrome is inherited as an autosomal dominant trait. The penetrance of the gene is high. The course is benign. The syndrome of conjunctival and oral lesions was first found in a tri-racial isolate of Halifiax County, N. C. The disease is present also in possibly collateral Caucasian descendants in general population. Histopathology of the ocular and oral lesions is similar. Conjunctival smears stained with Papanicolaou technique show waxy eosinophilic cells and a 'cell within cell' pattern, diagnostic for this disease.

OCULAR FINDINGS:

Orbit	
Lids	
Motility	
Lacr. App.	
Vision	Decreased vision due to possible corneal pathologic condition
Vis. Fields	
Intraoc. Ten.	
Ant. Segm. and Sclera	Foamy gelatinous plaques located in a typical horseshow fashion at 3 and 9 o'clock positions of the perilimbal area. The lesions are very superficial, more so than pterygia, and with hyperemia of the bulbar conjunctiva about the extent of these lesions. The lateral part of the tarsal conjunctiva shows papillary hypertrophy. These clinical features become usually apparent during the 1st year of life. Photophobia (mainly in children)
Ocul. Media	The cornea may be involved within the dyskeratotic process with corneal vascularization and consequential visual decrease
Retina and Choroid	
Optic Nerve	

OTHER CLINICAL FINDINGS:
1. Thickening of oral mucosa with whitish plaques and folds of a spongy character, (asymptomatic) with slow progression from birth into second decade of life. Commisural areas are more involved. Dorsal tongue, gingiva, uvula and pharynx are not involved

BIBLIOGRAPHY:
1. von Sallmann, L. and Paton, D.: Hereditary benign intraepithelial dyskeratosis: 1. Ocular Manifestations, Arch. Ophth. *63:*421, 1960.
2. Witkop, C. J., Jr.; Shankle, C. H.; Graham, J. B.; Murray, M. R.; Rucknagel, D. L. and Byerly, B. H.: Hereditary benign intraepithelial dyskeratosis: II. Oral manifestations and hereditary transmission, Arch. Path. *70:*696, 1960.

SYNDROME: Waardenburg

SYNONYMS: van der Hoeve-Halbertsma-Waardenburg syndrome, Waardenburg-Klein syndrome, embryonic fixation syndrome, Interoculo-irido-dermato-auditive dysplasia.

GEN. INFORMATION:
Irregular dominant inheritance. Penetrance of the different characteristics varies considerably in different pedigrees. Persistance of embryonal development 8 to 10 weeks. The complete syndrome is rare. A recessive autosomal gene for the combination of albinism and deaf-mutism, and different genes for the association of leucism and deaf mutism, one X-linked and one possibly autosomally dominant may lead to different phenotypes. The more generalized anomalies were attributed to a developmental fault in the neural crests which could account for the absence of the organ of Corti, the aplasia of the spiral ganglion, and the pigmentary changes (Fisch, 1959).

OCULAR FINDINGS:

Orbit	Hyperplasia of the medial portions of the eyebrows (45%): Widened interpupillary distance (Hypertelorism). Underdevelopment of the orbits (less frequently)
Lids	Lateral displacement of the medial canthia and lacrimal puncta. Blepharophimosis (99%). Caruncle hypoplasia. Thickening of the tarsus and epicanthus (less frequently)
Motility	Convergent squint*
Lacr. App.	Lengthening of the lacrimal canaliculi (puncta opposite the cornea)
Vision	Strabismic amblyopia*
Vis. Fields	
Intraoc. Ten.	
Ant. Segm. and Sclera	Heterochromia iridum (partial or total) (25%). Aniridia
Ocul. Media	Microcornea, cornea plana, microphakia
Retina and Choroid	Abnormal fundus pigmentation. Retinal hypoplasia
Optic Nerve	Hypoplasia of optic nerve

OTHER CLINICAL FINDINGS:
1. Congenital deafness, unilateral deafness or deaf mutism (20%)
2. Broad and high nasal root with absent nasofrontal angle (78%)
3. Brachycephaly (less frequently)
4. Albinotic hair strain (unilateral) (17%)
5. Faint patches of skin pigmentation (17%)

*Isolated findings

BIBLIOGRAPHY:
1. van der Hoeve, J.: Kl. Mbl. Augenhk. *56:*232, 1916.
2. Halbertsma, K. T. A.: Two apparently similar but essentially different congenital anomalies of the eye, Med. T. Geneesk. *73:*13, 1647, (1929); *83:*4985, (1939).
3. Waardenburg, P. J.: A new syndrome combining development anomalies of the eyelids, eyebrows and nose root with pigmentary defects of the iris and head and with congenital defects, Am. J. Hum. Genet. *3:*195, 1951.
4. Goldberg, M. F. Waardenburg's syndrome with fundus and other anomalies, Arch. Ophth. *76:*797, 1966.

SYNDROME: Waldenström
SYNONYMS: Macroglobulinemia syndrome
GEN. INFORMATION:
The disease occurs mainly in males (2:1) and usually above 50 years of age (with exceptions). Chromosomal abnormalities were reported most with of the cells having 47 chromosomes (range 45 to 49) and with an abnormally large chromosome, though apparently not as a constant finding. Chronic course over years without serious complications, but more severe progress with complications may develop. Laboratory findings: Elevated serum globulin fraction with globulins of abnormally high molecular weight (demonstrable with ultracentrifugation—in clinical practice this technique has been used to remove the macroglobulins from the patient's serum). Bone marrow changes. High sedimentation rate. Positive formol-gel reaction. Spontaneous gelification of blood serum at room temperature (occasional findings). Myeloma-like protein component on electrophoretic analysis. Normal white blood cell count. Normal bleeding and clotting time.

Orbit	
Lids	
Motility	
Lacr. App.	
Vision	Visual disturbances have been reported, however, without given explanations, these findings will have to be considered as a result of the fundus pathology
Vis. Fields	
Intraoc. Ten.	
Ant. Segm. and Sclera	
Ocul. Media	
Retina and Choroid	Hemorrhages, exudates—(in both retina and choroid)
Optic Nerve	Papilledema (occasional findings)

OTHER CLINICAL FINDINGS:
1. Adenopathy including salivary gland enlargements and slight hepatosplenomegaly
2. Weakness, fatigue
3. Pallor
4. Dyspnea
5. Weight loss
6. Nasal and oral hemorrhages and ulcerations
7. Subarachnoidal hemorrhages
8. Vasospasm of limbs
9. Anemia

BIBLIOGRAPHY:
1. Waldenström, J.: Incipient myelomatosis or essential hyperglobulinemia with fibrinogenopenia: A new syndrome? Acta Med. Scand. *117:*216, 1944.
2. Zlotnick, A.: Macroglobulinemia of Waldenstrom, A. J. Med., *24:*461, 1958.
3. Bottura, L.; Ferrari, I. and Veiga, A. A.: Chromosome abnormalities in Waldenström's macroglobulinemia, Lancet, *1:*1170, 1961.
4. Patau, K.: Chromosomal abnormalities in Waldenström's macroglobulinemia, Lancet, **2**:600, 1961.
5. Goldstein, R.: Pathologic bleeding, pages 592–593, in: McBryde, L. M.: *Signs and Symptoms,* 4th Ed., Philadelphia, J. B. Lippincott Co., 1964.

SYNDROME: Wallenberg
SYNONYMS: Dorsolateral medullary syndrome, lateral bulbar syndrome
GEN. INFORMATION:
Occlusion of the posterior inferior cerebellar artery. The disease is not uncommon and occurs usually above the age of 40 years. Complete recovery usually over months, but residuals possible. Clinical findings are similar to those present in Babinski-Nageotte syndrome but crossed hemiparesis is absent. The nystagmus is produced by involvement of the vestibular nuclei or the posterior longitudinal bundle.

OCULAR FINDINGS:

Orbit	Enophthalmos*
Lids	Ptosis*
Motility	Spontaneous homolateral or contralateral horizontal or rotating nystagmus, this is in contrast to syringobulbia with typical rotary nystagmus always ipsilateral (Jung and Kornhuber). Optokinetic nystagmus usually normal. Ipsilateral abducens paralsis may occur with involvement of the ambiguus nucleus
Lacr. App.	
Vision	
Vis. Fields	
Intraoc. Ten.	
Ant. Segm. and Sclera	Miosis*
Ocul. Media	
Retina and Choroid	
Optic Nerve	

OTHER CLINICAL FINDINGS:
1. Nausea, vertigo
2. Difficulty in swallowing and speaking
3. Ipsilateral ataxia
4. Muscular hypotonicity
5. Ipsilateral loss of pain and temperature sense of the face
6. Contralateral hypoesthesia for pain and temperature of extremities and trunk

*Horner's syndrome may appear with involvement of descending sympathetic fibers.

BIBLIOGRAPHY:
1. Wallenberg, A.: Antaomische Befunde in einem als "acute Bulbäraffektion (Embolie der Arteria cerebellar. post. inf. sinist.?)" beschriebenen Falle, Arch. f. Psychiat. *34,* 1901.
2. Wallenberg, A.: Klinische Beiträge zur Diagnostik acuter Herderkrankungen des verlängerten Marks und der Brücke, Dtsch. Ztschr. f. Nervenh. *19:*227, 1901.
3. Lewis, G.: Syndrome of thrombosis of posterior inferior cerebellar artery, report of 28 cases, Ann. Int. Med., *36:*592, 1952.
4. Jung, R. and Kornhuber, M. H.: Results of electronystagmography in man, in Bender, M. B. (Edit.), *The Oculomotor System,* New York, Harper & Row, 1964, p. 428.

SYNDROME: Weber

SYNONYMS: Weber-Gubler syndrome; cerebellar peduncle syndrome; alternating oculomotor syndrome

GEN. INFORMATION:

Lesion of the peduncle (crus) pons, medulla, which interrupts the 3rd nerve before it emerges from the peduncle and interrupts fibers in the pyramidal tract above the level of their nuclei. Hemorrhage and thrombosis most frequent cause, but tumor of the pituitary region, extending posteriorly, might cause similar findings. Differential diagnosis: Syphilitic vascular disease. Aneurysm of the circle of Willis.

OCULAR FINDINGS:

Orbit	
Lids	Ptosis
Motility	Homolateral third nerve palsy (usually complete)
Lacr. App.	
Vision	
Vis. Fields	
Intraoc. Ten.	
Ant. Segm. and Sclera	Fixed, dilated pupil
Ocul. Media	
Retina and Choroid	
Optic Nerve	

OTHER CLINICAL FINDINGS:

1. Contralateral hemiplegia
2. Contralateral paralysis of face and tongue (supranuclear type)
3. Polyuria } due to pressure in the region of the floor
4. Polydipsia } of the third ventricle

BIBLIOGRAPHY:

1. Weber, H. D.: A contribution to the pathology of the crura cerebri, Med.-Chir. Trans., *46*:121, 1863.
2. Walsh, F. B.: *Clinical Neuro-Ophthalmology,* 2nd Ed., Baltimore, The Williams & Wilkins Co., 1957.
3. Bender, M. B.: *The Oculomotor System,* New York, Harper & Row, 1964.

SYNDROME: Werner
SYNONYMS: Progeria of adults
GEN. INFORMATION:
Etiology is unknown (aberration of hepatic metabolism of steriod compounds). The disease may be transmitted according to the simple recessive mode of inheritance. Irregular dominance with signs of aggravation may be possible (Maeder). Consanguinity of parents is frequent. Males are somewhat more frequently affected. Appearance after puberty, most frequently in the second and third decade of life. Prognosis: poor life expectancy beyond 40 years of age. Differential diagnosis mainly against Rothmund's syndrome. Atrophic changes of distal limbs more pronounced in Werner's syndrome along with later appearance of symptoms.

OCULAR FINDINGS:

Orbit	
Lids	Absence of eye lashes and scanty eyebrows*
Motility	
Lacr. App.	
Vision	
Vis. Fields	
Intraoc. Ten.	
Ant. Segm. and Sclera	Blue sclerotics (Oppenheimer and Kugl: Tr. A. Am. Physicians, 1934)
Ocul. Media	Juvenile cataracts, usual onset between 20 and 35 years of age progressing slowly over a few years.* Bullous keratitis (Kleiber: Kl. Mbl. Augenhk., 1920), trophic corneal defects (Flandin et al.: Bull. Soc. méd. hôp., Paris, 1936)
Retina and Choroid	Paramacular retinal degeneration (Franceschetti and Maeder: Schw. med. Wschr. 1949)
Optic Nerve	*Typical eye findings for this syndrome

OTHER CLINICAL FINDINGS:
1. Leanness, short stature (160 cm max.)
2. Very thin limbs
3. Short, deformed fingers
4. Small mouth
5. Gray hairs and early baldness
6. Stretched, atrophic skin (scleropoikiloderma) of hyperpigmentation and deficient pigmentation
7. Telangiektasia and trophic indulent ulcers on toes, heels and ankles
8. Hypogonadism
9. Tendency to insulin resistant diabetes (10%)
10. Osteoporosis
11. Thyroid dysfunction
12. Arteriosclerosis with secondary heart failure

BIBLIOGRAPHY:
1. Werner, C. W. O.: Über Katarakt in Verbindung mit Sklerodermie, Inaug. Dissert., Kiel, 1904.
2. Agatston, S. A. and Gartner, S.: Precocious cataracts and scleroderma (Rothmund's syndrome: Werner's syndrome), Arch. Ophth. 41:492, 1939.
3. Thannhauser, S. J.: Werner's syndrome (Progeria of the adult) and Rothmund's syndrome. Two types of closely related heredofamilial atrophic dermatoses with juvenile cataracts and endocrine features, Ann. Int. Med., 23:559, 1945.
4. François, J.: Heredity in Ophthalmology, St. Louis, C. V. Mosby Co., 1961, p. 643.

SYNDROME: Wernicke

SYNONYMS: Superior hemorrhagic polioencephalopathic syndrome, hemorrhagic polioencephalitis superior syndrome, encephalitis hemorrhagica superioris.

GEN. INFORMATION:
Nutritional deficiecny with secondary lack of vitamin B_1 or thiamine. Focal vascular lesions in the gray matter around third and fourth ventricles and Sylvian aqueduct. The median fillet and pyramidal tracts may also be involved. Destruction of nerve cells and fibers with glial and vascular proliferation. Most in alcoholics (adults). In the Orient, in patients with beriberi of all age groups. The prognosis is poor. The course is usually rapid and fatal. Laboratory findings: Increased level of pyruvic acidin the blood.

OCULAR FINDINGS:

Orbit	
Lids	Ptosis, sometimes incomplete (50%)
Motility	Ophthalmoplegia (at first usually only one of the oculomotor group involved with progression to complete ophthalmoplegia (usually bilateral). The levator palpebrae are often spared. It has been suggested that the ophthalmoplegia is directly the result of the thiamine deficiency (Jolliffe: Arch. Neurol. & Psychiat., 1941). Horizontal and vertical nystagmus
Vision	Diplopia
Vis. Fields	
Intraoc. Ten.	
Ant. Segm. and Sclera	'Agyll Robertson' pupil occasionally. More frequently normal or a somewhat slow pupil reaction
Ocul. Media	
Retina and Choroid	Retinal hemorrhages (Ecker and Woltman: Proc. Staff Meet., Mayo Clin, 1939)
Optic Nerve	Papilledema (Wernicke), pallor of discs

OTHER CLINICAL FINDINGS:
1. Early prostration
2. Lethargy or irritability
3. Stupor and delirium
4. Mental disturbances to Korsakovs psychosis
5. Ataxia and tremor
6. Peripheral neuritis

The clinical symptomatology has been classified into 5 groups (Bender and Schilder): (1) Typical picture of polioencephalitis hemorrhagica with clouding of consciousness; (2) those with prominent cerebellar disturbances; (3) mental and neurological features resembling acute catatonia; (4) delirious symptoms more pronounced than neurological; (5) polyneuritis associated with signs of polioencephalitis

BIBLIOGRAPHY:
1. Wernicke, C.: Quoted in Bumke, O. and Kent, F.: *Handbuch der Neurologie,* Vol. 13, Berlin, Julius Springer, 1936, pp. 828–915.
2. Jolliffe, N.; Wortis, H. and Fein, H.: The Wernicke Syndrome, Arch. Neurol. & Psychiat. *46:*569, 1941.
3. De Wardener, H. E. and Lennox, B.: Cerebral Beri-Beri (Wernicke's encephalopathy) Review of 52 cases in Singapore Prisoner-of-War Hospital, Lancet, *1:*11, 1947.
4. Cogan, G., and Victor, M.: Ocular signs of Wernicke's disease, Tr. Am. Ophth. Soc., *51:*103, 1953.

15

SYNDROME: Wilson
SYNONYMS: Hepatolenticular degeneration
GEN. INFORMATION:
Lesion in the putamen and lenticular nucleus (Familial occurrence.). Most frequent in first decade of life, but also described in later age groups. Laboratory findings: Liver function tests show often reduced functioning capacity. Resting of urinary copper output and increase in copper content in tissue have been described. Shrinking of the corpus striatum. Tract degeneration from putamen to nucleus ruber and corpus luysii, to the posterior longitudinal bundles and superior cerebellar peduncles(Greenfield). Cirrhosis of the liver. Death usually within 2 to 5 years after first symptoms. Differential diagnosis: Phenothiazine toxicity. Paralysis agitans. Treatment with penicillamine have in some patients caused a decrease in intensity of the Kayser-Fleischer ring (Kearns, T. P., Arch. Ophth. *74*:708-709, 1965). Copper deposition in tissue may be due to a deficiency in synthesis of ceruloplasmin (Walshe)

OCULAR FINDINGS:

Orbit	
Lids	
Motility	Ocular movements affected late
Lacr. App.	
Vision	Night blindness might occasionally exist
Vis. Fields	
Intraoc. Ten.	
Ant. Segm. and Sclera	
Ocul. Media	Corneal ring (Kayser-Fleischer ring) on posterior surface of the cornea of golden appearance or grayish-green or ruby-red. Narrow ring of normal cornea peripheral to it
Retina and Choroid	
Optic Nerve	

OTHER CLINICAL FINDINGS:
1. Liver cirrhosis
2. Jaundice (early)
3. Difficulties in speaking (early)
4. Difficulties in swallowing and mastication
5. CNS involvement (not always)
6. Extensive muscular rigidity
7. Mouth usually open with salivation ("Fixed grin")
8. Coarse tremor
9. Hematemesis and ascites in late stages

BIBLIOGRAPHY:
1. Wilson, S. A. K.: Progressive lenticular degeneration. A familial nervous disease associated with cirrhosis of the liver, Brain *34*:295,1912.
2. Pillat, A.: Changes in the eyegrounds in Wilson's disease, A. J. O., *16*:1, 1933.
3. Eckhardt, R. E.; Stolzar, T. M.; Adam, A. B.; and Johnson, L. V.: The pigment of the Kayser-Fleischer ring, A. J. O., *26*:151, 1943.
4. Denny-Brown, D.,; and Porter, M.: The effect of BAL (2,3 dimercapto-propanol) on hepatolenticular degeneration (Wilson's disease), New Engl. J. Med., *245*:917, 1951.
5. Ravin, H. A.: Wilson's disease, an inborn error of metabolism and a model of degenerative central nervous system disease, Bull. Detroit Sinai Hosp. *12*:25 ,1964.
6. Richmond, J., *et al.:* Hepato-lenticuiar degeneration (Wilson's disease) treated by penicillamine, Brain, *87*:619, 1964.
7. Walshe, J. M.:The physiology of copper in man and its relation to Wilson's disease, Brain, *90*:149, 1967.

SYNDROME: Zinsser-Engman-Cole
SYNONYMS: Dyskeratosis congenita with pigmentation, Cole-Rauschkolb-Toomey syndrome
GEN. INFORMATION:
The syndrome has been suggested of being a variant of Fanconi's familiar aplastic anemia (Ref. 4). The syndrome here described is suggestive of being recessively inherited with possible male linkage. Parental consanguinity has also been observed (Castello and Bunke: Arch Derm., 1956). Onset of skin changes around puberty. Histopathological findings: Capillary hyperplasia with atrophy of epidermis and subcutaneous tissue. Dense melanin deposits mainly along vessels.

OCULAR FINDINGS:

Orbit	
Lids	Ectropion, chronic blepharitis, loss of eyelashes (single report;- Pastinszky *et al.*: Derm. Wschr., 1957)
Motility	
Lacr. App.	Obstruction of lacrimal puncta with subsequent profuse tearing
Vision	
Vis. Fields	
Intraoc. Ten.	
Ant. Segm. and Sclera	Conjunctival keratinization, bullous conjunctivitis
Ocul. Media	
Retina and Choroid	
Optic Nerve	

OTHER CLINICAL FINDINGS:
1. Congenital dyskeratosis with pigmentation of 'marble' configuration, or gun metal appearance, atrophic areas and telangiectasis.
2. Dystrophy of nails
3. Vesicular and bullous lesion of oral cavity followed by ulceration, mucosal atrophy; leukoplakia
4. Aplastic anemia
5. Hypersplenism
6. Arocyanosis upper and lower limbs
7. Hyperhidrosis palms and soles
8. Bullous skin lesions (not common)
9. Mental retardation*
10. Dysphagia*
11. Diverticula of esophagus*

*Occasional findings (Garb and Rubin: Arch. Derm. and Syph., 1944)

BIBLIOGRAPHY:
1. Zinsser, F.: Atrophica cutis reticularis cum pigmentatione, dystrophia unguinum et leukoplakia oris., Ikonographia Dermat. Kioto., 1906.
2. Engman, M. F.: A unique case of reticular pigmentation of the skin with atrophy, Arch. Dermat. & Syph. *13*:685, 1926.
3. Cole, H. N.; Rauschkolb, J. E. and Toomey, J.: Dyskeratosis congenita with pigmentation, dystrophia unguis and leukokeratosis oris, Arch. Dermat. & Syph. *21*:71, 1930.
4. Cole, H. N.; Cole, H. N., Jr. and Lascheid, W. P.: Dyskeratosis congenita; Relationship to poikiloderma atrophicans vasculare and to aplastic anemia of Fanconi, Arch. Dermat. *76*:712, 1957.
5. Gorlin, R. J. and Pindborg, J. J. *Syndromes of the Head and Neck;* New York, McGraw-Hill Book Co. (Blakiston Division), 1964.

Cross Reference of Syndromes
Based on Ocular Manifestations

ANTERIOR SEGMENT
Conjunctiva

Addison: Conjunctivitis, keratitis, cataracts, retinopathy, papilledema, ptosis—moniliasis, tetany, weakness, skin pigmentation, seizures

Angelucci: Conjunctivitis—tachycardia, vasomotor lability, excitability

Charlin: Pseudopurulent conjunctivitis, keratitis, iritis—rhinorrhea, pain ala nasi

Cogan: Congested conjunctiva, subconjunctival hemorrhage, keratitis, blepharospasm—nausea, vertigo, deafness, periarteritis

Degos: Conjunctival telangiectasia, choroiditis, atrophic skin of lids—white skin lesion, anorexia, gastrointestinal involvement

Fabry-Anderson: Conjunctival varicositis, corneal opacities, aneurysmal dilatations of retinal vessels—angiokeratoma of the skin, elevated blood pressure, albuminuria

Feer: Conjunctival injection and itching, photophobia, keratitis, lacrimation. proptosis, optic nerve involvement—restlessness, irritability, sleeplessness, sweating, muscle hypotony, exanthema

Fuchs II: Conjunctivitis—headache, fever, swelling of face, cyanosis, ulcers of mucous membranes

Gaucher: Pinguecula, macular infiltration—infantile form: hypertonia, opisthotonus, cachexia; chronic form: hepatosplenomegaly, skin pigmentation, lymphadenopathy

Goldenhar: Epibulbar dermoid, lid coloboma—micrognathia, preauricular fistulae, auricular appendices, vertebral anomalies

Goldscheider: Conjunctival shrinkage, symblepharon, bullous keratitis, blepharitis—skin lesions, growth and mental retardation

Herrick: Conjunctival telangiectasis, scleral icterus, vitreous hemorrhages, retinopathy—anemia, bone and joint aches, jaundice, hepatosplenomegaly, cardiomegaly, enlarged lymph nodes

Hutchinson: Subconjunctival hemorrhages, exophthalmos, lid hematoma, papilledema—severe anemia, increased sedimentation rate, occasional abdominal tumor

Louis-Bar: Conjunctival telangiectasia, pseudoophthalmoplegia, fixational nystagmus—cerebellar ataxia, scanning speech, hypotonia, cutaneous telangiectasis

Oculo-oro-genital syndrome: Conjunctivitis, keratitis, optic atrophy—stomatitis, glossitis, exfoliating dermatitis of scrotum, erythema pharynx and soft palate, ulcers buccal membranes

Parinaud's oculoglandular syndrome: Conjunctivitis—preauricular and cervical lymphadenitis, fever

Recklinghausen von: Conjunctival nodules, iris nodules, nodular corneal swelling, cataract, proptosis, ptosis, muscle palsies, hydrophthalmos, optic nerve involvement, fundus changes—café-au-lait skin pigmentation, fibromata, growth abnormalities, spontaneous fractures, facial hemihypertrophy

Reiter: Purulent conjunctivitis, iritis, keratitis—skin erythema, genital ulcerations, arthritis, pleuritis

Sallmann von-Paton-Witkop: Foamy perilimbal conjunctival lesions—thickening of oral mucosa

Stevens-Johnson: Conjunctivitis, conj. ulcers, chemosis, hypopyon, iritis—acute respiratory infection, skin and mucous membrane eruptions, rhinitis, urethritis

Uyemura: Conjunctival xerosis, Bitôt' spots, transient nightblindness, white spots of the ocular fundus

Zinsser-Engman-Cole: conjunctival keratinization, bullous conjunctivitis, obstruction of lacrimal puncta, ectropion—congenital dyskeratosis, oral lesions, anemia, hypersplenism, hyperhidrosis palms and soles

Cornea

Addison: Keratitis, conjunctivitis, cataracts, retinopathy, papilledema, ptosis—moniliasis, tetany, weakness, skin pigmentation, seizures

Apert: Exposure keratitis, cataract, exophthalmos, ptosis, strabismus, nystagmus, decreased vision, field defect, optic atrophy—tower skull, syndactyly, synostoses, brevicollis, headaches, convulsions

Axenfeld: Ring-like corneal opacity, changes in chamber angle, glaucoma

Barré-Liéou: Corneal hypesthesia, corneal ulcers—headaches, vasomotor disturbances of face, ear noises, impaired memory

Behcet: Keratitis, hypopyon, iritis, conjunctivitis, uveitis, retinal changes, muscle palsies, visual loss—aphthous lesions of mucous membranes, symptoms of CNS, skin erythema, urethritis

Charlin: Keratitis, corneal ulcers, pseudopurulent conjunctivitis, iritis, orbital pain—rhinorrhea, pain of ala nasi

Chediak-Higashi: Corneal edema, decreased uveal pigmentation, optic nerve involvement—hepatosplenomegaly, lymphadenopathy, oculo-cutaneous albinism

Cogan: Interstitial keratitis, subconjunctival hemorrhage, blepharospasm, lacrimation, blurred vision—vestibulo-auditory symptoms, nausea, vertigo, deafness

Congenital epiblepharon-inferior oblique insufficiency: Keraitits, narrow PD, entropion, inferior oblique insufficiency—chubby cheeks

Crouzon: Exposure keratitis, cataract, exophthalmos, nystagmus, strabismus, visual loss, field defects, optic atrophy—prognathism, maxillary hypoplasia, hydrocephalus interus, headaches, subnormal mentality

Cushing (2): Decreased corneal reflex, paresis VI, VII, nystagmus—deafness, tinnitus, hyperesthesia of face, facial nerve paralysis

Eaton-Lambert: Corneal haziness, decreased vision, ocular myoclonus—weakness, peripheral anesthesia, poor response to neostigmin.

Ehlers-Danlos: Thin cornea, microcornea, keratoconus, subluxated lens, bluish sclera, hypotony of lid skin, ptosis, strabismus, retinopathy—cutaneous hyperelasticity, thin skin, pseudomolluscoid tumors, articular laxity, luxations.

Fabry-Anderson: Corneal opacities, conjunctival varicositis, aneurysmal dilatations of retinal vessels—angiokeratoma of the skin, elevated blood pressure, albuminuria

Feer: Keratitis, photophobia, conjunctival irritation—restlessness, irritability, sweating, rapid pulse, exanthema of palms and soles, muscle hypotony.

Felty: Keratitis, scleritis—rheumatoid arthritis, splenomegaly, leukopenia, oral lesions

Foix: Paralysis V, chemosis, paresis III, IV, VI, lid edema proptosis, optic atrophy—postauricular edema

Goldscheider: Keratitis with ulcers, symblepharon, conjunctival shrinkage, blepharitis— skin lesions, growth and mental retardation

Gorlin-Goltz: Corneal leukoma, congenital cataract, glaucoma, strabismus, hypertelorismus—basal cell nevi, cysts of the jaws, vertebral and other skeletal anomalies

Gradenigro: Reduced corneal sensitivity, pain V, photophoba paraliysis III, IV, VI, optic nerve involvement— inner ear infection, mastoiditis

Groenblad-Strandberg: Corneal degeneration, fundus changes—pseudoxanthoma elasticum, flattening of pulse curve

Hand-Schüller-Christian: Corneal degeneration, exophthalmos, xanthelasma, ophthalmoplegia, optic nerve involvement, retinopathy—xanthoma of the skin, skull defects, lung fibrosis, gingival ulcers, hepatosplenomegaly, growth and sexual retardation

Hoeve, van der: Thin cornea, keratoconus, cataract, blue sclera—brittle bones, deafness, hyperflexibility of ligaments

Hunt: Absence of corneal reflex, decreased lacrimation—facial palsy, hearing defect, decreased salivation

Hunter: Deposition of abnormal mucopolyssacharides in corneal endothelium, iris, ciliary body and sclera, retinal pigment degeneration, nightblindness—dwarfism, hepatosplenomegaly, deafness, gargoylelike facies

Hurler: Opaque cornea, glaucoma, ptosis, strabismus, optic atrophy, macular edema—kyphosis, head deformities, retarded development, hepatosplenomegaly, infantilism

Jacod: Trigeminal neuralgia, ophthalmoplegia, optic atrophy—trigeminal neuralgia, enlarged cervical lymph nodes

Jadassohn-Lewandowski: Corneal dyskeratosis—keratosis and hyperhidrosis of palms and soles, leukokeratosis of oral mucosa, congenital pachyonychia, follicular keratosis

Laurence-Moon-Bardet-Biedl: Keratoconus, cataract, nystagmus, strabismus, visual loss, field defects, optic atrophy, retinopathy—obesity, hypogenitalism, polydactyly, mental retardation

Melkersson-Rosenthal: Keratitis, corneal ulcers, crocodile tear phenomenon—chronic facial edema, facial palsy, furrowed tongue

Meyer-Schwickerath-Weyers: Microcornea, iris anomalies, glaucoma, microphthalmos, short lid aperture—hypoplastic alae nasi, skeletal anomalies of hands and feet, sparse hair growth

Morquio-Brailsford (MPS—IV): Hazy Corneal, Horner's trias—dwarfism, skeletal deformities, decreased muscle tone

Oculo-oro-genital syndrome: Keratitis, conjunctivitis, optic atrophy—glossitis, stomatitis, exfoliating dermatitis of scrotum, buccal ulcers

Recklinghausen, von: Nodular swelling of corneal nerves, iris nodules, cataract, ptosis—café-au-laît spots, fibromata, growth abnormalities, spontaneous fractures

Reiter: Keratitis, purulent conjunctivitis, iritis—genital ulcerations, urethritis, arthritis, lymphadenopathy

Riegers: Microcornea, corneal opacities, dislocated lens, congenital glaucoma, iris hypoplasia, optic atrophy—broad face, suppression of dentation, underdeveloped maxilla

Riley-Day: Keratitis, corneal ulcers and anesthesia, absent tear production—excessive salivation, failure to thrive, respiratory infection, skin blotching, hyporeflexia

Rochon-Duvigneaud: Decreased corneal sensitivity, optic nerve involvement, visual loss, ophthalmoplegia, lid edema—decreased sensitivity area V

Rollet: Corneal anesthesia, pain V, exophthalmos, ptosis, ophthalmoplegia, optic nerve involvement—hyperesthesia or anesthesia of forehead, vasomotor disturbances

Romberg: Keratitis, cataract, heterochromia irides, choroiditis, ptosis, paralysis ocular muscles—atrophy soft tissue one side of face, neuralgia V, seizures

Rubella: Corneal opacities, cataract, glaucoma, optic atrophy—low birth weight, diarrhea, urinary infection, involuntary movements

Schaumann: Band shaped keratitis, granulomatous uveitis, retinopathy—fatigue, lymphadenopathy

Scheie: Diffuse corneal clouding, possible retinopathy with nightblindness and ring scotoma—broad facies, limited motion, thickened joints, aortic valvular disease

Sjögren: Keratoconjunctivitis sicca, photophobia, blurred vision, decreased lacrimation—dryness of mucous membranes, polyarthritis, muscle weakness

Trisomy—18: Unilateral ptosis, corneal opacities—mental retardation, small mandible, low set ears, flexion of fingers

Turner: Oval cornea, exophthalmos, ptosis, strabismus, retinal pigment disturbances—webbed neck, diminished growth, mental retardation, deafness

Uveitis-rheumatoid arthritis syndrome: Band Shaped keratopathy, uveitis, scleritis, choroiditis—rheumatoid arthritis

Wilson: Corneal ring, nightblindness—liver cirrhosis, jaundice, muscular rigidity, tremor

Iris

Adie: Enlarged pupil with diminished reaction—loss of tendon reflexes

Argyll Robertson: Absent pupil reaction, absent lid reflex—syphilis of CNS, general paresis, tabes dorsalis

Babinski-Nageotte: Miosis, enophthalmos, ptosis, nystagmus—hemiparesis, disturbance of sensibility, hemiataxia

Behcet: Iritis, kerato-conjunctivitis, recurrent uveitis, visual loss—aphthous lesions of mucous membranes, erythema, urethritis, CNS symptoms

Cestan-Chenais: Miosis, enophthalmos, ptosis, nystagmus—pharyngolaryngeal paralysis, cerebellar hemiataxia

Charcot-Marie-Tooth: Pupillary disturbances, nystagmus, decreased visual acuity, optic atrophy—atrophy of small muscles of hands and feet

Chediak-Higashi: Decreased uveal pigmentation, corneal edema, elevated optic disc—hepatosplenomegaly, lymphadenopathy, oculo-cutaneous albinism

Déjerine-Klumpke: Miosis, enophthalmos, ptosis—paralysis and atrophy of small muscles of hand and forearm

de Lange: Anisocoria, myopia, antimongoloid fissure slant, telecanthus—mental retardation, skeletal abnormalities, hirsutism

Ellis-van Crefeld: Iris coloboma, congenital cataract, strabismus—polydactyly, skeletal anomalies, congenital heart defects (50%), genital anomalies

Frenkel: Mydriasis, iridoplegia, subluxated lens, retinal pigmentary changes

Fuchs (1): Heterochromia, cyclitis, cataract, ant. chamber activity, corneal opacities, choroiditis

Guillain-Barré: Dilated pupils, facial nerve palsy, ophthalmoplegia, optic nerve involvement—polyneuritis, absent tendon reflexes, paralysis, facial diplegia

Hemifacial microsomia: Iris coloboma, strabismus, microphthalmos—microtia, macrostomia, failure of development of mandibular ramus and condyle

Herrenschwand, von: Heterochromia, enophthalmos, miosis, ptosis—decrease of sweating ipsilateral side of face

Horner: Miosis, decreased iris pigmentation, lacrimation, enophthalmos, ptosis—anhidrosis, facial hemiatrophy

Hunter: Deposition of abnormal mucopolysaccharides in iris, ciliary body, corneal endothelium and sclera, retinal pigment degeneration, nightblindness—dwarfism, hepatosplenomegaly, deafness, gargoyle-like facies

Lowe: Absent pupil reaction, nystagmus, cong. glaucoma—mental retardation, osteomalacia, acidosis

Meyer-Schwickerath-Weyers: Iris anomalies, glaucoma, microphthalmos, microcornea, short lid aperture—hypoplastic alae nasi, skeletal anomalies of hands and feet, sparse hair growth

Naffziger: Small pupil, ptosis—weakness ipsilateral hand grip, reduced biceps reflex

Pancoast: Miosis, ptosis, enophthalmos—pulmonary apical tumor, paresthesias

Parinaud: Displaced pupils, ptosis, nystagmus, muscle palsies, papilledema—vertigo, ataxia

Parkinson: Sluggish pupil reaction, mydriasis, anisocoria, nystagmus, diplopia, blepharospasm—rhythmical tremor, slowness of movements, 'cog wheel' rigidity of arms, loss of facial expression

Raeder: Miosis, enophthalmos, ptosis, diplopia, epiphora, scotoma, hypotony—facial pain

Recklinghausen von: Iris nodules, corneal and conjunctival nodules, cataract, retinopathy—café-au-laît spots, fibromata, spontaneous fractures

Reiter: Iritis, purulent conjunctivitis, keratitis—genital ulcerations, urethritis, lymphadenopathy, anorexia

Riegers: Iris hypoplasia, microcornea, corneal opacities, dislocated lens, congenital glaucoma, optic atrophy—broad face, supression of dentation, undeveloped maxilla

Romberg: Heterochromia irides, iritis, absent pupil reflex, keratitis, cataract, ptosis, paralysis ocular muscles—atrophy soft tissue one side of face, neuralgia V, seizures

Sylvian: Pupillary disturbances, nystagmus, muscle palsies

Takayasu: Iris atrophy, cataract, retinal microaneurysms, optic atrophy—decreased pulsation arteries, facial atrophy, seizures, fatigue

Trisomy 13–15 (D-Trisomy): Iris coloboma, optic nerve coloboma, shallow orbits, microphthalmia—hemangiomata, polydactyly, cerebral defects, horizontal palm creases

Waardenburg: Heterochromia, wide PD, epicanthus—congenital deafness, broad nasal root

Wallenberg: Miosis, enophthalmos, ptosis, nystagmus, diplopia—nausea, ataxia, muscular hypotonicity, hypoesthesia

Weber: Fixed, dilated pupil, ptosis, palsy III—hemiplegia, paralysis of face and tongue

Lens

Addison: Cataracts, keratoconjunctivitis, retinopathy, papilledema, ptosis—moniliasis, tetany, weakness, skin pigmentation, seizures

Alport: Subcapsular cataracts, anterior lenticonus, thinning of lens capsule, fundus albi punctatus—hemorrhagic nephritis, progressive deafness

Apert: Cataract, keratitis, ptosis, optic atrophy, nystagmus—tower skull, syndactyly, synostoses headaches, convulsions

223

Bloch-Sulzberger: Cataract, orbital mass, nystagmus, strabismus, optic atrophy, pseudoglioma—skin pigmentation, alopecia, dental anomalies

Bonnevie-Ullrich: Congenital cataract, absent lacrimal glands and carunculae, ocular muscle palsies, ptosis—hyperelastic skin, pterygium colli, hypertrichosis, skeletal anomalies

Cockayne: Cataract, pigmentary degeneration of retina, optic atrophy—dwarfism, deafness, mental retardation

Crouzon: Cataract, keratitis, nystagmus, optic atrophy—maxillary hypoplasia, hydrocephalus internus, short a—p skull diameter

Down: Lens opacities, myopia, nystagmus, slanted eyelid fissures, epicanthus—mental retardation, heart anomalies, skeletal abnormalities

Ehlers-Danlos: Subluxated lens, thin cornea and sclera, keratoconus, ptosis, strabismus, retinopathy—cutaneous hyperelasticity, thin skin, articular laxity, luxations

Ellis—van Crefeld: Congenital cataract, iris coloboma, strabismus—polydactyly, skeletal and gential anomalies, congenital heart defect (50%)

Frenkel: Subluxated lens, retinal pigmentary changes, mydriasis

Fuchs (1): Cataract, heterochromia, cyclitis

Gorlin-Goltz: Congenital cataract, leukoma, glaucoma, strabismus, hypertelorism—basal cell nevi, cysts of the jaws, vertebral and other skeletal anomalies

Hallermann-Streiff: Congenital cataracts, nystagmus, microphthalmos—malformations of skull, facial skeleton, dental anomalies, mental retardation

Hallgren: Cataract, retinitis pigmentosa, optic atrophy, nightblindness to complete blindness, visual field contraction—deafness, ataxia, mental and skeletal deficiencies

Homocystinuria: Dislocated lens—mental retardation, arachnodactyly, sparseness of hair

Laurence-Moon-Bardet-Biedl: Cataract, keratoconus, nystagmus, retinopathy, visual loss—obesity, hypogenitalism, polydactyly, turricephalia

Marchesani: Lens dislocation, myopia, glaucoma—brachydactyly, reduced growth, short neck, hearing defect

Marfan: Lens dislocation, coloboma, myopia, strabismus, nystagmus—arachnodactyly, congenital heart disease, muscular underdevelopment

Riegers: Dislocated lens, corneal opacities, microcornea, congenital glaucoma, iris hypoplasia, optic atrophy—broad face, suppression of dentation, underdeveloped maxilla

Romberg: Cataract, keratitis, iritis, choroiditis, ptosis, paralysis ocular muscles—atrophy soft tissue one side of face, neuralgia V, seizures

Rothmund: Bilateral cataracts— hypogenitalism, telangiectasia, skin pigmentation

Rubella: Cataract, corneal opacities, glaucoma, optic atrophy—low birth weight, diarrhea, urinary infections, involuntary movements

Takayasu: Cataract, iris atrophy, retinal micro aneurysms, optic atrophy—decreased arterial pulsation, facial atrophy, seizures, fatigue

Werner: Cataract, absent eye lashes—leanness, short fingers, atrophic skin, osteoporosis, thyroid dysfunction

Sclera

Crouzon: Bluish sclera, exophthalmos, strabismus, papilledema—prognathism, maxillar atrophy, deformity anterior fontanel

Ehlers-Danlos: Bluish thin sclera, keratoconus, subluxated lens, strabismus,

224

hypotony of extraocular muscles, increased intraocular tension, ptosis, retinopathy—cutaneous hyperelasticity, skin atrophy, excessive articular laxity

Felty: Scleritis, keratitis—rheumatoid arthritis, splenomegaly, leukopenia, oral lesions

Herrick: Scleral icterus, conjunctival telangiectasis, vitreous hemorrhages, retinopathy—severe anemia, joint pain, hepatosplenomegaly, cardiomegaly

Hoeve, van der: Bluish sclera, keratoconus—brittle bones, deafness, hyperflexible ligaments,

Recklinghausen, von: Nodular swelling of ciliary nerves, proptosis, ptosis, muscle palsies, hydrophthalmos—nodular swellings, café-au-laît spots, spontaneous fractures, fibromata

Uveitis-rheumatoid arthritis: Scleritis, uveitis, band-shaped keratopathy, choroidal inflammation—rheumatoid arthritis

Uveitis

Harada: Uveitis, visual loss, choroiditis, retinal detachment—headaches, vomiting, deafness

Heerfordt: Granulomatous uveitis—parotid gland swelling, lymphadenopathy, slight fever

Schaumann: Uveitis, keratitis, retinopathy—lymphadenopathy, fatigue

Uveitis-rheumatoid arthritis syndrome: Uveitis, keratitis, scleritis, choroiditis—rheumatoid arthritis

Vogt-Koyanagi: Uveitis, glaucoma, retinal detachment, choroiditis—alopecia, vitiligo, hearing defect

FUNDUS

Choroid

Bing: Chorioretinitis, glaucoma, ptosis, paralysis extraocular muscles

Degos: Choroiditis, atrophic skin of eye lids, conjunctival telangiectasis—white skin lesions, anorexia, gastrointestinal involvement

Fuchs(1): Choroiditis, heterochromia, cataract

Harada: Choroiditis, retinopathy, uveitis—headaches, deafness, meningeal irritation

Hemifacial microsomia: Choroidal coloboma, iris coloboma, strabismus, microphthalmos—microtia, macrostomia, failure of development of mandibular ramus and condyle

Laurence-Moon-Bardet-Biedl: Choroiditis, retinitis pigmentsoa, optic atrophy, nystagmus, strabismus, visual loss, scotoma, ant. segm. involvement—obesity, hypogenitalism, polydactyly, mental retardation

Romberg: Choroiditis, keratitis, iritis, cataract, ptosis, paralysis ocular muscles—atrophy soft tissue one side of face, neuralgia V, seizures

Sabin-Feldman: Chorioretinal degenerative changes—cerebral calcifications, convulsions

Siegrist: Choroiditis, exophthalmos—hypertension, albuminuria

Uveitis-rheumatoid arthritis syndrome: Choroiditis, uveitis, keratitis—rheumatoid arthritis

Vogt-Koyanagi: Exudative choroiditis, uveitis, retinal detachment, glaucoma—alopecia, hearing defect

Optic Nerve

Addison: Papilledema, retinopathy, cataract, keratoconjunctivitis—moniliasis, tetany, weakness, skin pigmentation, seizures

Albright: Papilledema, optic atrophy, proptosis, field defects—osteo fibrosa cystica, skin pigmentations, endocrine dysfunctions

Apert: Optic atrophy, exophthalmos, ptosis, strabismus, nystagmus, visual loss, field defects, keratitis—tower skull, syndactyly

Arnold-Chiari: Papilledema, nystagmus, diplopia, field defects—spina bifida, hydrocephalus, cerebral ataxia, pyramidal tract signs

Batten-Mayou: Optic atrophy, retinal pigment disturbance, decreasing vision—mental disturbances, palsies, convulsions

Behr: Temporal optic nerve atrophy, nystagmus—pyramidal tract signs, mental deficiency

Bloch-Sulzberger: Optic atrophy, papillitis, retinal pseudoglioma, orbital mass, nystagmus, cataract—alopecia in females, dental anomalies, skin pigmentations

Carotid artery-cavernous sinus fistula syndrome: Papilledema (see Fundus— Retina)—unilateral headaches, carotid artery sign

Central nervous system deficiency syndrome: Bitemporal pallor of the disc, reduced vision—deafness, tinnitus, numbness in legs

Charcot-Marie-Tooth: Optic atrophy, nystagmus, decreased visual acuity, pupillary disturbanecs —atrophy of small muscels

Cockayne: Optic atrophy, retinal pigmentary degeneration—dwarfism, deafness, mental retardation

Crouzon: Papilledema, optic atrophy, exophthalmos, nystagmus, strabismus, visual loss, field defects, keratitis—synostosis of skull suture lines, subnormal mentality, widening temporal fossa

Cushing (1): Optic atrophy, ocular muscle palsy, visual field changes—obesity, hirsutism, hypertension, skin pigmentation

Cushing (3): Optic atrophy, field defects

Dandy-Walker: Papilledema, ptosis, paralysis VI

Devic: Optic neuritis, optic atrophy, visual loss, field defects—ascending myelitis, weakness

Empty sella: Optic atrophy, visual field defects, reduced vision—acromegalic features

Feer: Choked disc, optic neuritis, proptosis, lacrimation, keratitis, conjunctivitis—irritability, muscle hypotony, rapid pulse, exanthema with exfoliation of palms and soles

Foix: Optic atrophy, proptosis, lid edema, paresis III, IV, V, VI, chemosis— less distended external jugular vein on affected side

Foster Kennedy: Optic atrophy, contralateral papilledema, central scotoma— anosmia

Frankl-Hochwart: Choked disc, limitation upward gaze, field defects— bilateral deafness, ataxia, hypopituitarism

Fröhlich: Papilledema, optic atrophy, impaired scotopic vision, field defects— adiposity, genital hypoplasia, polydypsia

Gradenigro: Optic nerve involvement, spasm III, IV, paralysis VI, pain V— inner ear infection, mastoiditis

Greig: Optic atrophy, enophthalmos, epicanthus, palsy VI, astigmatism— skull malformations, mental impairment

Guillain-Barré: Optic neuritis, papilledema, paralysis V, ophthalmoplegia, fixed pupil—polyneuritis, facial diplegia

Hallgren: Optic atrophy, retinitis rigmentosa, cataract, nightblindness to complete blindness, visual field contraction—deafness, ataxia, mental and skeletal deficiencies

Hand-Schüller-Christian: Papilledema, optic atrophy, exophthalmos, xanthelasma, nystagmus, retinal pathology—xanthoma of skin, skull defects, lymph adenopathy, hepatosplenomegaly

Hunter: Optic atrophy, macular edema, retinal pigmentary degeneration—dwarfism, hepatosplenomegaly

Hurler: Optic atrophy, macular edema, ptosis, strabismus, glaucoma, corneal opacity—kyphosis, abdominal pretuberance, infantilism

Hutchinson: Papilledema, subconjunctival hemorrhage, exophthalmos, lid hematoma—anemia, increased sedimentation rate, occasional abdominal tumor

Jacod: Optic atrophy, ophthalmoplegia, trigeminal neuralgia—trigeminal neuralgia, lymph node swelling

Kloepfer: Optic atrophy—blistering in sunlight, dementia

Laurence-Moon-Bardet-Biedl: Optic atrophy, retinitis pigmentosa, choroidal atrophy, nystagmus, strabismus, visual loss, scotoma, ant. segm. involvement—obesity, hypogenitalism, reduced intelligence

Leber: Optic neuritis, optic atrophy, retinopathy, visual loss—headaches, vertigo

Morgagni: Optic nerve injury, field loss—hyperostosis, obesity, headache, vertigo

Naegeli: Papillitis, optic atrophy, pseudoglioma, nystagmus, strabismus—skin changes, dental abnormalities, keratosis

Oculo-oro-genital syndrome: Optic atrophy, conjunctivitis, keratitis—stomatitis, dermatitis

Parinaud: Papilledema, ptosis, diplopia, displaced pupils—vertigo, ataxia

Pelizaeus-Merzbacher: Optic atrophy, retinitis pigmentosa, nystagmus—retarded development, athetosis, abnormal reflexes, spastic paralysis, hearing and speech disturbances

Recklinghausen von: Optic atrophy, papilledema, retinal nodules, choroiditis, proptosis, ptosis, muscle palsies, hydrophthalmos, ant. segm. involvement—café-au-lait skin pigmentation, fibromata, spontaneous fractures

Retinohypophysary syndrome: Optic neuritis, optic atrophy, narrow retinal vessels, reduced vision, field defects—glycosuria, headaches, vertigo, psychic disturbances

Riegers: Optic atrophy, congenital glaucoma, dislocated lens, microcornea, corneal opacities, iris hypoplasia—broad face, supression of dentation, underdeveloped maxilla

Rochon-Duvigneaud: Optic atrophy, visual loss, decreased corneal sensitivity, ophthalmoplegia, lid edema—decreased sensitivity area V

Rollet: Optic atrophy, optic neuritis, papilledema, exophthalmos, ptosis, ophthalmoplegia, visual loss, pain V—vasomotor disturbances, hyperesthesia of the forehead

Rubella: Optic atrophy, corneal opacities, cataract, glaucoma—low birth weight, diarrhea, urinary infections, involuntary movements

Schilder: Papilledema, optic atrophy, nystagmus, visual loss, hemianopsia—spastic paralysis, irritability, scanning speech

Symonds: Papilledema, optic atrophy, retinal hemorrhages, diplopia—mastoiditis, meningitis, drowsiness

Takayasu: Optic atrophy, retinal micro aneurysms, cataract, iris atrophy—decreased pulsation of arteries, facial atrophy, seizures, fatigue

Tay-Sachs: Optic atrophy, retinal pigmentary changes, macular cherry red spot, visual loss, nystagmus, strabismus—mental retardation, convulsions, flaccid muscles becoming spastic with progression

Temporal arteritis: Optic atrophy, retinal detachment, choroidal exudates, diplopia, visual loss, photophobia—headache, painful temporal area, malaise

Tolosa-Hunt: Optic atrophy with visual loss, scotomata, sluggish pupil reaction, ptosis, ophthalmoplegia

Trisomy-13-15: Optic atrophy, retinal dysplasia, lens opacities, microphthalmia—hemangiomata, cerebral defects, cleft lip and palate

Waldenström: Papilledema, retinopathy—adenopathy, dyspnoe, vasospasm

Retina

Addison: Retinal hemorrhages, papilledema, cataract, keratocojunctivitis—moniliasis, tetany, weakness, skin pigmentation, seizures

Alport: Fundus albi punctatus, bilateral cataracts, anterior lenticonus—hemorrhagic nephritis, progressive nerve deafness

Amaurosis fugax: Retinal arterial spasm, partial to complete blindness—hypertension

Bassen-Kornzweig: Retinitis pigmentosa—steatorrhea, acanthocytosis, neuropathy

Batten-Mayou: Retinal pigment disturbances, optic atrophy, decreasing vision—amaurotic idiocy, convulsions

Behcet: Retinal thrombophlebitis, muscle palsies, visual loss, ant. segment involvement—skin lesions, ulcerations of mucous membranes

Bonnet-Dechaume-Blanc: Angiomatosis, arteriovenous-angiomas—angiomata of mesencephalon and thalamus

Bourneville: Retinal tumor, hemorrhages, cystic changes, cloudy vitreous—adenoma sebaceum, epilepsy, mental deficiency

Carotid artery—cavernous sinus fistula syndrome: Retinal edema, hemorrhages, papilledema, exophthalmos, ophthalmoplegia, glaucoma—unilateral headache, subjective buzzing intracranial noise

Cockayne: Retinal pigmentary degeneration, optic atrophy—dwarfism, deafness, mental retardation

Cone dysfunction syndrome: Macular degenerative changes, field defects, decreased visual acuity

de Lange: Pallor of optic disc, anisocoria, myopia, telecanthus, antimongoloid fissure slant—mental retardation, skeletal abnormalities, hirsutism

Dialinas-Amalric: Atypical retinitis pigmentosa—deaf mutism

Ehlers-Danlos: Angioid streaks, retinitis, chorioretinal hemorrhages, retinitis proliferans with secondary ablatio, thin sclera and cornea, ptosis, strabismus, hypotonic skin of the lids, subluxated lens—cutaneous hyperelasticity, atrophic skin, excessive articular laxity

Fabry-Anderson: Aneurysmal dialtations of retinal vessels, conjunctival varicositis, corneal opacities—angiokeratoma of the skin, elevated blood pressure, albuminuria

Frenkel: Retinal pigment disturbance, hyphema, lens subluxation

Gaucher: Macular infiltration, pinguecula—infantile form: hypertonia, opisthotonus, cachexia; chronic form: hepatosplenomegaly, skin pigmentation, lymphadenopathy

Groenblad-Strandberg: Angioid streaks, macular involvement, corneal involvement—pseudoxanthoma elasticum

Hallgren: Retinitis pigmentosa, retinal atrophy, optic atrophy, nightblindness to complete blindness, visual field contraction, cataract—deafness, ataxia, mental and skeletal deficiencies

Hand-Schüller-Christian: Retinal hemorrhages and exudates, papilledema, expohthalmos, xanthelasma, ophthalmoplegia—skin xanthomatosis, diabetes insipidus, skull defects

Harada: Retinal detachment, retinal edema, retinal pigment changes, choroiditis, uveitis, visual loss—meningeal irritation

Herrick: Retinal neovascularization, microaneurysms, retinitis proliferans, hemorrhages and exudates, scleral icterus, conjunctival telangiectasis, vitreous hemorrhages—severe anemia, joint pain, hepatosplenomegaly, cardiomegaly

Hippel-Lindau, von: Retinal angiomatosis, vitreous hemorrhages, secondary glaucoma—cerebral angiomatosis, epilepsy, psychic disturbances

Hunter: Retinal pigment degeneration, nightblindness, ERG and EOG changes, deposition of abnormal mucopolysaccharides in iris, ciliary body and corneal endothelium—dwarfism, hepatosplenomegaly, deafness, gargoyle-like facies

Laurence-Moon-Bardet-Biedl: Retinitis pigmentosa choroiditis, optic atrophy, nystagmus, strabismus, visual loss, scotoma, ant. segm. involvement—obesity, hypogenitalism, polydactyly, mental deficiency

Leber: Retinal hemorrhages, exudates and edema, optic neuritis and atrophy, visual loss—vertigo, headaches

Marfan: Retinal detachment, strabismus, nystagmus, myopia, glaucoma, lens involvement—arachnodactyly, congenital heart defects, relaxed ligaments

Niemann-Pick: Red macular spot, reduced vision, optic atrophy—mental retardation, epileptic seizures, hepatosplenomegaly, deafness, skin pigmentation

Ophthalmoplegic-retinal degeneration: Retinitis pigmentosa, ptosis, ocular myopathy—progressive muscular dystrophy (possible)

Pelizaeus-Merzbacher: Tapetoretinal degeneration, optic atrophy, nystagmus—retarded development, athetosis, abnormal reflexes, spastic paralysis, hearing and speech disturbances

Pierre Robin: Retinal disinsertion, myopia, glaucoma—micrognathia, cleft palate

Refsum: Retinal degeneration, constricted fields, nightblindness, pupillary changes—ataxia, polyneuritis, deafness, CNS degeneration

Sanfillipo-Good: Retinal pigmentary changes, nightblindness may exist—mental deficiency, seizures

Schaumann: Inflammatory retinal exudates, uveitis, vitreous floaters, keratitis—hilar nodes, lymphadenopathy

Sjögren-Larsson: Chorioretinitis with macular pigment degeneration, reduced visual acuity—oligophrenia, ichthyosis, epilepsy, osseous dysplasia, speech defect, hyperreflexia

Sturge-Weber: Retinal glioma, choroidal angioma, hydrophthalmos—skin vascular nevi, symptoms of CNS involvement

Takayasu: Retinal micro aneurysms, cataract, iris atrophy, optic atrophy—decreased arterial pulsation, facial atrophy, seizures, fatigue

Tapetal-like reflex: Retinitis pigmentosa, bright reflex from posterior fundus, ring scotoma

Tay-Sachs: Retinal pigmentary changes, macular cherry red spot, optic atrophy, visual loss, nystagmus, strabismus—mental retardation, convulsions, flaccid muscles becoming spastic with progression

Temporal arteritis: Retinal detachment, choroidal exudates and hemorrhages, optic atrophy, diplopia, visual loss, photophobia—hyperalgesia of the scalp, pain temporal region

Turner: Deficiency of retinal pigment, oval corneae, exophthalmos, ptosis, strabismus—webbed neck, deafness, diminished growth

Unverrichts: Retinopathy, amaurosis—myoclonus, epilepsy, dementia, pseudobulbar palsy
Usher: Retinitis pigmentosa (atypical), possible visual field constriction—deaf mutism
Uyemura: White spots of the retina, nightblindness, conjunctival xerosis, Bitot' spots
Vermis: Papilledema, nystagmus—vomiting, enlarged head, incoordination
Vogt-Koyanagi: Serous retinal detachment, exudative choroiditis, uveitis, glaucoma—alopecia, poliosis, hearing defect
Waldenström: Retinal hemorrhages and exudates, papilledema—adenopathy, vasospasm of extremities, dyspnea

INTRAOCULAR TENSION

Glaucoma

Axenfeld: Glaucoma, angle pathology, corneal changes
Bing: Glaucoma, chorioretinitis, ptosis, paralysis extraocular muscles
Carotid artery-cavernous sinus fistula syndrome: Sec. glaucoma, exophthalmos, ophthalmoplegia, optic nerve involvement, retinopathy—unilateral headache, subjective buzzing intracranial noise
Ehlers-Danlos: Increased intraocular tension, bluish sclera, keratoconus, microcornea, strabismus, subluxated lens, hypotony of lid skin, ptosis, retinopathy—cutaneous hyperelasticity atrophic skin, excessive articular laxity
Gorlin-Goltz: Glaucoma, congenital cataract, leucoma, strabismus, hypertelorism—basal cell nevi, cysts of the jaws, vertebral and other skeletal anomalies
Hippel-Lindau, von: Secondary glaucoma, retinal angiomatosis, vitreous hemorrhages—cerebral angiomatosis, epilepsy, psychic disturbances
Hurler: Glaucoma, ptosis, strabismus, corneal opacities, optic atrophy, macular edema—retarded normal development, dorso lumbar kyphosis, head deformities
Lowe: Cong. glaucoma, nystagmus, ant. segment involvement, a. o.—mental retardation, acidosis, osteomalacia
Marchesani: Glaucoma, myopia, lens involvement—brachydactyly, reduced growth
Marfan: Glaucoma, nystagmus, strabismus, myopia, anterior segm. involvement—arachnodactyly, congenital heart defects, relaxed ligaments
Meyer-Schwickerath-Weyers: Glaucoma, iris anomalies, microphthalmos, short lid aperture—thin nose with hypoplastic alae, skeletal anomalies of hands and feet, sparse hair growth
Pierre Robin: Cong. glaucoma, myopia, retinal disinsertion—micrognathia, cleft palate
Posner-Schlossman: Glaucomatocyclitic crisis, anisocoria, blurring of vision—allergy
Recklinghausen, von: Hydrophthalmos, proptosis, ptosis, muscle palsies, ant. segment involvement, optic atrophy, retinopathy—nodular swelling, café-su-laît spots, spontaneous fractures, fibromata
Riegers: Congenital glaucoma, dislocated lens, microcornea, corneal opacities, iris hypoplasia, optic atrophy—broad face, suppression of dentation, underdeveloped maxilla
Rubella: Glaucoma, cataract, corneal opacities, optic atrophy—low birth weight, diarrhea, urinary infections, involuntary movements

Sturge-Weber: Hydrophthalmos, fundus changes—skin vascular nevi, symptoms of CNS involvement

Vogt-Koyanagi: Sec. glaucoma, uveitis, retinal detachment, choroiditis—hearing defects, alopecia, poliosis

Hypotony

Horner: Hypotony, enophthalmos, ptosis, lacrimation, miosis—anhidrosis, facial hemiatrophy

Raeder: Hypotony, enophthalmos, ptosis, diplopia, epiphora, scotoma, miosis—facial pain

LACRIMAL APPARATUS

Ascher: Protrusion lacrimal gland, lack of tone of orbital fascia, blepharochalasis—goiter, reduplication upper lip

Bogorad: Lacrimation while eating—excessive salivation

Bonnevie-Ullrich: Absent lacrimal glands and carunculae, congenital cataract, ocular muscle palsies, ptosis—hyperelastic skin, pterygium colli, hypertrichosis, skeletal anomalies

Cogan: Lacrimation, blepharospasm, keratitis, subconj. hemorrhages—vestibuloauditory symptoms

Crouzon: Develop. anomalies of lacrimal apparatus, exophthalmos, oblique lid fissures, nystagmus, strabismus, visual loss, field defects, anterior segment involvement, papilledema, sec. optic atrophy—prognathism, maxillar atrophy, deformity anterior fontanel

Feer: Lacrimation, proptosis, photophobia, keratitis, optic nerve involvement—muscle hypotony, irritability, profuse sweating, skin exfoliation palms and soles

Horner: Lacrimation, enophthalmos, ptosis, hypotony, miosis—anhidrosis, facial hemiatrophy

Hunt: Decreased lacrimation, decreased corneal reflex—facial palsy, hearing defect, decreased salivation

Melkerson-Rosenthal: Crocodile tear phenomenon, keratitis, corneal ulcer—chronic facial edema, facial palsy, furrowed tongue

Mikulicz-Radecki: Decreased lacrimation, bilateral enlarged lacrimal glands—enlargement of salivary glands

Morquio-Brailsford (MPS IV): Excessive lacrimation, Horner's trias, hazy cornea—dwarfism, skeletal deformities, decreased muscle tone

Page: Lacrimation—hypotension, hot flashes, tachycardia

Raeder: Lacrimation, enophthalmos, ptosis, diplopia, hypotony, miosis, field defects—facial pain

Riley-Day: Absent tear production, keratitis, corneal ulcers—excessive salivation, failure to thrive, respiratory infections, skin blotching, hyporeflexia

Sjögren: Decreased lacrimation, photophobia, keratoconjunctivitis—polyarthritis, dryness of mucous membranes

Zinsser-Engman-Cole: Obstruction lacrimal puncta, conjunctival keratinization, bullous conjunctivitis, ectropion—congenital dyskeratosis, oral lesions, anemia, hypersplenism, hyperhidrosis palms and soles

LIDS

Anomalies

Argyll Robertson: Lid reflex absent, absent pupil reaction, iris atrophy—involvement of CNS

Ascher: Blepharochalasis, lack of tone of orbital fascia, protrusion lacrimal gland—goiter, reduplication of upper lip

Crouzon: Oblique canthus, exophthalmos, nystagmus, visual loss, field defects, optic nerve involvement—prognathism, maxilla atrophy, deformity of anterior fontanel

Degos: Atrophic skin of eye lids, diplopia, conjunctival telangiectasis, choroiditis—white skin lesions, anorexia, gastrointestinal involvement

Down: Epicanthus, oblique eyelid fissures, nystagmus, myopia, lens opacities, blepharitis—mental retardation, skeletal abnormalities, heart anomalies

Duane: Narrow palpebral fissure, global retraction, motility disturbances

Elhers-Danlos: Hypotony of palpebral skin, epicanthus, ptosis, thin sclera and cornea, keratoconus, subluxated lens, retinopathy, strabismus—cutaneous hyperelasticity, atrophic skin, excessive articular laxity

Franceschetti: Lid colobomata, oblique eye position—fish-like face, high palate, abnormal dentation

Gänsslen: Epicanthus, microphthalmia, increased P.D.—splenomegaly, hemolytic crises, polydactyly, a.o.

Glodenhar: Lid coloboma, epibulbar dermoid—micrognathia, preauricular fistulae, auricular appendices, vertebral anomalies

Greig: Epicanthus, enophthalmos, 6th nerve paralysis, astigmatism, optic atrophy—mental deficiency, skull deformation

Parkinson: Fluttering eyelids, blepharospasm, nystagmus, mydriasis—loss of facial expression, "cog wheel" rigidity, tremor

Pseudo-Graefe: Delayed upper lid movement

Rubinstein-Taybi: Antimongoloid slant of lid fissure, epicanthus, highly arched brows, strabismus, refractive error—broad thumbs and toes, abnormal facial features, motor and mental retadation

Treacher Collins: Lid coloboma, lack of cilia—micrognathia, hypoplastic zygomatic arc, absence ext. ear

Waardenburg: Canthal displacement, wide P. D., heterochromia—deafness, broad nasal root, albinotic hair strain

Werner: Absence of eye lashes, cataracts—thin limbs, leanness, small mouth, stretched atrophic skin

Ectropion

Guillain-Barré: VII nerve paralysis, ectropion, pupillary disturbances, possible external ophthalmoplegia—polyneuritis, absent tendon reflexes

Zinsser-Engman-Cole: Ectropion, obstruction of lacrimal puncta, conjunctival keratinization, bullous conjunctivitis—congenital dyskeratosis, oral lesions, anemia, hypersplenism, hyperhidrosis palms and soles

Edema

Foix: Lid edema, proptosis, paralysis III, IV, VI., Chemosis, optic atrophy—external jugular vein less distended on affected side, postauricular edema

Hutchinson: Lid hematoma, subconjunctival hemorrhage, exophthalmos, papilledema—anemia, increased sedimentation rate, occasional abdominal tumor

Entropion

Congenital epiblepharon-inf. obl. insufficiency: Narrow PD, epicanthus, spastic entropion, motility disturbance, keratitis—chubby cheeks

Ptosis

Addison: Ptosis, blepharospasm, keratoconjunctivitis, cataract, retinopathy, papilledema—moniliasis, tetany, weakness, skin pigmentation, seizures

232

Apert: Ptosis, slant canthus, exophthalmos, squint, field defects, keratitis, optic atrophy—syndactyly

Babinski-Nageotte: Ptosis, enophthalmos, nystagmus, miosis—cerebellar hemiataxia, hemiparesis

Bing: Bilateral ptosis, chorioretinitis, glaucoma, paralysis extraocular muscles

Cestan-Chenais: Ptosis, enophthalmos, nystagmus, miosis—flaccid paralysis of soft palate and vocal cord, contralateral hemiplegia, ataxia

Cushing (2): Paresis VII and VI, nystagmus, decreased corneal reflex—tinnitus, deafness, defect in labyrinth function

Dandy-Walker: Ptosis, six nerve palsy, optic nerve involvement—hydrocephalus

Déjerine-Klumpke: Ptosis, enophthalmos, miosis—paralysis and atrophy of small muscles of upper extremities

Ehlers-Danlos: Hyperelasticity of palpebral skin, ptosis, epicanthus, hypotony extraocular muscles, glaucoma, thin sclera and cornea, keratoconus, subluxated lens, retinopathy—cutaneous hyperelasticity, atrophic skin, excessive articular laxity

Erb-Goldflam: Ptosis, strabismus, diplopia—myasthenia gravis, muscle weakness

Herrenschwand, von: Ptosis (sympathetic), enophthalmos, miosis, heterochromia—decreased sweating ipsilateral side of face

Horner: Ptosis, enophthalmos, lacrimation, miosis—anhidrosis, facial hemiatrophy

Hurler: Ptosis, squint, corneal involvement, optic nerve involvement—retarded development, dorso-lumbar kyphosis ,head deformities

Marcus Gunn: Ptosis, VI nerve palsy, lid elevates with movement of the mandible

Moebius: Ptosis, proptosis, muscle involvement—facial diplegia, deafness, digital defects

Naffziger: Ptosis, miosis—reduced strength of hand grip

Noonan: Ptosis, hypertelorism, exophthalmos—valvular pulmonary stenosis, short stature, webbed neck, cubitus valgus, micrognathia

Ophthalmoplegic-retinal degeneration: Ptosis, ocular myopathy, retinitis pigmentosa—progressive muscular dystrophy (possible)

Pancoast: Ptosis, enophthalmos, miosis—shoulder pain, paresthesia arm and hand

Parinaud: Ptosis, diplopia, displaced pupils, papilledema—vertigo

Raeder: Ptosis, enophthalmos, diplopia, scotoma, miosis—facial pain

Recklinghausen, von: Ptosis, proptosis, muscle palsies, hydrophthalmos, ant. segm. and uveal involvement, optic nerve involvement—nodular swellings, café-au-laît spots, spontaneous fractures, fibromata

Rollet: Ptosis, exophthalmos, diplopia, optic nerve involvement—vasomotor disturbances, hyperaesthesias

Romberg: Ptosis, paralysis ocular muscles, keratitis, iritis, choroiditis, cataract—atrophy soft tissue one side of face, neuralgia V, seizures

Tolosa-Hunt: Ptosis, ophthalmoplegia, retroorbital pain, scotomata, visual loss, sluggish pupil reaction

Trisomy—18: Unilateral ptosis, corneal opacities—mental retardation, face anomalies, failure of flexion of fingers

Turner: Ptosis, exophthalmos, squint, retinal involvement—webbed neck, deafness, diminished growth

Wallenberg: Ptosis, enophthalmos, diplopia, miosis—nausea, difficulty in speaking and swallowing

Weber: Ptosis, 3rd nerve palsy, fixed pupil—hemiplegia, paralysis face and tongue

Wernicke: Ptosis, ophthalmoplegia—peripheral neuritis, ataxia, mental disturbances

Spasm

Cogan: Blepharospasm, lacrimation, blurred vision, conj. congestion, keratitis—vestibuloauditory symptoms

Koerber-Salus-Elschnig: Lid retraction, nystagmus, muscle palsies—headaches, hypertension, hemiparesis, ataxia

Parkinson: Blepharospasm, nystagmus, diplopia, sluggish pupil reaction—rhythmical tremor, 'cog wheel' rigidity of arms, loss of facial expression

Xanthelasma

Hand-Schüller-Christian: Xanthelasma, exophthalmos, nystagmus, corneal degeneration, optic nerve involvement, retinal exudates—skin xanthomatosis, diabetes insipidus, skull defects

MOTILITY

Anomalies

de Lange: Antimongoloid fissure slant, telecanthus, myopia, anisocoria, pale optic disc—mental retardation, skeletal abnormalities, hirsutism

Duane: Global retraction, narrowing of palpebral fissure

Nystagmus and Strabismus

Apert: Strabismus, nystagmus, exophthalmos, slant fissure, field defect, keratitis, optic atrophy—syndactyly

Arnold-Chiari: Nystagmus, diplopia, hemianopsia, papilledema—pyramidal tract signs, vertebral malformations

Babinski-Nageotte: Nystagmus, enophthalmos, ptosis, miosis—cerebellar hemiataxia, hemiparesis

Behr: Nystagmus, partial optic atrophy—abortive hereditary ataxia, mental deficiency

Bielschowsky-Lutz-Cogan: Dissociated nystagmus, unilateral or bilateral ext. ocular muscle palsies

Bing: Paralysis extraocular muscles, ptosis, chorioretinitis, glaucoma

Bloch-Sulzberger: Nystagmus, strabismus, cataract, optic nerve involvement—bullous skin eruptions and pigmentations

Cestan-Chenais: Nystagmus, ptosis, enophthalmos, miosis—flaccid paralysis of soft palate and vocal cord, ataxia, contralateral hemiplegia

Charcot-Marie-Tooth: Nystagmus, visual loss, optic atrophy—progressive muscular atrophy

Crouzon: Nystagmus, strabismus, exophthalmos, visual loss, anterior segment involvement—prognathism, maxillar atrophy, deformity anterior fontanel

Cushing (I): Ocular muscle palsy, visual field changes, optic atrophy—obesity, hirsutism, hypertension, skin pigmentation

Down: Nystagmus, myopia, slanted eyelid fissures, lens opacities, epicanthus—mental retardation, skeletal and heart anomalies

Ehlers-Danlos: Hypotony extraocular muscles, strabismus, ptosis, hyper-

234

elastic skin, thin sclera and cornea, keratoconus, subluxated lens, retino-pathy—cutaneous hyperelasticity, atrophic skin, excessive articular laxity

Ellis—van Crefeld: Internal strabismus, congenital cataract, iris coloboma—polydactyly, skeletal and genital anomalies, congenital heart defects (50%)

Erb-Goldflam: Strabismus, ptosis, diplopia—myasthenia gravis, muscle weakness

Hallermann-Streiff: Nystagmus, strabismus, cataract, microphthalmia—malformations of skeleton, teeth anomalies, mental retardation

Hemifacial microsomia: Strabismus, microphthalmos, iris and choroidal colobomata—microtia, macrostomia, failure of development of mandibular ramus and condyle

Hennebert: Otitic nystagmus—vertigo

Hurler: Strabismus, ptosis, corneal opacity, optic nerve and retinal involve-ment—retarded development, dorso-lumbar kyphosis, head deformities

Klippel-Feil: Congenital squint—platybasia, brevicollis

Koerber-Salus-Elschnig: Nystagmus, muscle palsies, lid retraction—head-aches, hypertension, hemiparesis, ataxia

Laurence-Moon-Bardet-Biedl: Nystagmus, strabismus, ophthalmoplegia, vis. field defect, optic nerve and retinal involvement—obesity, hypogenitalism, polydactyly, mental deficiency

Lenoble-Aubineau: Nystagmus—head and limb tremor, myoclonia

Louis-Bar: Pseudoophthalmoplegia, fixation nystagmus, conjunctival tel-angiectasia—ataxia, scanning speech, hypotonia, cutaneous telangiectasis

Lowe: Nystagmus, cong. glaucoma, ant. segment involvement, a.o.—mental retardation, acidosis, osteomalacia

Marfan: Nystagmus, strabismus, anterior segment and lens involvement—arachnodactyly, congenital heart defect, relaxed ligaments

Ménière: Nystagmus—vertigo, tinnitus, progressive deafness

Millard-Gubler: Paralysis VI, diplopia, strabismus—hemiplegia of arm and leg

Naegeli: Nystagmus, strabismus, papillitis, pseudoglioma—keratosis, pig-mentary skin changes

Parkinson: Nystagmus, diplopia, blepharospasm, sluggish or absent pupil reaction—rhythmical tremor, 'cog wheel' rigidity of arms, loss of facial expression

Pelizaeus-Merzbacher: Nystagmus, retinitis pigmentosa, optic atrophy—retarded development, athetosis, abnormal reflexes, spastic paralysis, hearing and speech disturbances

Pseudohypoparathyroidism: Strabismus—obesity, short stature, tetany, mental retardation

Rubinstein-Taybi: Strabismus, antimongoloid slant of lid fissure, epicanthus, highly arched brows, refractive error—broad thumbs and toes, abnormal facial features, motor and mental retardation

Schilder: Nystagmus, extraocular palsy, visual loss, vis. field defect, optic nerve involvement—spastic paralysis, mental deficiency, tremor

Sylvian: Central nystagmus, muscle palsy, pupillary disturbances, tonic con-vergence spasm, clonic convergence movements

Tay-Sachs: Nystagmus, strabismus, optic atrophy, macular cherry red spot and retinal pigmentary changes, visual loss—mental retardation, convul-sions, flaccid muscles becoming spastic with progression

Vermis: Nystagmus, papilledema—vomiting, enlarged head, incoordination

Wallenberg: Nystagmus, diplopia, enophthalmos, ptosis, miosis—nausea, difficulty in speaking and swallowing

235

Paralysis

Axenfeld-Schürenberg: Cyclic oculomotor paralysis

Balint: Psychic paralysis of visual fixation—loss of body coordination

Behcet: Muscle palsies, nystagmus, visual loss, anterior segm. involvement, uveitis, retinopaty—ulcerations of mucous membranes, skin lesions

Benedikt: Paralysis III—contralateral hemichorea

Bielschowsky-Lutz-Cogan: Unilateral or bilateral ext. ocular muscle palsies, dissociated nystagmus

Bonnevie-Ullrich: Ocular muscle palsies, ptosis, congenital cataracts, absent lacrimal glands and curunculae—hyperelastic skin, pterygium colli, skeletal anomalies

Carotid artery—cavernous sinus fistula: Ophthalmoplegia, exophthalmos, retinal and optic nerve involvement—unilateral headache, subjective buzzing intracranial noise

Claude: Paralysis III, IV—contralateral hemianesthesia and hemiataxia

Congenital epiblepharon-inf. oblique insufficiency: Narrow PD, keratitis, epicanthus—chubby cheeks

Cushing (2): Paralysis VI, VII, nystagmus, decreased corneal reflex—tinnitus, deafness, defect in labyrinth function

Dandy-Walker: Paralysis VI, ptosis, papilledema—hydrocephalus

Dejean: Diplopia, exophthalmos—superior maxillary pain, numbness V 1 and 2

Eaton-Lambert: Ocular myoclonus, decreased visual acuity, corneal haziness—weakness, peripheral anesthesia, poor response to neostigmin

Fisher: Ophthalmoplegia (internal and external)—ataxia, loss of deep reflexes

Foix: Paralysis III, IV, V, VI, proptosis, lid edema, chemosis, optic atrophy—external jugular vein less distended on affected side, postauricular edema

Foville: Paralysis VI, nystagmus—peripheral facial palsy, Contralateral hemiplegia

Frankl-Hochwart: Limitation upward gaze, field defect, choked disc—hypopituitarism, ataxia, bilateral deafness

Gradenigro: Paralysis VI, pain V, photophobia, lacrimation—inner ear infection, mastoiditis

Greig: Paralysis VI, enophthalmos, epicanthus, astigmatism, optic atrophy—mental deficiency, skull deformation

Guillain-Barré: Ophthalmoplegia, dilated pupils—polyneuritis, absent tendon reflexes

Hand-Schüller-Christian: Ophthalmoplegia, exophthalmos, corneal degeneration, retinopathy, optic nerve involvement—skin xanthomatosis, diabetes insipidus, skull defects

Jacod: Ophthalmoplegia, neuralgia V, optic atrophy—cervical lymphadenopathy

Johnson: Pseudoparalysis of lateral or superior rectus muscle

Marcus Gunn: Paralysis VI, ptosis, lid elevates with movement of mandible

Moebius: Weakness of adductor muscles, ptosis, proptosis—facial diplegia, deafness, digital defects

Nothnagel: Oculomotor paresis—cerebellar ataxia

Oculocerebellar-tegmental syndrome: Paralysis of associated movements—hemiplegia

Ophthalmoplegic-migraine: Transitory oculomotor paralysis, supraorbital pain—migraine headache possible

Ophthalmoplegic-retinal degeneration: Ocular myopathy, ptosis, retinitis pigmentosa—progressive muscular dystrophy (possible)

Parinaud: Paralysis of conjugate upward movement, diplopia, nystagmus, displaced pupils, ptosis, papilledema—vertigo

Raeder: Diplopia, ptosis, enophthalmos, vis. field defect, hypotony, miosis—facial pain

Raymond: Paralysis VI—hemiplegia, anesthesia

Recklinghausen, von: Muscle palsies, ptosis, proptosis, hydrophthalmos, ant. segment involvement, fundus and optic nerve involvement—nodular swellings, café-au-lait spots, fibromata, spontaneous fractures

Rochon-Duvigneaud: Ophthalmoplegia, optic atrophy, visual loss, decreased corneal sensitivity—decreased sensitivity area V

Rollet: Ophthalmoplegia, exophthalmos, ptosis, vis. field defect, pain V, optic nerve involvement—vasomotor disturbances, hyperesthesias

Romberg: Paralysis extraocular muscles, ptosis, keratitis, iritis, choroiditis, cataract—atrophy soft tissue on side of face, neuralgia V, seizures

Sphenocavernous: External ophthalmoplegia, proptosis—paresis 5th nerve

Symonds: Paralysis VI, diplopia, retinal hemorrhages, optic nerve involvement—drowsiness, otitis media, meningeal involvement, headaches

Temporal arteritis: Diplopia, visual loss, photophobia, optic atrophy, retinal detachment, choroidal involvement—hyperalgesia of the scalp, pain temporal region

Tolosa-Hunt: Ophthalmoplegia (III, IV, VI), ptosis, visual loss depending on optic nerve involvement

Turner: Squint, exophthalmos, ptosis, retinal pigment deficiency—webbed neck, deafness, diminished growth

Weber: Paralysis III, ptosis, dilated pupil—hemiplegia, paralysis of face and tongue

Wernicke: Ophthalmoplegia, nystagmus—peripheral neuritis, ataxia, mental disturbances

ORBIT

Anomalies

Apert: Bilateral shallow orbits, wide PD, ptosis, squint, nystagmus, decr. vision, keratitis, optic atrophy—syndactyly

Ascher: Herniation orbital fat, blepharochalasis, protrusion lacrimal glands—goiter, reduplication upper lip

Congenital epiblepharon-inf. oblique insufficiency: Narrow PD, epicanthus, epiblepharon, entropion, inf. oblique insufficiency, keratitis, trichiasis—chubby cheeks

Franceschetti: Oblique position of eyes, lid coloboma—fish-like face, high paalte, abnormal dentation

Gänsslen: Increased PD, microphthalmia, epicanthus—splenomegaly, hemolytic crises, polydactyly

Hallermann-Streiff: Microphthalmos, nystagmus, strabismus, cataract—malformations of skeleton, teeth anomalies, mental retardation

Hemifacial microsomia: Microphthalmos, congenital cystic ophthalmia, iris and choroidal colobomata, strabismus—microtia, macrostomia, failure of development of mandibular ramus and condyle

Meyer-Schwickerath-Weyers: Microphthalmos, glaucoma, iris anomalies, short lid aperture—thin nose with hypoplastic alae skeletal anomalies of hands and feet, sparse hair growth

237

Noonan: Hypertelorism, exophthalmos, antimongoloid slanting palpebral fissures, ptosis—pulmonary stenosis, short stature, webbed neck, cubitus valgus, micrognatia

Trisomy 13–15 (D Trisomy): Microphtalmia, shallow orbits, iris coloboma, optic nerve coloboma—hemangiomata, polydactyly, cerebral defects, harelip, finger and hand anomalies

Waardenburg: Hyperplasia medial eyebrows, wide PD, lateral displacement medial canthi, heterochromia iridis—deafness, broad nasal root, albinotic hair strain

Enophthalmos

Babinski-Nageotte: Enophthalmos, ptosis, miosis, nystagmus—cerebellar ataxia, hemiparesis

Cestan-Chenais: Enophthalmos, ptosis, nystagmus, miosis—flaccid paralysis of soft palate and vocal cord, ataxia, controalateral hemiplegia

Déjerine-Klumpke: Enophthalmos, ptosis, miosis—paralysis and atrophy of small muscles of upper extremities

Greig:Enophthalmos, wide PD, epicanthus, 6th nerve palsy, astigmatism, Optic atrophy—mental deficiency, skull deformation

Herrenschwand, von: Enophthalmos, ptosis, miosis, heterochromia—decreased sweating ipsilateral side of face

Horner: Enophthalmos, ptosis, lacrimation, hypotony, miosis—anhidrosis, facial hemiatrophy

Pancoast: Enophthalmos, ptosis, miosis—shoulder pain, paresthesia arm and hand

Raeder: Mild enophthalmos, ptosis, diplopia, epiphora, scotoma, hypotonia, miosis—facial pain

Wallenberg: Enophthalmos, ptosis, miosis—nausea, difficulty in swallowing and speaking

Exophthalmos

Albright: Unilateral proptosis, vis, field defect, optic disc changes—osteitis fibrosa, skin pigmentations, endocrine dysfunction

Bloch-Sulzberger: Orbital mass, nystagmus, squint, cataract, disc changes, retinal pseudo glioma—bullous skin eruptions and pigmentations

Carotid artery-cavernous sinus fistula: Progressive exophthalmos, ophthalmoplegia, sec. glaucoma, disc changes, retinal edema and hemorrhages—unilateral headache, subjective buzzing intracranial noise

Crouzon: Bilateral exophthalmos, wide PD, oblique palpebral fissure, nystagmus, squint, visual loss, visual field defects, bluish sclera—prognathism, maxillar atrophy, defomity anterior fontanel a. o.

Dejean: Exophthalmos, diplopia—superior maxillary pain, numbness in region of 1st and 2nd branch of V.

Feer: Exophthalmos (rare), lacrimation, photophobia, conj. injection, dilated pupil, keratitis, optic disc changes—muscle hypotony, irritability, skin exfoliation on palms and soles

Foix: Proptosis, lid edema, paresis III, IV. VI, chemosis, optic atrophy—jugular vein less distended on affected side, post-auricular edema

Hand-Schüller-Christian: Exophthalmos, xanthelasma, ophthalmoplegia, corneal degeneration, optic nerve and retinal involvement—skin xanthomata, diabetes insipidus, skull defects, a.o.

Hutchinson: Exophthalmos, lid hematoma, subconjunctival hemorrhage, papilledema—anemia, increased sedimentation rate, occasional abdominal tumor

Moebius: Proptosis, ptosis, disturbance in motility—facial diplegia, deafness, digital defects

Recklinghausen, von: Proptosis, ptosis, muscle palsies, glaucoma, ant. segm. involvement, fundus changes—café-au-laît spots, nodular swelling, fibromata, spontaneous fractures

Rollet: Exophthalmos, ptosis, diplopia, visual field changes, optic nerve involvement—hyperesthesias, vaso-motor disturbances

Siegrist: Exophthalmos, choroidal changes—hypertension, albuminuria

Spheno-cavernous: Proptosis, external ophthalmoplegia—paresis 5th nerve

Turner: Exophthalmos, ptosis, squint, retinal involvement—webbed neck, deafness, diminished growth

Pain

Charlin: Severe orb. pain, pseudopurulent conj., keratitis, ant. uveitis—rhinorrhea

Ophthalmoplegic-migraine: Unilateral supraorbital pain, transitory oculomotor paralysis—migraine headache possible

Tolosa-Hunt: Retroorbital pain, ptosis, ophthalmoplegia, scotomata, visual loss depending on optic nerve involvement, sluggish rupil reaction

VISUAL ACUITY

Amaurosis fugax: Partial to complete blindness, retinal arteriolar spasm—hypertension

Anton: Blindness-confabulation, allocheiria

Apert: Decreased vision, exophthalmos, ptosis, strabismus, nystagmus, field defect, keratitis, optic atrophy—syndractyly

Arnold-Pick: Apperceptive blindness—progressive dementia, cerebral atrophy

Barré-Liéou: Transitory reduced vision, corneal hypesthesia—headaches, vasomotor disturbances of face, ear noises, impaired memory

Batten-Mayou: Progressive to total blindness, optic atrophy, retinal pigment disturbances—amaurotic idiocy, convulsions

Behcet: Gradual loss of vision, muscle palsies, nystagmus, ant. segment involvement, retinopathy—ulcerations of mucous membranes, skin lesions

Central nervous system deficiency: Reduced vision, bitemporal pallor of disc—deafness, tinnitus, unsteady gait, tingling in legs

Charcot-Marie-Tooth: Reduced vision, optic atrophy, nystagmus—progressive muscular dystrophy

Charcot-Wilbrand: Visual agnosia, loss of ability to revisualize images

Cogan: Blurred vision, blepharospasm, lacrimation, anterior segment involevment—vestibuloauditory symptoms

Cone dysfunction syndrome: Reduced or absent color vision, decreased vision, retinopathy

Crouzon: Decreased vision, exophthalmos, nystagmus, strabismus, field defects, ant. segment and optic nerve involvement—prognathism, maxillary atrophy, deformity anterior fontanel, a.o.

Devic: Progressive visual loss to complete blindness, field defects, optic neuritis—ascending myelitis

Down: High myopia, lens opacities, nystagmus, oblique eyelid fissures, epicanthus—mental retardation, skeletal and heart anomalies.

Eaton-Lambert: Decreased vision, ocular myoclonus, corneal haziness—weakness, peripheral anethesia, poor response to neostigmine

Empty sella: Reduced vision, visual field defects, optic atrophy—acromegalic features

Espildora-Luque: Unilateral blindness, ophthalmic artery emboly—contralateral temporary hemiplegia

Fröhlich: Impaired scotopic vision, field defects, optic nerve involvement—adiposity, genital hypoplasia

Greig: High astigmatism, enophthalmos, epicanthus, paralysis VI, optic atrophy—mental deficiency, skull deformation

Groenblad-Strandberg: Decreased vision with macular lesion, retinopathy—pseudoxanthoma elasticum

Harada: Reduced vision in acute state, uveitis, choroiditis, retinopathy and detachment—meningeal irritation

Heidenhain: Rapid loss of vision, cortical blindness—presenile dementia, ataxia, rigidity

Klüver-Bucy: Visual agnosia—changes in emotional behavior, deficiency of memory, hypersexuality, oral tendencies

Laurence-Moon-Bardet-Biedl: Progressive visual loss, nystagmus, strabismus, field defect, optic atrophy, retinopathy—obesity, hypogenitalism, polydactyly mental deficiency

Leber: Visual loss, optic neuritis and atrophy, retinopathy—vertigo, headaches

Marchesani: Myopia, glaucoma, lens involvement—brachydactyly, reduced growth

Marfan: Myopia, anterior slgment involvement, strabismus, nystagmus—arachnodactyly, congenital heart defects, relaxed ligaments

Pierre Robin: High myopia, glaucoma, retinal disinsertion—micrognathia, cleft palate

Refsum: Nightblindness, retinal degeneration, visual field constriction—ataxia, polyneuritis, deafness, CNS degneration

Retinohypophysary syndrome: Reduced central vision, field defects, optic neuritis and atrophy—glycosuria, vertigo, psychic disturbances

Rochon-Duvigneaud: Reduced visual acuity depending on optic nerve involement, ophthalmoplegia, decreased corneal sensitivity—decreased sensitivity area V

Schilder: Progressive visual loss, nystagmus, muscle palsy, field defect, optic nerve involvement—spastic paralysis, mental deficiency, tremor

Sjögren: Blurred vision, decreased lacrimation, photophobia, keratoconjunctivitis sicca—polyarthritis, dryness of mucous membranes

Sjögren-Larsson: Reduced vision, chorioretinal degeneration—oligophrenia, ichthyosis, epilepsy, osseous dysplasia, speech defect, hyprereflexia

Tay-Sachs: Visual loss, optic atrophy, macular cherry red spot, retinal pigmentary changes, nystagmus, strabismus—mental retardation, convulsions, flaccid muscles becoming spastic with progression

Temporal arteritis syndrome: Partial to complete visual loss, diplopia, photophobia, optic atrophy, retinopathy—pain temporal region, hyperalgesia of the scalp

Tolosa-Hunt: Visual loss depending on optic nerve involvement, scotomata, ptosis, ophthalmoplegia, retroorbital pain, sluggish pupil reaction

Trisomy 22: High myopia—schizophrenia, micrognathia, large nostrils, flat occiput, overextension of elbows

Unverrichts: Amaurosis, retinopathy—myoclonus, epilepsy, dementia, pseudobulbar palsy

Uyemura: Nightblindness (transient), white spots in the retina, conjunctival xerosis, Bitôt' spots

Wilson: Nightblindness, corneal ring—liver cirrhosis, muscular rigidity, ascites in late stages

VISUAL FIELDS

Albright: Irregular field defect, proptosis, optic atrophy—osteitis fibrosa, skin pigmentations, endocrine dysfunction

Apert: Upper field defects, exophthalmos, ptosis, strabismus, nystagmus, exposure keratitis, optic atrophy—syndactyly

Arnold-Chiari: Bitemporal hemianopsia, diplopia, nystagmus, papilledema—pyramidal tract signs, vertebral malformations

Cone dysfunction syndrome: Peripheral field loss, decreased vision, retinopathy

Crouzon: Upper field defects, exophthalmos, nystagmus, strabismus, visual loss, optic atrophy—prognathism, maxillar atrophy, deformity anterior fontanel. a. o.

Cushing (1): Abnormal visual field defects, optic atrophy, ocular muscle palsy—obesity, hirsutism, hypertension, skin pigmentation

Cushing (3): Bitemporal hemianopsia (progressive), optic atrophy

Déjerine-Roussy: Hemianopsia—transient hemiplegia, ataxia, choreoathetotic movements

Devic: Field loss, visual impairment, optic neuritis and atrophy—ascending myelitis

Empty sella: Hemianopsia, quadranopsia or irregular field defects, reduced vision, optic atrophy—acromegalic features

Foster Kennedy: Central scotoma, optic atrophy, contralateral papilledema—anosmia (frontal lobe tumor)

Frankl-Hochwart: Concentric field defect, choked disc, limitation upward gaze—hypopituitarism, ataxia, bilateral deafness

Fröhlich: Bitemporal hemianopsia, decreased scotopic vision, papilledema—adiposity, genital hypoplasia, a. o.

Laurence-Moon-Bardet-Biedl: Ring scotoma, nystagmus, strabismus, visual loss, optic atrophy, retinopathy—obesity, hypogenitalism, polydactyly, mental deficiency

Morgagni: Varies field defects, optic nerve changes—hyperostosis frontalis interna

Raeder: Scotoma, enophthalmos, ptosis, diplopia, epiphora, hypotony, miosis—facial pain

Retinohypophysary syndrome: Atypical field defects, reduced central vision, optic atrophy—vertigo, glycosuria, psychic disturbances

Rollet: Field defects according to nerve involvement, exophthalmos, ptosis, ophthalmoplegia, diplopia, pain V, optic nerve involvement—hyperesthesias, vaso-motor disturbances

Schilder: Hemianopsia, nystagmus, muscle palsy, visual loss, optic nerve involvement—spastic paralysis, tremor, mental deficiency

Tapetal-like reflex syndrome: Ring scotoma, retinal changes

Cross Reference of Syndromes
Based on Systemic Manifestations

CARDIOVASCULAR SYSTEM

Amaurosis fugax: Hypertension—partial to total blindness, retinal arteriolar spasm

Angelucci: Tachycardia, vasomotor lability—conjunctivitis

Bonnet-Dechaume-Blanc: Angiomas of thalamus and mesencephalon— retinal angiomata

Cogan: Periarteritis nodosa, vestibuloauditory symptoms, deafness—blepharospasm, interstitial keratitis, lacrimation

Ellis-van Crefeld: Congeital heart defect (50%), polydactyly, skeletal and genital anomalies—congenital cataract, iris coloboma, strabismus

Fabry-Anderson: Hypertension, cardiomegaly, angiokeratoma, prominent lower jaw and lips—conjunctival varicositis, corneal opacities

Foix: Less distended ext. jugular vein, postauricular edema— proptosis, lid edema paresis III, IV, VI, chemosis, optic atrophy

Gorlin-Chaudhry-Moss: Patent ductus arteriosus, skull anomalies—microphthalmia, lid anomalies

Groenblad-Strandberg: Flat puls, aneurysms, intestinal hemorrhages—angioid streaks, macular changes

Hippel-Lindau, von: Cerebral angiomatosis, epilepsy, psychic disturbances— retinal angiomata, vitreous hemorrhages, sec. glaucoma

Hypothalamique-carrefour: Hypertension, hemianesthesia, apraxia—visual loss

Koerber-Salus-Elschnig: Hypertension, ataxia, hemitremor, positive Babinski sign—lid retraction, ocular muscle palsies

Louis-Bar: Telangiectasis, scanning speech, cerebellar ataxia—conjunctival telangiectasia

Noonan: Pulmonary stenosis, multiple skeletal anomalies, pterygium colli, mental retardation—hypertelorism, exophthalmos, ptosis

Page: Vasomotor blush, tachycardia, hypertension, salivation, frigidity— excessive lacrimation

Rubella: Heart disease, urinary infection, pneumonia, hearing loss, low birth weight, a.o.—glaucoma, iritis, hazy corneae, cataract, optic atrophy

Rubinstein-Taybi: Heart murmurs, urinary infection, skeletal anomalies, mental retardation—refractive error, strabismus, epicanthus

Scheie: Aortic valvular disease, broad facies, thickened joints—corneal haziness, visual field changes

Siegrist: Hypertension, albuminuria—exophthalmos, visual loss, choroidal pigmentary changes

Sturge-Weber: Vascular nevi, neurological signs depending on location of intracranial angiomas, endocrine dysfunction—glaucoma, retinopathy, conjunctival telangiectasis

Takayasu: Diminished or absent pulsation of arteries—cataracts, retinal microaneurysms, optic atrophy

Temporal arteritis syndrome: Headache, temporal pain, malaise, fever— diplopia, visual loss, retinopathy, optic atrophy

Waldenström: Vasospasm of limbs, hepatosplenomegaly, nasal and oral hemorrhages—retinal and choroidal hemorrhages and exudates

Werner: Arterioclerosis with sec. heart failure, endocrine dysfunctions, skeletal anomalies—cataracts, lack of eye lashes

17   245

DIGESTIVE SYSTEM

Bassen-Kornzweig: Steatorrhea, hyposcholesteremia, acanthocytosis—retinitis pigmentosa

Bogorad: Excessive salivation—unilateral lacrimation while eating

Chediak-Higashi: Hepatosplenomegaly, lymphadenopathly, cutaneous albinism— decreased fundus and iris pigmentation, edema basal cells of corneal epithelium

Degos: Gastrointestinal lesions, peritonitis, white skin lesions, CNS involvement—diplopia, conjunctival telangiectasia and atrophy, chorioretinitis, papillitis

Felty: Splenomegaly, rheumatoid arthritis, lenkopenia—keratitis

Hand-Schüller-Christian: Hepatosplenomegaly, endocrine disturbances, bone defects, lung fibrosis, skin xanthoma—exophthalmos, ophthalmoplegia, retinopathy, optic nerve changes

Heerfordt: Parotid gland swelling, submaxillary and sublingual glands may be involved, lymphadenopathy, cutaneous nodules—bilateral uveitis

Hurler: Hepatosplenomegaly, abdominal protuberans, bone anomalies, infantilism—ptosis, strabismus, corneal pathology, macular edema

Mikulicz-Radecki: Enlargement of salivary glands, dryness of mouth and larynx—enlarged lacrimal glands with decreased lacrimation

Niemann-Pick: Hepatosplenomegaly, mental and physical deterioration, seizures, skin pigmentation—retinopathy, red macular spot, optic atrophy, reduced vision

Oculo-oro-genital syndrome: Stomatitis, glossitis, ulcers of buccal membranes, erythema of pharynx and soft palate, dermatitis of scrotum—keratoconjunctivitis, optic atrophy

Rubella: Diarrhea, low birth weight, urinary infection, pneumonia, hearing loss, heart disease—glaucoma, iritis, cataract, hazy corneae, optic atrophy

Waldenström: Hepatosplenomegaly, adenopathy, nasal and oral hemorrhages, vasospasm of limbs—retinal and choroidal hemorrhages and exudates.

Wilson: Difficulties in swallowing and mastication, increased salivation, hematemesis, liver cirrhosis, jaundice, ascites—greenish corneal ring (Kayser-Fleischer)

ENDOCRINE SYSTEM

Addison: Hypoparathyroidism, adrenal insufficiency, moniliasis, anorexia— cataract, keratoconjunctivitis, papilledema, ptosis

Albright: Endocrine dysfunction, osteitis fibrosa cystica, brown skin spots— proptosis, visual field defect, optic nerve pathology

Ascher: Goiter, reduplication upper lip—blepharochalasis

Cockayne: Dwarfism, precocious senile appearance, deafness, mental retardation sensitivity to sunlight—cataract, retinal pigmentary changes, optic atrophy

Cushing (1): Adrenal hyperplasia, osteoporosis, diabetes, obesity, hirsutism, skin pigmentation—ocular muscle palsies, visual field changes, optic nerve invlovement

Empty-Sella: Acromegalic features—decreased vision, optic atrophy, visual field defects

Fröhlich: Genital hypoplasia, disturbances in sec. sexual manifestations, adiposity, retarded growth possible, polyuria, polydypsia—impaired scotopic vision, hemianopsia, optic nerve changes

Gänsslen: Hypogenitalism, infantilismus, splenomegaly, polydactyly, hip luxation— epicanthus, increased interpupillary distance

Hand-Schüller-Christian: Diabetes insipidus, growth and sexual retardation, bone defects, lung fibrosis, xanthoma of the skin, hepatosplenomegaly— exophthalmos, ophthalmoplegia, retinopathy, optic nerve changes

Hutchinson: Suprarenal tumor, anemia—subconjunctival hemorrhage, papilledema, exophthalmos, muscle pasly
Klinefelter: Sterility, small testes, gynecomastia, eunuchoid physique, mental retardation
Laurence-Moon-Bardet-Biedl: Hypogenitalism, obesity, polydactyly, short stature, metabolic disturbances—ptosis, nystagmus, nightblindness, retinopathy
Recklinghausen, von: Growth anomalies, spontaneous fractures, facial hemihypertrophy, skin changes—proptosis, ptosis, hydrophthalmos, retinopathy, iris nodules
Retinohypophysary syndrome: Glycosuria, psychic disturbances, vertigo, headache—reduced central vision, visual field defects, optic nerve changes
Rothmund: Endocrine disorder usually confined to hypogenitalism, telangiectases, skin pigmentation—bilateral cataracts
Sjögren: Endocrine dysfunction, skin and mucous membrane changes, polyarthritis—deficient lacrimation, keratoconjunctivitis sicca
Sturge-Weber: Acromegaly, adipositas, neurological signs depending on location of intracranial angiomas, vascular nevi—glaucoma, retinopathy, conjunctival telangiectases
Turner: Diminished growth, failure in sex organs development, congenital deafness, mental retardation—ptosis, retinal pigmentary changes
Werner: Thyroid dysfunction, hypogonadism, osteoporosis, skeletal anomalies, atrophic skin, arteriosclerosis—cataracts, lack of eye lashes

MUSCULOSKELETAL SYSTEM

Addison: Progressive weakness, skin pigmentation, hypoparathyroidism, moniliasis—cataract, keratoconjunctivitis, papilledema, ptosis
Albright: Osteitis fibrosa cystica, brown skin spots, endocrine dysfunction—proptosis, visual field defects, pathologic condition of opitc nerve
Apert: Tower skull, synostoses, brevicollis, CNS symptoms, syndactyly—orbital anomalies, ocular motility disturbances, visual field defects, corneal and lens changes, pathologic condition of optic nerve
Barré-Liéou: Cervical arthritis, vasomotor disturbances of face—corneal ulcers
Bonnevie-Ullrich: Cubitus valgus, skeletal anomalies, muscular hypotrophy, pterygium colli, hyperelastic skin—cataracts, absent lacrimal puncta, epicanthus, ocular paralysis
Cartilagenous-arthritis-ophthalmic-deafness syndrome: Rheumatoid arthritis, joint dislocations, deafness—uveitis
Cockayne: Dwarfism, mental retardation, deafness, sensitivity to sunlight—cataract, retinal pigmentary changes, optic atrophy
Crouzon: Skull changes, headaches, subnormal mentality, loss of hearing—exophthalmos, oblique lid fissures, nystagmus, loss of vision, visual field defects, optic nerve changes
Cushing (1): Osteoporosis, adipositas, skin pigmentation, hirsutism, diabetes—ocular muscle palsies, visual field changes, optic nerve involvement
Dejean: Lesion in orbital floor, numbness area of lst and 2nd trigeminal branch—exophthalmos, diplopia
de Lange: Multiple skeletal anomalies, muscular hypertrophy, growth and mental retardation—myopia, blue sclerae, pale discs
Down: Skull and long bone anomalies, short 5th finger, overextention of joints, mental retardation, heart anomalies—hypertelorism, epicanthus, nystagmus, myopia, lens opacities

Duane: Malformation of face, ears, teeth—primary global retraction

Eaton-Lambert: Weakness, fatigue, peripheral paresthesia—hazy cornea, conjunctival injection, decreased vision, ocular myoclonus

Ellis-van Crefeld: Polydactyly, genu valgum, talipes, thoracic constriction, dental anomalies, congenital heart defect (50%), genital anomalies—congenital cataract, iris coloboma, strabismus

Empty sella syndrome: Acromegalic features—visual field loss, optic atrophy

Erb-Goldflam: Myasthenia gravis—ptosis, strabismus, diplopia

Felty: Rheumatoid arthritis, splenomegaly, leukopenia—keratitis

Franceschetti: Skull and face malformations—oblique positions of the lid fissures, lid coloboma

Fröhlich: Open epiphyses, retarded growth possible, endocrine disturbances—impaired scotopic vision, optic nerve changes

Gänsslen: Congenital hip dislocation, splenomegaly, polydactyly, hypogenitalism—epicanthus, increased pupillary distance

Gaucher: (infantile form) Hypertonia, opisthotonus, dysphagia, (chronic form) hepatosplenomegaly osteolytic lesions, skin pigmentation—pinguecula, macular infiltration

Goldenhar: Multiple skeletal anomalies, preauricular fistulae, deafness—epibulbar dermoids, lid coloboma

Gorlin-Chaudhry-Moss: Craniofacial dysostosis, dental anomalies, patent ductus arteriosus—microphthalmia, lid anomalies

Gorlin-Goltz: Skeletal anomalies, basal cell nevi, mental retardation—glaucoma, cataracts, leukoma

Greig: Skull malformation, mental impairment—epicanthus, 6th nerve paralysis, astigmatism, optic nerve changes

Hallermann-Streiff: Multiple skeletal anomalies, dwarfism, mental retardation—microphthalmos, nystagmus, cataracts

Hallgren: Skeletal anomalies, mental retardation, deafness, ataxia—retinitis pigmentosa, night blindness, visual field contraction, optic atrophy

Hand-Schüller-Christian: Skull defects, defects in long bones, pelvis, ribs and spine, endocrine disturbances, lung fibrosis, hepatosplenomegaly—exophthalmos, ophthalmoplegia, retinopathy, optic nerve changes

Hemifacial microsomia: Numerous facial anomalies—microphthalmos, strabismus, iris and choroidal colobomata

Herrick: Joint pain, hemarthros, cortical thickening, skull changes, anemia, hepatosplenomegaly, lymph node swelling—retinopathy, conjunctival vascular changes

Hoeve, van der: Brittle bones, dental defects, hyperflexibility of ligaments, deafness—bluish sclera, thin cornea

Homocystinuria: Arachnodactyly, genu valgum, mental retardation—optic atrophy, lens anomalies

Hunter: Dwarfism, gargoylelike face, deafness, hepatosplenomegaly—retinal pigmentary degeneration, night blindness, corneal changes

Hurler: Kyphosis, skull anomalies, short cervical spine, wide clavicles, short limbs, hepatosplenomegaly, abdominal protuberans, infantilism—ptosis, strabismus, corneal pathology, macular edema

Klippel-Feil: Platybasia, upward displacement of the scapula, brevicollis, mirror movement—strabismus

Laurence-Moon-Bardet-Biedl: Turricephaly, shortness of stature, genu valgum, obesity, hypogenitalism, metabolic disturbances—ptosis, nystagmus, night blindness, retinopathy

Marchesani: Brachydactyly, reduced growth, short neck, decreased joint flexibility, hearing defects—myopia, lens anomalies

Marfan: Arachnodactyly, spina bifida, congenital heart disease—nystagmus, strabismus, myopia, miosis, lens anomalies, retinopathy

Meyer-Schwickerath-Weyers: Multiple skeletal anomalies, sparse hair growht—microphthalmia, short lid fissure, glaucoma, iris anomalies, microcornea

Moebius: Supernumerary digits, club foot, webbed fingers and toes, muscle defects of chest and neck, facial diplegia, deafness—proptosis, ptosis, weakness of adductor muscles

Morgagni: Hyperostosis frontalis interna, obesity, mental incapacity, hirsutism—visual field loss, optic nerve atrophy

Morquio-Brailsford (MPS IV): Dwarfism, multiple skeletal anomalies—corneal haziness

Noonan: Many skeletal anomalies, pulmonary stenosis, pterygium colli, mental retardation—hypertelorism, exophthalmos, ptosis

Ophthalmoplegic-retinal degeneration syndrome: Possible muscular dystrophy—ocular myopathy, ptosis, retinitis pigmentosa

Pierre Robin: Micrognathia, cleft palate, dyspnea—myopia, glaucoma, retinal disinsertion

Pseudohypoparathyroidism syndrome: Short stature, short extremities, obesity, tetany, mental retardation—strabismus

Recklinghausen, von: Growth anomalies, spontane fractures, skin pigmentations, fibroma and sebaceous adenoma—proptosis, ptosis, hydrophthalmos, retinopathy, iris nodules

Reiter: Arthritis, urethritis, erythema, pleuritis—keratoconjunctivitis, iritis

Riegers: Facial deformities—iris changes, glaucoma, corneal and lens involvement, optic atrophy

Riley-Day: Hyporeflexia, spontaneous fractures, failure to thrive, skin blotching, respiratory infection—congenital failure of tear production, keratitis

Romberg: Atrophy soft tissue one side of face, neuralgia V—ptosis, paresis extern. ocular muscles, iritis, keratitis

Rubinstein-Taybi: Skeletal anomalies, heart murmurs, urinary infection, mental retardation—refractive error, strabismus, epicanthus

Scheie: Thickened joints, broad facies, aortic valvular disease—corneal haziness, visual field changes

Treacher Collins: Absence ext. auditory canal and ext. ear, hypoplastic zygomatic arc, absence of normal malar eminences—lid coloboma, absence of lower puncta lacrimalia, oblique palpebral fissure

Trisomy-13-15: Polydactyly, cleft palate, hemangiomata, cerebral defects—hypertelorism, small orbits, microphthalmia, iris coloboma, cataracts

Trisomy-18: Small mandible, hyperflexion of fingers, low set ears, mental retardation—ptosis,' corneal opacities

Trisomy-22: Overextension of elbows, flat occiput, micrognathia, schizophrenia—high myopia

Turner: Diminished growth, pterygium colli, congenital deafness, mental retardation—ptosis, retinal pigmentary changes

Uveitis-rheumatoid arthritis syndrome: Rheumatoid arthritis—uveitis, iridocyclitis, choroiditis, keratopathy

Vermis: Enlargement of head, stiffness of neck and shoulders, incoordination, disturbances in equilibrium—nystagmus, papilledema

Waardenburg: Brachycephaly, broad nasal root, congenital deafness—caruncle hypoplasia, widened interpupillary distance, blepharophimosis, heterochromia iridum

Werner: Short stature, thin extremities, short fingers, osteoporosis, endocrine dysfunctions, skin changes, arteriosclerosis—cataracts, lack of eye lashes

NERVOUS SYSTEM (Central *and* Peripheral)

Adie: Loss of tendon reflexes—enlarged pupils, disturbance in pupil reaction

Alport: Progressive nerve deafness, hemorrhagic nephritis—anterior lenticonus, subcapsular cataracts, fundus albi punctatus

Anton: Confabulation, denial of blindness, allocheiria—blindness

Apert: Convulsions, loss of hearing and smell, bone anomalies—orbital anomalies, ocular motility changes, visual field defects, corneal and lens changes, pathology condition of optic nerve

Argyll Robertson: Syphilis of CNS, general paresis, tabes dorsalis—abnormalities of pupil reaction

Arnold-Chiari: Spina bifida, meningocele, hydrocephalus, cerebellar ataxia, bilateral pyramidal tract sign—nystagmus, visual field defects, papilledema

Arnold Pick: Dementia, aphasia, apraxia, apathy, patient is unaware of his surroundings—apperceptive blindness

Babinski-Nageotte: Hemiparesis, sensibility disturbances, cerebellar hemiataxia, adiadochokinesis, analgesis—ptosis, nystagmus, miosis

Balint: Tonic and motor phenomena (upper extremities) loss of body coordination, optic ataxia—psychic paralysis of visual fixation

Bassen-Kornzweig: Ataxia, areflexia, positive Babinski sign, steatorrhea, acanthocytosis—retinitis pigmentosa

Batten-Mayou: Mental disturbances, convulsions, apathy, irritability, ataxia, palsies, rigidity, dementia—partial to total blindness, retinopathy, optic atrophy

Behcet: CNS symptoms, skin anomalies, urethritis—ocular muscular paralysis, visual loss, keratoconjunctivitis, retinopathy

Behr: Pyramidal tract signs, ataxia, mental deficiency, vesical sphincter weakness—nystagmus, optic nerve atrophy

Benedict: Hyperkinesis, ataxia, paresis, tremor—paralysis III

Bonnet-Dechaume-Blanc: Angiomas of thalamus and mesencephalon—retinal angiomata

Bonnevie-Ullrich: Facial paralysis, hyperelastic skin, pterygium colli, skeletal anomalies—congenital cataracts, ocular muscle palsies, absent lacrimal glands and carunculae

Bourneville: Epilepsy, mental changes, neurologic symptoms, spina bifida, skin changes, kidney tumors—retinopathy, optic nerve changes

Carotid artery-cavernous sinus fistula: Headache, buzzing noise—ophthalmoplegia, retinopathy, papilledema

Cartilaginous-arthritic-ophthalmic-deafness syndrome: Deafness, bone changes —uveitis

Central nervous system deficiency: Deafness, tinnitus, numbness of legs— reduced vision

Cestan-Chenais: Pharyngolaryngeal paralysis, cerebellar ataxia, disturbance of sensibility—ptosis, enophthalmos, nystagmus, miosis

Charcot-Marie-Tooth: Atrophy of small muscles of hands and feet (degeneration of muscular branches of motor fibers supplying the limbs—nystagmus, reduced vision, optic atrophy

Charlin: Neuritis nasal branch of trigeminal nerve—orbital pain, keratoconjunctivitis

Claude: Ataxia, hemianesthesia—paralysis oculomotor nerve

Cockayne: Mental retardation, deafness, dwarfism, sensitivity to sunlight— cataract, retinal pigmentary changes, optic atrophy

Cushing (2): Hyperesthesia of the face, facial nerve paresis, deafness, tinnitus—paresis orbicularis muscle, paresis ext. rectus muscle, decreased corneal sensitivity

Dandy-Walker: Hydrocephalus—ptosis, six nerve paralysis, papilledema

Degos: Paresthesias, progressive cerebral and cerebellar atrophy, white skin lesions, gastrointestinal ulcers—conjunctival telangiectasia and atrophy, chorioretinitis, papillitis

Dejean: Numbness in area of 1st and 2nd branch of trigeminal nerve, severe pain superior maxillary region—exophthalmos, diplopia

de Lange: Mental and growth retardation, multiple skeletal anomalies, muscular hypertrophy—myopia, blue sclerae, pale discs

Déjerine-Klumpke: paralysis of small muscles of forearm and hand—enophthalmos, ptosis, miosis

Déjerine-Roussy: Sensory disturbances, hemiataxia, hemiplegia, choreoathetotic movements, partial facial paresis, bladder disturbances—hemianopsia

Devic: Ascending myelitis, pain, weakness, paralysis—loss of vision, visual field changes, optic neuritis

Dialinas-Amalric: Deaf-mutism—atypical retinitis pigmentosa

Down: Mental retardation, skeletal abnormalities, heart anomalies—hypertelorism, epicanthus, nystagmus, myopia, lens opacities

Feer: Disturbance of autonomous nervous system with restlessness, irritability, sweating, rapid pulse, exanthema of palms—lacrimation, photophobia, keratitis, proptosis

Fisher: Ataxia, loss of deep reflexes—external and internal ophthalmoplegia

Foster Kennedy: Anosmia—scotomata, optic atrophy

Foville: Facial palsy, hemiplegia —paralysis VI

Frankl-Hochwart: Ataxia, deafness, hypopituitarism—limitation of upward gaze, visual field defects, choked optic disc

Goldscheider: Mental and growth retardation, skin lesions—conjunctival shrinkage and symblepharon, blepharitis

Gorlin-Goltz: Mental retardation, basal cell nevi, skeletal anomalies—glaucoma, cataracts, leukoma

Gradenigro: Ear involvement, facial paresis—paralysis VI, pain in area ophthalmic branch V, optic nerve may be involved

Greig: Mental impairment, skull malformation—epicanthus, 6th nerve paralysis, astigmatism, optic nerve changes

Guillain-Barré: Polyneuritis, tendon reflexes absent, paralysis, bladder incontinence—ectropion lower lid, ophthalmoplegia

Hallermann-Streiff: Mental retardation, multiple skeletal anomalies, dwarfism—nystagmus, cataracts, microphthalmos

Hallgren: Deafness, vestibulo-cerebellar ataxia, mental deficiency, skeletal anomalies—retinitis pigmentosa, night blindness, visual field contraction, optic atrophy.

Harada: Headaches, deafness, meningeal irritation—visual loss, bilateral uveitis, retinal detachment, diffuse exudative choroiditis

Heidenhain: Ataxia, athetoid movements, presenile dementia—visual loss

Hennebert: Vertigo, labyrinth fistula—nystagmus

Hippel-Lindau, von: Epilepsy, psychic disturbances, cerebral angiomatosis—retinal angiomata, vitreous hemorrhages, sec. glaucoma

Homocystinuria: Mental retardation, genu valgum, arachnodactyly—optic atrophy, lens anomalies

Horner: Facial hemiatrophy, anhidrosis hemilateral side of face—enophthalmos, ptosis, miosis

251

Hypothalamique-carrefour: Hemianesthesia, apraxia, hypertension—visual loss
Jacod: Trigeminal neuraglia, enlargement of cervical lymph nodes—ophthalmoplegia, trigeminal neuralgia, optic atrophy
Kloepfer: Dementia, blistering in sunlight—blindness
Klüver-Bucy: Changes in emotional and psychic behavior—visual agnosia
Koerber-Salus-Elschnig: Ataxia, hemitremor, positive Babinski sign, hypertension—lid retraction, ocular muscle palsies
Leber: Headaches, vertigo—loss of vision, retinopathy, optic neuritis
Lenoble-Aubineau: Tremor, overactive reflexes—nystagmus
Louis-Bar: Cerebellar ataxia, mental retardation, scanning speech, telangiectasia skin and conjunctiva
Ménière: Vertigo, deafness, nausea—nystagmus
Millard-Gubler: Paralysis one side of the face, hemiplegia—diplopia, squint
Moebius: Facial diplegia, deafness, loss vestibular response, anomalies of hands and feet, muscle defects chest and neck—proptosis, ptosis, weakness of adductor muscles
Morgagni: Mental incapacity, somnolence, hirsutism, obesity, hyperostosis frontalis interna—visual field loss, optic nerve atrophy
Naffziger: Weakness of hand grip, reduced biceps reflex—ptosis, miosis, absent ciliospinal reflex
Niemann-Pick: Mental retardation, epileptic seizures, deafness, physical deterioration, skin pigmentation, hepatosplenomegaly—retinopathy, red macular spot, reduced vision, optic atrophy
Nothnagel: Cerebellar ataxia—oculomotor paresis
Oculocerebellar-tegmental syndrome: Hemiplegia—paralysis of associated ocular movements
Ophthalmoplegic-migraine syndrome: Migraine headaches—supraorbital pain, oculomotor paralysis
Parinaud: Ataxia, vertigo—ptosis, paralysis of conjugate movements of the eyes, pupil anomalies, papilledema
Parkinson: Rhythmical tremor, slowness of movements, rigidity of arms, loss of facial expression—fluttering eyelids, blepharospasm, nystagmus, pupillary disorders
Pelizaeus-Merzbacher: Ataxia, tremor, abnormal reflexes, seizures, spastic paralyis, retarded mental and physical development—retinal pigmentary degeneration, optic nerve involvement with visual impairment, nystagmus
Raeder: Facial pain, weakness of jaw muscles—ptosis, epiphora, ocular hypotony, miosis
Raymond: Hemiplegia, anethesia of face, limbs and trunk—paralysis of lateral conjugate gaze
Refsum: Spinocerebellar ataxia, polyneuritis, deafness, CNS degeneration—retinal degeneration, nightblindness, visual field constriction, pupillary changes
Rochon-Duvigneaud: Decreased sensitivity V—lid edema, ophthalmoplegia, optic nerve involvement possible
Rollet: Hyperesthesia or anesthesia of forehead—exophthalmos, ptosis, optic nerve changes
Romberg: Epileptic seizures, neuralgia V, atrophy soft tissue one side of face—ptosis, paresis ocular muscles, choroiditis, iritis, keratitis
Sabin-Feldman: Cerebral calcifications, convulsions, microcephaly—atrophic chorioretinal changes
Sanfillipo-Good: Mental deficincy, seizures—retinal pigment anomaly, possible night blindness

252

Schilder: Spastic paralysis, mental deterioration, deafness, tremore, scanning speech—nystagmus, visual loss, visual field defects, optic nerve changes

Sjögren-Larsson: Oligophrenia, epilepsy, tremor, spastic disorders, speech defect, ichthyosis—chorioretinitis, reduced vision

Spheno-cavernous syndrome: Paresis Vth nerve—proptosis, lid edema, paresis IV, V, VI, visual impairment, chemosis

Sturge-Weber: Paresis, atrophy etc. depending on localization of intracranial angiomas, vascular nevi, endocrine dysfunction—glaucoma, retinopathy, conjunctival telangiectases

Symonds: Meningitis, headaches, drowsiness, otitis media—diplopia, retinal hemorrhages, papilledema, optic atrophy

Tay-Sachs: Mental retardation, convulsions, flaccid muscles becoming spastic wtith progressing disease—retinopathy, cherry red macular spot, progressive visual loss, nystagmus

Trisomy-13–15: Cerebral defects, polydactyly, cleft palate—microphthalmia, small orbit, coloboma of iris and optic nerve, cataracts

Trisomy-18: Mental reardation, low set ears, small mandible, hyperflexion of fingers—ptosis, coneal opacities

Trisomy-22: Schizophrenia, overextension of elbows, flat occiput, micrognathia—high myopia

Turner: Mental retardation, endocrine dysfunction, congenital deafness, diminished growth—ptosis, retinal pigmentary changes

Unverrichts: Epilepsy, myoclonus, dementia, tetraplegia, pseudobulbar palsy—amaurosis

Usher: Deaf mutism—retinitis pigmentosa, concentric visual field constriction

Vermis: Vomiting, incoordination, equilibratory disturbances, enlarged head—nystagmus, papilledema

Wallenberg: Ataxia, muscular hypotonicity, hypoesthesia for pain and temperature, nausea—ptosis, nystagmus, diplopia, miosis

Weber: Hemiplegia, paralysis of face and tongue—ptosis, IIIrd nerve palsy, fixed pupil

Wernicke: Ataxia, mental distubances, peripheral neuritis—ptosis, nystagmus, ophthalmoplegia

RESPIRATORY SYSTEM

Hand-Schüller-Christian: Lung fibrosis, cardiac insufficiency, endocrine disturbances, bone defects, skin xanthoma, hepatosplenomegaly—exophthalmos, ophthalmoplegia, retinopathy, optic nerve changes

Louis-Bar: Pulmonary infections, cerebellar ataxia, mental retardation, scanning speech, talangiectasia skin and conjunctiva

Pancoast: Pulmonary apical tumor, severe shoulder pain, anesthesia and atrophy homolateral arm and hand—ptosis, miosis, enophthalmos

Pierre Robin: Acute dyspnea, cyanosis, cleft palate—myopia, glaucoma, retinal disinertion

Posner-Schlossman: Allergy—glaucomato cyclitc crisis, no visual loss

Riley-Day: Respiratory infections, failure to thrive, emotional instability, skin blotching, hyporeflexia, spontaneous fractures—congenital failure of tear production, keratitis

Schaumann: Enlarged hilar nodes, lymphadenopathy, fatigue—uveitis, retinopathy, vitreous floaters

Stevens-Johnson: Acute respiratory infection, rhinitis, urethritis, skin and mucous membrane eruptions—visual loss, conjunctivitis, keratitits

SKIN AND MUCOUS MEMBRANE

Addison: Skin pigmentation, brittle finger and toe nails, sparse pubic and axillary hair, moniliasis, tetany—cataract, keratoconjunctivitis, papilledema ptosis

Albright: Brown pigmented skin spots, osteitis fibrosa, endocrine dysfunction—proptosis, visual field defect, pathologic condition of optic nerve

Ascher: Reduplication upper lip, goiter—blepharochalasis

Behcet: Aphthous lesions of mucous membranes, skin erythema, CNS symptoms, arthritis, urethritis—ocular muscle palsies, visual loss, kerato-conjunctivitis, retinopathy

Bloch-Sulzberger: Skin pigmentation, alopecia, dental anomalies— nystagmus cataract, retinopathy, optic nerve pathology

Bonnevie-Ullrich: Hyperelastic skin, pterygium colli, muscular hypotrophy, skeletal anomalies—cataracts, absent lacrimal puncta, epicanthus, ocular paralysis, ptosis

Bournevill: Adenoma sebaceum, CNS symptoms, kidney tumors—retinopathy, optic nerve changes

Chediak-Higashi: Oculo-cutaneous albinism, hepatosplenomegaly, lymphadeno-pathy—edema basal cells of corneal epithelium

Cockayne: Sensitivity to sunlight, dwarfism, mental retardation, deafness—cataract, retinal pigmentary changes, optic atrophy

Cushing (1): Skin pigmentation, hirsutism, obesity, hypertension, diabetes, osteoporosis—ocular muscle palsies, visual field defects, optic nerve involvement

Degos: White skin lesion, oral mucosa lesions, gastrointestinal ulcers, CNS involvement—conjunctival telangiectasia and atrophy, chorioretinitis, papillitis

Fabry-Anderson: Angiokeratoma of the skin, pain in arms and legs, cardiomegaly, hypertension, conjunctival varicositis, corneal opacities

Feer: Exfoliation of skin on palms and soles, irritability, hyperflexibility of joints—proptosis, photophobia, lacrimation

Fuchs (2): Cyanosis, swelling of face, ulcers of mucous membranes—conjunctivitis

Goldscheider: Skin lesions, grwoth and mental ratardation—conjunctival shrinkage and symblepharon, blepharitis

Gorlin-Goltz: Multiple basal cell nevi, skeletal anomalies, mental retardation—glaucoma, cataract, corneal leukoma

Goernblad-Strandberg: Pseudoxanthoma elasticum, flat puls, vascular disturbances—angioid streaks, macular changes

Hand-Schüller-Christian: Xanthoma of the skin, bone defects, lung fibrosis, endocrine disturbances, hepatosplenomegaly—exophthalmos, ophthalmoplegia retinopathy, optic nerve changes

Heerfordt: Cutaneous and subcutaneous nodules, salivary gland swelling, lymphadenopathy—bilateral uveitis

Hunt: Zoster lesions of face and neck, reduced hearing and taste, vertigo—loss of motor corneal reflex, reduced lacrimation

Jadassohn-Lewandowski: Keratosis and hyperhidrosis palms and soles, leuko-keratosis oral mucosa, pachyonychia—corneal dyskeratosis

Kloepfer: Severe blistering in sunlight, dementia—blindness

Melkersson-Rosenthal: Facial edema, glossitis, furrowed tongue, facial palsy—excessive lacrimation, keratitis, conjunctival irritation

Naegeli: Pigmentary skin changes, keratosis, hands and feet, dysfunction of sweat glands, dental abnormalities—nystagmus, retinal pseudoglioma, optic nerve changes

Noonan: Webbed neck, pulmonary stenosis, mulitiple skeletal defects—hypertelorism, ptosis, exophthalmos, antimongoloid slant of palpebral fissure

Oculo-oro genital syndrome: Exfoliating dermatitis of scrotum, stomatitis—keratoconjunctivitis, optic atrophy

Recklinghausen, von: Café-au-laît spots, fibroma, adenoma, growth abnormalities, spontaneous fractures—proptosis, ptosis, hydrophthalmos, retinopathy urethritis—keratoconjunctivitis, iritis

Reiter: Skin erythema, genital ulcers, lymphadenopathy, pleuritis, arthritis,

Rothmund: Brownish skin pigmentation, telangiectases, endocrine disorder—bilateral cataracts

Sallmann, von-Paton-Witkop: Thickened oral mucosa with whitish plaques—conjunctival perilimbal foamy lesions

Sjögren: Scleroderma, alopecia, purpura, dryness of mucous membranes, polyarthritis, weakness, endocrine dysfunction—blepharo conjunctivitis, deficient lacrimation, keratitis sicca

Stevens-Johnson: Erythema multiforme, rhinitis, urethritis, respiratory infection—visual loss, keratitis, conjunctivitis

Vogt-Koyangi: Alopecia, poliosis, vitiligo, hearing defect—reduced vision, secondary glaucoma, steamy cornea, retinopathy

Werner: Atrophic skin ulcers lower limbs, endocrine dysfunctions, skeletal anomalies, arteriosclerosis—cataracts, lack of eye lashes

Zinsser-Engman-Cole: Dyskeratosis with pigmentation, oral lesions, hypersplenism, anemia—obstruction lacrimal puncta, conjunctival keratinization

URINARY SYSTEM

Alport: Hemorrhagic nephritis, progressive nerve deafness—anterior lenticonus, subcapsular cataracts, fundus albi punctatus

Behcet: Urethritis, CNS symptoms, skin anomalies—ocular muscular paralysis, visual loss, keratoconjunctivitis, retinopathy

Behr: Vesical sphincter weakness, CNS sign—nystagmus, optic nerve atrophy

Bourneville: Kidney tumors, CNS symptoms, skin changes—retinopathy, nerve changes

Déjerine-Roussy: Bladder disturbance, hemiataxia, hemiplegia, choreoathetotic movements, sensory disturbances—hemianopsia

Ellis-van Crefeld: Genital anomalies, multiple skeletal anomalies, congenital heart defect—cataract, strabismus, iris coloboma

Guillain-Barré: Bladder incontinence, polyneuritis, paralysis, absent tendon reflexes—ectropion, ophthalmoplegia

Reiter: Urethritis, genital ulcers, erythema, arthritis, pleuritis—keratoconjunctivitis, iritis

Riley-Day: Ureteric malformations, failure to thrive, respiratory infections, skin blotching—congenital failure of tear production, keratitis

Rubella: Urinary infection, diarrhea, pneumonia, hearing loss, a.o.—glaucoma, cataract, iritis, hazy corneae, optic atrophy

Rubinstein-Taybi: Urinary infection, skeletal anomalies, heart murmurs, mental retardation—refractive error, strabismus, epicanthus

Stevens-Johnson: Urethritis, erythema multiforme, respiratory infection—conjunctivitis, keratitis, visual loss

Cross Reference of Syndromes Based on Etiological Factors and on Age, Sex and Ethnic Groups

ETIOLOGY
Brain Lesion

Arnold Pick: Cerebral atrophy, manifest between 40 and 70 years, more often in females

Babinski-Nageotte: Lesion in pontobulbar transitional region

Blaint: Lesion of the parieto-cocipital region

Batten-Mayou: Cerebellar atrophy, most common in Jewish families, onset between 5 and 8 years of life

Behcet: Occurs in adults, more frequent in males, virus infection (?)

Benedict: Lesion of inferior nucleus ruber (vascular, traumatic, neoplastic)

Bonnet-Dechaume-Blanc: Vascular lesions (angiomata) of thalamus and mesencephalon

Bourneville: Sclerotic patches lateral ventricles, sclerotic convolutions, irregular dominant inheritance, occurs in childhood—less frequent in adults

Cestan-Chenais: Lesion in lateral portion of the medulla oblongata (thrombosis vertebral artery)

Charcot-Marie-Tooth: Changes in motor cells of spinal gray matter, pyramidal tracts and posterior columns, onset between 5 to 15 years or early middle age, heredo familiar occurrence

Dandy-Walker: Malformation and stenosis of foramina Luschka and Magendie, dilation of the fourth ventricle, anomaly of rostral portion of the vermis, manifestations in infants

Cushing (3): Suprasellar meningioma or primary intrasellar tumor. Possible posterior fossa lesion

Cushing (2): Tumor involving V, VI, VII, VIII and brain stem

Déjerine-Roussy: Posterior thalamic lesion, lesion in ventral part of optic thalamus (hemorrhage, thrombosis, tumor)

Devic: Ophthalmoencephalomyelopathy. Etiology unknown (toxic? virus? vascular?). Occurs at any age but most frequently between age 20 and 50years

Espildora-Luque: Emboly of the ophthalmic artery with reflectory spasm of the middle cerebral artery

Foix: Tumor lateral sinus wall or sphenoid bone: other causes inntracranial aneurysm, cavernous and lateral sinus thrombosis, inflammatory lesion

Foster Kennedy: Tumor or other lesion in the base of the frontal lobe or sphenoidal meningioma

Foville: Pontine area tumor; other causes: hemorrhage, MS, tuberculoma, unilateral obstruction of paramedian branches

Frankl-Hochwart: Pineal gland tumor

Fröhlich: Chromophobe adenoma of the pituitary, Rathke pouch tumor, craniopharyngeoma, suprasellar tumors, encephalitis, trauma etc. More frequent in Jews, manifestations in childhood

Heidenhain: Cortical degeneration, mainly occipital

Horner: Hypothalamic lesion with first neuron involved or many other causes leading to paralysis of cervical sympathetic

Leber: Distortion of sella turcica; male linkage (?) recessive, has been observed in females too, most frequent in third decade of life

Millard-Gubler: Unilateral lesion in the base of the pons affecting VI and VII and pyramidal tract

Nothnagel: Lesion superior cerebellar peduncle, red nucleus and emerging oculomotor fibers.

Page: Irritation of parasympathetic and sympathetic centers in the diencephalon

Parinaud: Pineal tumor, nuclear lesions, vascular lesions, inflammation, hemorrhages, midbrain lesion etc.

Parkinson: Late stages of epidemic encephalitis with widespread destruction in the substantia nigra.

Pelizaeus-Merzbacher: Congenital extracortical aplasia involving white matter of CNS. Symptoms in infancy and childhood

Pseudo-Graefe: Short circuit of impulses from one cranial nucleus into another. After trauma, tabes, tumor, vascular lesions, etc., misdirection of regenerating oculomotor nerve fibers

Raymond: Nuclear lesion and involvement of pyramidal tract. Most frequently lesion of small branches of the basilar artery, tumor and vascular thrombosis possible

Schilder: Lesions in subcortical white matter; Demyelinization of the hemispheres of the brain and the cerebellum; Occurs at any age.

Sjögren-Larsson: Enlargement of ventricular system as result of shrinkage of gray matter

Sphenocavernous syndrome: Lesion in the carvernous sinus

Sylvian: Tumor or inflammation in region of the Sylvian aqueduct, third and fourth ventricle, or corpora quadrigemina

Wallenberg: Occlusion of posterior inferior cerebellar artery; occurs usually above age 40 years

Weber: Lesion of the peduncle, pons, medula; hemorrhage and thrombosis most frequent cause, but tumor of the pituitary region may cause similar signs

Wernicke: Focal vascular lesions around third and fourth ventricles and Sylvian aqueduct; nutricial deficiency with secondary lack of vitmain B_1

Wilson: Lesion in the putamen and lenticular nucleus; most frequent in first decade of life, but also described in later age groups

Hemorrhage

Déjerine-Roussy: Lesion posterior thalamus, lesion ventral part of optic thalamus (hemorrhage, thrombosis, tumor)

Déjerine-Klumpke: Lesion involving inferior roots of brachial plexus (see, Tumor)

Foville: Hemorrhage, MS, vascular lesion or pontine area tumor

Parinaud: See Barin lesions

Weber: Lesion of the peduncle, pons, medulla; hemorrhage and thrombosis most frequent cause; tumor of the pituitary region possible

Infections and Inflammations

Alport: Hemorrhagic nephritis, increase of $\alpha 2$ fraction of serum protein, early death in males, normal life span in females

Argyll Robertson: Syphilis (most frequently), rare: epidemic encephalitis, disseminated sclerosis, diabetes, brain tumor, syringomyelia, syringobulbia, chronic alcoholism, injury

Arnold-Chiari: Adhesive arachnoiditis around herniated cerebellar tonsils, brain stem or cerebellum

Behcet: Virus infection (?), more frequent in males, occurs in adults, brain lesions

Bloch-Sulzberger: Virus infection of mother duing pregnancy (?), manifestations present at birth

Charlin: Neuritis nasal branch of trigeminal nerve

Fisher: Acute idiopathic polyneuritis

Foix: Inflammatory lesion, vascular lesion or tumor of the lateral sinus wall or sphenoid bone

Gradenigro: Extradural abscess of the petrosus portion of the temporal bone (trauma, meningitis, hemorrhage, mastoiditis)

Guillain-Barré: Polyneuritis: etiology unknown; occurs in children and adolescents (16 to 50 years of age)

Hennebert: Congenital syphilis; manifestations in childhood

Hunt: Herpes zoster infection of the geniculate, or sensory ganglion

Koerber-Salus-Elschnig: Inflammation or tumor in region of the aqueduct, third and fourth ventricle or corpora quadrigemina

Parinaud: SEE Brain lesions

Parinaud's oculoglandular syndrome: Tularemia, leptothrix, sporotrichosis, lymphogranuloma venerum, etc.

Parkinson: Late stage of epidemic encephalitis, after manganese and carbon monoxide posisoning. Widespread destruction in substatia nigra

Rochon-Duvigneaud: Inflammation (arachnoiditis, tuberculosis, syphilis) involving superior orbital fissure, trauma, tumor and vascular lesions may also produce the syndrome

Rollet: Lesion in the apex of the orbit

Rubella syndrome: Rubella infection in the mother duing first trimester of pregnancy

Sylvian: Inflammation or tumor in region of the Sylvian aqueduct, third and fourth ventricle, or corpora quadrigemina

Symonds: Serous meningitis; occurs in children and adolescents

Takayasu: (2 types), non-specific arteritis or occlusive vascular disease without inflammation

Temporal arteritis syndrome: Inflammation temporal artery; occurs in caucasians at age 55 to 80 years

Tolosa-Hunt: Inflammatory lesion of the cavernous sinus

Vogt-Koyanagi: Virus infection?; Italians and Japanese more frequently affected than other groups; usually in young adults

Tumor

Benedict: Neoplastic lesion, vascular, traumatic, (lesion of inferior nucleus ruber)

Cushing (1): Adrenal neoplasm or adrenocortical hyperplasia and piluitary tumors

Cushing (2): Tumor involving V, VI, VII VIII cranial nerve and brain stem, possible vascular lesion

Cushing (3): Suprasellar meningioma or primary intrasellar tumor. Possible posterior fossa lesion

Déjean: Lesion involving the orbital floor. Extension into cranial cavity may occur

Déjerine-Klumpke: Lesion involving inferior roots of brachial plexus (Pancoast's tumor, menigeal or spinal tumor), other causes include birth trauma, Pott's disease, hemorrhage, shoulder dislocation, myelitis

Dejerine-Roussy: Posterior thalamic lesion, lesion in ventral part of optic thalamus (tumor, hemorrhage, thrombosis)

Eaton-Lambert: Myasthenic syndrome often associated with intrathoracic tumors

Empty sella syndrome: Condition after sugical or radiation treatment of sella tumors, progressing visual field loss probably due to constriction by scar formation and ischemia; enlarged sella on x-ray examination

Foix: Tumor lateral sinus wall or sphenoid bone, other causes intracranial aneuryms, cavernous, and lateral sinus thrombosis, inflammatory lesions

18

Foster Kennedy: Tumor in the base of the frontal lobe or sphenoidal meningioma. (Aneuryms, abscess, sclerosis etc. possible)

Foville: Pontine area tumor; other causes hemorrhage, MS, tuberculoma, unilateral obstruction of paramedian branches

Frankl-Hockwart: Pineal gland tumor

Fröhlich: Chromophobe ademona of the pituitary, Rathke pouch tumor, craniopharyngeoma, suprasellar tumors, encephalitis, trauma etc. More frequent in Jews. Manifestations in childhood (most often during puberty)

Gorlin-Goltz: Multiple basal cell nevi, jaw cysts and skeletal anomalies, autosomal dominant inheritance

Hutchinson: Infraorbital neuroblastoma

Jacod: Most frequently malignant nasopharyngeal tumor oringinating in lateropharyngeal area involving nerve II through VI.

Koerber-Salus-Elschnig: Tumor or inflammation in region of the aqueduct, third and fourth ventricle or corpora quadrigemina

Pancoast: Tumor in pulmonary apex. Primary bronchogenic carcinoma most frequent cause (50%).

Raeder: Meningioma or aneurysm of internal carotid artery involving the fifth nerve and sympathetic fibers

Rochon-Duvigneaud: Meningioma of sphenoid frequent cause of the syndrome but trauma, vascular and inflammatory etiology possible

Rollet: Lesion in the apex of the orbit

Sylvian: Tumor or inflammation in region of the Sylvian aqueduct, third and fourth ventricle or corpora quadrigmina

Vermis: Tumor of the fourth ventricle; more frequent in children

Vascular

Amaurosis fugax: Hypertension, other causes—tabagism

Bielschowsky-Lutz-Cogan: Lesion in the medial longitudinal fasciculus causing internuclear ophthalmoplegia

Bonnet-Dechaume-Blanc: Angiomatosis of retina, thalamus and mesencephalon

Carotid artery-cavernous sinus fistula syndrome

Cestan-Chenais: Thrombosis vertebral artery, lesion in lateral portion of the medula oblongata

Charcot-Wilbrand: Partial occulsion of posterior cerebral artery

Claude: Occlusion of terminal branches of paramedian arteries supplying the inferior portion of the nucleus ruber

Cushing (2): Vascular lesion involving V, VI. VII, VIII carnial nerve and brain stem, but usually caused by tumor

Degos: Multiple cerebral infarcts and/or thrombosis of small arteries, white skin lesions, male preponderance

Déjerine-Roussy: Posterior thalamic lesion, lesion in ventral part of optic thalamus, (thrombosis, hemorrhage, tumor)

Espildora-Luque: Emboly of the ophthalmic artery with reflectory spasm of the middle cerebral artery

Fabry-Anderson: Angiokeratosis most likely caused by lipoid storage disorder

Foix: Intracranial aneurysm, cavernous and lateral sinus thrombosis, inflammatory lesions or tumor lateral sinus wall or sphenoid bone

Foville: Unilateral obstruction of paramedian branches, hemorrhage, MS or pontine area tumor

Hippel-Lindau, von: Angiomata of the cerebellum and the walls of the fourth ventricle; familial disease, dominantly transmitted

Melkersson-Rosenthal: Disturbance in blood supply to facial nerve (viral?)

Oculocerebellar-tegmental: Vascular lesion of the mesencephalon

Parinaud: (SEE Brain lesion)

Raeder: Aneurysm of internal carotid artery or meningioma involving the fifth nerve and sympathetic fibers

Raymond: Nuclear lesion and involvement of the pyramidal tract; most frequently lesion of small branches of the basilar artery

Rochon-Duvigneaud: Vascular lesion involving superior orbital fissure; tumor, trauma and inflammation may also produce the syndrome

Takayasu: (2 types) non-specific arteritis or occlusive vascular disease without inflammation

Wallenberg: Occlusion of posterior inferior cerebellar artery; occurs usually above age 40 years

Weber: Lesion of the peduncle, pons, medulla; hemorrhage and thrombosis most frequent cause

Wernicke: Focal vascular lesions around third and fourth ventricles and Sylvian aqueduct; nutricial deficiency with secondary lack of vitamin B_1

Others

Addison: Atrophy of adrenal cortex, hypoparathyroidism, moniliasis, onset 1st or 2nd decade of life

Alport: Congenital hemorrhagic nephritis

Amaurosis fugax: Tabagism; other causes-hypertension

Angelucci: Etiology unknown, lymphatic condition

Argyll Robertson: Most frequently syphilis (See Infections and contagious diseases)

Ascher: Possibly related to develpoment of the thyroid gland, questionable inheritance for the entire syndrome,-struma, double lip, blepharochalasis

Barré-Liéou: Trauma or arthritic changes of cervical spine causing irritation of the vertebral nerve with resulting circulatory disturbances in area of cranial nuclei

Bassen-Kornzweig: A-β Lipoproteinemia, inability to absorb and transport lipids

Batten-Mayou: Possible disturbance in lipoid metabolism. Heredofamiliar disorder—mainly in Jewish families

Benedict: Lesion of inferior nucleus ruber, (traumatic, vascular, neoplastic)

Bonnevie-Ullrich: Pterygolymphangiectasia, hereditary factor has not been established, more frequent in females (4:1)

Central nervous system deficiency: Dietary deficiency (?), etiology unknown

Dialinas-Amalric: Deaf-mutism and retinitis pigmentosa

Ellis-von Crefeld: Ectodermal and chondro dysplasia, congenital heart defects. Parental consanguinity in about 25%

Erb-Goldflam: Myasthenia gravis,—defect at myoneural junction with involvement or disturbance of acetylcholin metabolism

Frenkel: Blunt trauma to anterior segment of the globe

Fröhlich: Increased sugar tolerance; reduction or absence of urinary gonadotropins in both sexes

Gänsslen: Decreased osmotic resistance of erythrocytes, spherocytes

Gaucher: Glucocerebroside storage disorder with infantile and chronic form

Goldenhar: Oculo-auriculo-vertebral dysplasia,—epibulbar dermoids or lipodermoids

Goldscheider: Dystrophic changes with scar formation

Gradenigro: Trauma with following extradural abscess or hemorrhage of the petrosus portion of the temporal bone

Hallermann-Streiff: Familial occurrence, multiple skeletal anomalies, mental retardation

Hand-Schüller-Christian: Granulomatous lesions of the RES with lipoid cell hyperplasia and proliferation of histiocytes. Etiology unknown; onset before age of 6 years

Herrick: Sickle shaped erythrocytes; only in negroes with possibly few exceptions; inherited as a Mendelian dominant

Homocystinuria: Disorder of amino acid metabolism, increased urinary excretion of homocystine

Hunter: Systemic mucopolysaccharidosis (II), increased excretion of chondroitin sulfate B and heparitin sulfate

Jadassohn-Lewandowski: Congenital pachyonychia inherited autosomal dominant with low penetrance

Klüver-Bucy: Syndrome caused after removal of temporal lobe

Niemann-Pick: Phosphatide lipidosis and lipid storage

Oculo-oro-genital: Vitamin B deficiency and possible vitamin A deficiency

Ophthalmoplegic-retinal degeneration: Ocular myopathy, nuclear ophthalmoplegia

Parkinson: Late stage of epidemic encephalitis after manganese and carbon monoxide poisoning

Refsum: Disorder of lipid metabolism, interstitial hypertrophic polyneuropathy has been suggested as cause

Romberg: Irritation in peripheral trophic sympathetic system possibly after trauma

Sanfillipo-Good: Heparitinuria, systemic mucopolysaccharidosis (III)

Scheie: Systemic mucopolysaccharidosis (V)

Sjögren: Possible disturbance in endocrine function; occurs almost exclusively in women above 40 years of age

Tay-Sachs: Disorder with storage of ganglioside, familial amaurotic idiocy

Turner: Ovarian or gonadal agenesis; females are generally involved, rarely in males (See Noonan syndrome)

Uyemura: Vitamin A deficiency

Werner: Aberration of hepatic metabolism of steroid compounds; the disease may be transmitted according to the simple recessive mode of inheritance; occurs mainly in second and third decade of life

Zinsser-Engman-Cole: Congenital dyskeratosis with pigmentation, capillary hyperplasia and atrophy of epidermis and subcutaneous tissue

Unknown

Adie: Onset 2nd and 3rd decade, more frequent in females

Albright: Hereditary for bone lesions (?), manifest in childhood and young adults

Angelucci: (lymphatic condition)

Anton: Isolation of diencephalon from occipital lobe would be necessary to result in the features of the syndrome

Batten-Mayou: Most common in Jewish families, possible disturbance in lipoid metabolism

Bonnevie-Ullrich: Status lymphaticus? More frequent in females (4:1). Similarities to Turner's syndrome

Chediak-Higashi: Anemia and albinism with typical ctyoplasmic inclusion bodies in many leukocytes. Occurs in infants and results in early death

Cartilaginous-arthritic-ophthalmic-deafness syndrome

Central nervous system deficiency: Dietary deficiency (?)

Cogan: Etiology unknown; occurs in young adults but also in older persons de Lange: Congenital muscle hypertrophy, extrapyramidal motor disturbances, mental deficiency

Devic: Etiology (toxic? virus? vascular?), most frequently between 20 and 50 years of age but occurs in all ages. Demyelinization of nerves with destruction of axis-cyclinders

Feer: Onset early childhood (4 months to 4 years). Etiology unknown (infections?)

Felty: Infection or allergies have been thought to cause the syndrome

Fuchs (1): Etiology unknown

Fuchs (2): Etiology unknown; mucocutaneous ocular syndrome

Greig: Etiology unknown; defect occurs in early embryonic development; spontaneous and familial occurrence; manifestations present at birth

Guillain-Barré: Etiology unknown; occurs in children and adults (16 to 50 years of age).

Hand-Schüller-Christian: Etiology unknown; onset in childhood (before age of 6 years); male preponderance (2:1)

Harada: Etiology unknown; Japanese and Italians more frequently affected than other groups

Heerfordt: Etiology unknown; occurs mainly in young female adults

Hemifacial microsomia: Deformations most likely caused by disturbance at an approximate 20 to 25 mm stage of fetal life

Louis-Bar: A thymic abnormality leading to an immunologic deficiency has been suggested for this syndrome

Morquio-Brailsford: Systemic mucopolysaccharidosis (IV)

Pierre Robin: Etiology unknown. Manifestations present at birth

Posner-Schlossman: Glaucomatocyclitic crisis, allergy has been suggested as cause

Pseudo hypoparathyroidism: Etiology unknown; manifestations present at birth. More frequent in females

Reiter: Etiology unknown; onset age 16 to 42 years; males more frequently affected

Riegers: Developmental defect possibly occurring during 5th and 6th week of fetal life

Riley-Day: Possible adrenal hypofunction and liver dysfunction, exact mechanism not known

Sabin-Feldman: Etiology unknown, symptoms similar to toxoplasmosis

Schaumann: Etiology unknown; predominantly occurring in negroes; onset mainly third and fourth decade of life

Stevens-Johnson: Etiology unknown (virus? allergy?); occurs in young adults; most frequently in males

Treacher Collins: Etiology unknown (arrest in fetal development)

AGE

Addison: 1st and 2nd decade of life

Adie: Onset 2nd and 3rd decade, etiology unknown, more frequently found in females

Albright: Manifestations in childhood and young adults, etiology unknown, hereditary for bone lesions (?)

Alport: Hereditary familial congenital hemorrhagic nephritis. Early death in males, normal life span in females

Apert: Manifestations congenital, defect in germ plasm (?), rarely hereditary or familial

Arnold-Chiari: Recognized in infants or adults

Arnold Pick: Manifest between 40 and 70 years, females more frequently affected, cerebral atrophy

Ascher: Symptoms start usually around puberty

Axenfeld: Apparent in adolescence or early adulthood, dominant inheritance

Barré-Liéou: Usually chronic course ourse. Most frequent in older patients

Batten-Mayou: Onset between 5 and 8 years of life, mostly in Jewish families, possible disturbance in lipoid metabolism, cerebellar atrophy

Behcet: Occurs in adults, more frequent in males, virus infection (?), brain lesions

Bloch-Sulzberger: Manifestations present at birth, virus infection of mother during pregnancy

Bonnevie-Ullrich: Congenital syndrome with females more frequently affected (4:1)

Bourneville: Occurs in childhood—less frequently in adults, more often in females, brain lesions irregular dominant inheritance

Charcot-Marie-Tooth: Onset between 5 and 15 years or early middle age, brain lesions, heredofamiliar occurrence

Chediak-Higashi: Occurs in infancy and early childhood. Usually early death

Cogan: Young adults but also in older persons, sudden onset, etiology unknown

Crouzon: Manifestations present at birth, dominant inherited

Cushing (1): Most common in females of childbearing age

Dandy-Walker: Manifestations in infants, stenosis of foramina Luschka and Magendie, dilation fourth ventricle, anomaly of rostral portion of the vermis

Degos: Malignant atrophic papulosis. Fatal disease usually few months after diffuse eruption of skin lesions

Devic: Most frequently between age 20 to 50 years but occurring in all ages

Duane: Congenital manifestations. More frequent in females, autosomal dominiant inherifance

Eaton-Lambert: Myoclonic syndrome, mainly in males after 40 years of age

Ehlers-Danlos: Manifestations present at birth, transmitted as regular or irregular autosomal dominant condition. May be recessive

Erb-Goldflam: Myasthenia gravis. Onset at all ages. Incidence in females vs. males about 3:2.

Feer: Onset in early childhood (4 months to 4 years), etiology unknown (infections ?)

Felty: The disease follows a chronic course. Onset usually in middle-aged patients

Fröhlich: Manifestations in childhood (most often during puberty) rarely in postadolescent period. More frequent in Jews. Tumor of the pituitary most frequent

Gaucher: Glucocerebroside storage disorder. Onset at any age. Infantile or chronic form. Mainly found in Jewish families

Gorlin-Goltz: Onset in childhood mainly about puberty

Greig: Manifestations present at birth, spontaneous and familial occurrence; etiology unknown; defect occurs in early embryonic development

Groenblad-Strandberg: All ages involved but usually manifest in youth and early middle age; familial occurrence, recessive inheritance, consanguinity of parents fequent

Guillain-Barré: Occurs in children and adults (16 to 50 years of age): etiology is unknown

Hand-Schüller-Christian: Onset in childhood (before age of 6 years); etiology unknown

Heerfordt: Occurs mainly in young adults, more often in females; etiology unknown

Hennebert: Manifestations in childhood; congenital syphilis

Hoeve, van der: Progressive from birth on; heredofamiliar disease

Hurler: Manifestations within first year of life; occurs sporadic or familial

Hutchinson: Onset usually in infancy and up to 6 years of age. Poor prognosis with life expectancy of few months to 1 year

Johnson: Most frequent onset in children below age 3 years; manifestations of congenital delayed development

Klippel-Feil: Manifestations present at birth (often not recognized until much later)

Kloepfer: Manifestations—2 months of age. Death 20 to 31 years of life

Leber: Most frequent onset in third decade of life but also described in other age groups. More frequent in males

Louis-Bar: Ataxia-telangiectasia syndrome, life expectancy usually not longer than 2 decades

Marchesani: Onset 9 months to 13 years of age; hyperplastic form of dystrophia mesodermalis congenita; mode of transmission not established

Morquio-Brailsford: Systemic mucopolysaccharidosis (IV). Usually apparent between ages 4 to 10 years

Niemann-Pick: Essential lipoid histocytosis. Poor prognosis. Mainly in Jewish families

Pelizaeus-Merzbacher: Onset of symptoms in infancy or childhood with rapid or protracted course. Death usually from intercurrent complications

Pierre Robin: Manifestations present at birth. Etiology unknown

Pseudohypoparatyroidism: Manifestations present at birth; etiology unknown

Recklinghausen, von: Present at birth but usually not recognized until early childhood; simple dominant.

Reiter: Onset 16 to 42 years of age; almost exclusively in males; etiology unknown (virus?)

Rothmund: Onset early childhood, often in siblings; recessive heredofamilial disorder

Rubella: Chinical manifestations present in infancy. Rubella infection of the mother during first trimester of pregnancy

Schaumann: Onset mainly third and fourth decade of life; predominantly occurring in Negroes; etiology unknown

Sjögren: Occures almost exclusively in women above 40 years of age; possibly endocrine dysfunction

Stevens-Johnson: Occurs in young adults; most frequent in males, etiology unknown (virus?, allergy ?)

Symonds: Occurs in children and adolescents; serous meningitis

Takayasu: Pulseless disease. Type 1 with non-specific arteritis more frequent in young Japanese women. Type 2, occlusive vascular disease without inflammation mainly in 5th and 6th decade of life

Tay-Sachs: Familial amaurotic idiocy (infantile form) occurs almost exclusively in Jewish infants. Death during first 2 years of life

Temporal arteritis: Occurs at age 55 to 80 years in Caucasians; inflammation of temporal artery. More frequent in females

Trisomy-13–15: Fatal in first few months of life; extra chromosome in the D-group

Unverrichts: Begin in late childhood. Diffuse neuronal disease

Uveitis-rheumatoid arthritis syndrome: Most frequently in children, but occurs also in adults; general collagen disorder

Vermis: More frequent in children; tumor of the fourth ventricle

Vogt-Koyanagi: Usually in young adults; Italians and Japanese more frequently affected than other groups; virus infection?

Waldenström: Occurs in males above 50 years of age

Wallenberg: Occurs usually above age 40 years; occlusion of posterior inferior cerebellar artery

Werner: Occurs mainly in second and third decade of life; abberation of hepatic metabolism of steroid compounds; simple recessive mode of inheritance

Wilson: Most frequent in first decade of life, but also described in later age groups; lesion in the putamen and lenticular nucleus

ETHNIC GROUPS

Batten-Mayou: Most common in Jewish families, etiology unknown, possible disturbance in lipoid metabolism

Fröhlich: More frequent in Jews, manifestations in childhood, tumor of the pituitary most frequent

Gaensslen: Occurs mainly in Caucasians; manifestation frequently in early childhood; dominant or recessive inheritance

Gaucher: Mainly in Jewish families, infantile and chronic form. Glucocerebroside storage disorder

Harada: Japanese and Italians more frequently affected than other groups; etiology unknown

Herrick: Only in Negroes with possible few exceptions; sickle shaped erythrocytes; inherited as a Mendelian dominant

Laurence-Moon-Bardet-Biedl: Predominantly in Caucasians but also in Japanese and Egyptians; onset in childhood; one dominant autosomal and one recessive sex-linked gene; male preponderance

Niemann-Pick: Essential lipoid histiocytosis, poor prognosis, Mainly in Jewish families

Riley-Day: Occurs in Jewish children. Inherited in autosomal recessive manner

Schaumann: Predominantly occurring in Negroes; onset mainly third and fourth decade of life; etiology unknown

Takayasu: Pulseless disease. Type 1 with non-specific arteritis more freqent in young Japanese women. Type 2, occlusive vascular disease without inflammation maily in 5th and 6th decade of life.

Tay- Sachs: Familial amaurotic idocy (infantile form) occurs almot exclusively in Jewish infants. Death during first 2 years of life

Temporal arteritis syndrome: Caucasians at age 55 to 80 years; inflammation of temporal artery

VogtKoyanagi: Italians and Japanese more commonly affected than other groups; occurs usually in young adults; virus infection?

SEX LINKAGE, PREPONDERANCE LIMITATION, a.o.

Female

Adie: More frequent in females, onset 2nd and 3rd decade, etiology unknown

Albright: Manifest in childhood and young adults, etiology unknown, hereditary for bone lesions (?), endocrine dysfunction

Arnold Pick: Females more frequently affected, manifest between 40 to 70 years, cerebral atrophy

Bonnevie-Ullrich: Etiology not known; females more frequently affected than males (4:1)

Bourneville: More frequent in females, occurs in childhood, irregular dominant inheritance, brain lesions

Cushing (1): Most common in females of child bearing age

268

Duane: Females more frequently affected, congenital manifestations, autosomal dominant inheritance

Erb-Goldflam: Myastenia gravis. Ratio of incidence of females vs males about 3:2. Onset at all ages

Heerfordt: More frequently in females: occurs mainly in young adults; etiology unknown—sarcoidosis most likely

Morgagni: Almost exclusively in females; onset middle age (45 years)

Pseudohypoparathyroidism: Higher frequency in females (2:1); manifestations present at birth; etiology unknown

Siegrist: Famale preponderance (2:1), malignant hypertension

Sjögren: Occurs almost exclusively in women above 40 years of age; congenital or familial, possibly endocrine dysfunction

Tay-Sachs: Familial amaurotic idiocy (infantile type). Occurs almost exclusively in Jewish infants and more frequently in females

Temporal arteritis syndrome: Apparently more frequent in females: occurrence in Caucasians at 55 to 80 years of age; inflammation of temporal artery

Turner: Female linkage (very rarely in males; see Noonan syndrome.) Ovarian or gonadal agenesis

Male

Alport: Autosomal dominant inheritance possibly modified by a sex linked suppressor gene. Early dath in males, normal life span in females

Behcet: More frequent in males, virus infection (?), occurs in adults, brain lesions

Cone dysfunction syndrome: Male linkage with female carrier. Congenital recessive inheritance

Degos: Rare cutaneovisceral disease. Definite male preponderance

Eaton-Lambert: Myasthenic syndrome. Predominantly found in males usually over 40 years of age

Fabry-Anderson: Diffuse angiokeratosis; inheritance by X-linked recessive trait. Some signs of the syndrome have been observed in a few heterozygous females

Hand-Schüller-Christian: males more frequently affected (2:1); onset in childhood (before age 6 years); etiology unknown

Hunter: Systemic mucopolysaccharidosis (II), sex linked recessive

Klinefelter: Occurrence in 1% of retarded males; phenotypically males with positive female sex chromatin; karyotype shows 47 chromosomes, 44 autosomes and 3 sex chromosomes

Laurence-Moon-Bardet-Biedl: Male preponderance; predominantly in Caucasinas but also in Japanese and Egyptians. Onset in childhood; one dominant-autosomal and one recessive sex-linked gene

Leber: Male preponderance (sex linked recessive ?); (Disease has been described in females, too.) Onset in third decade of life (but also in other age groups)

Ménière: More common in males (mainly age 40 to 60 years).

Morquio-Brailsford: Mucopolysaccharidosis (IV). Slight predilection for males

Pelizaeus-Merzbacher: Most often inherited as X-linked recessive-male members affected through normal-appearing carrier mothers. Some female cases have been reported

Reiter Occurs mainly in males; onset age 16 to 42 years; etiology unknown (virus infection?)

Schilder: Occurs more often in males; onset at any age; lesions in subcortical white matter

Stevens-Johnson: Occurs in young adults; etiology unknown (virus, allergy?)

Waldenstrom: Occurs mainly in males (2:1) above 50 years of age (with exceptions)

Zinsser-Engman-Cole: Dyskeratosis congenita, recessively inherited with possible male likage

HEREDITY

Addison: Familial occurrence in some cases though the pattern of a possible inheritance is not entirely clear

Adie: Myotonic pupil; more frequent in females. Some genetic factors involved

Albright: Osteodystrophia fibrosa; heredity for bone lesions (?), etiology unknown. Manifest in childhood and young adults.

Alport: Hereditary familial congenital hemorrhagic nephritis; autosomal dominant inheritance possibly modified by sex-linked suppressor gene. Early death in males, normal life span in females

Apert: Acrocephalosyndactylism; most often recessive, sometimes dominant inheritance, defect in germ plasm (?), manifestations congenital

Axenfeld: Posterior embrytoxon; doinant inheritance, glaucoma apparent in adolescence or early childhod; sporadic cases have been observed

Bassen-Konrzweig: A-β Lipoproteinemia. Genetically determined inability to absorb and transport lipids. Inherited as an autosomal recessive gene

Batten-Mayou: Juvenile amaurotic family idiocy; heredofamilial predispositon as a Mendelian recessive; most common in Jewish families; onset between 5 and 8 years of life; etiology unknown

Behr: Infantile form of heredofamilial optic atrophy and hereditary ataxia. Autosomal recessive

Bonnet-Dechaume-Blanc: Neuro-retinoangiomatosis; congenital manifestations: dominant inheritance

Bourneville: Tuberous sclerosis; irregular dominant transmission. Although penetrance of gene is high, its power of expression may be very variable. Occurs more frequent in females

Charcot-Marie-Tooth: Progressive neuritic muscular atrophy; heredofamiliar occurrence; onset between 5 and 15 years or early middle age, brain lesions

Cockayne: (Trisomy-20) Autosomal recessive. 47 chromosomes with an extra chromosome in the F group

Cone dysfunction syndrome: Congenital male linked recessive inheritance

Crouzon: Dysostosis craniofacialis, autosomal dominant inheritance; manifestations present at birth

Down: Mongolism; Trisomy chromosome 21, probably resulting from maternal primary nondisjunction

Duane: Retraction syndrome; autosomal dominant; more frequent in females

Ehlers-Danlos: Transmitted as a regular or irregular autosomal dominant condition with relative low penetrance. In certain cases inheritance may be recessive; manifestations present at birth (cutis hyperelastica)

Ellis-van Crefeld: Chondroectodermal dysplasia, inherited as an autosomal recessive trait. Parental consanguinity (approx. 25 %)

Fabry-Anderson: Diffuse angiokeratosis; inheritance by X-linked recessive trait

Franceschetti: Mandibulo-facial dysostosis; transmitted in an irregular dominant mode, incomplete penetrance and variable expressivity

Gänsslen: Familial hemolytic icterus; dominant or recessive inheritance; most frequent in Caucasians; manifestations in early childhood

Gaucher: Glucocerebroside storage disease; automal recessive inheritance (occasional dominant); more frequently in Jewish families

Goldscheider: Epidermolysis bullosa; inherited either autosomal dominant or recessive

Golin-Goltz: Multiple basal cell nevi syndrome; autosomal dominant inheritance with possibly poor penetrance

Greig: Hypertelorism; sporadic and familial occurrence; transmission as autosomal dominant trait and sex chromatin anomalies have been described. Defect occurs in early embryonic development; manifestations present at birth; etiology unknown

Groenblad-Starndberg: Familial autosomal recessive inheritance, consanguinity of parents frequent. All ages involved but usally manifest in youth and early middle age

Hallerman-Streiff: Oculomandibulodyscephaly; familial occurrence and parental consanguinity have been observed

Hallgren: Retinitis pigmentosa-deafness-ataxia; single autosomal recessive gene with complete penetrance in both sexes

Herrick: Inheritied as a Mendelian dominant; hemolytic dissorder with sickle shaped erythrocytes; only in Negroes with possible few exceptions

Homocystinuria: Hereditary disorder of amino acid metabolism; trait is transmitted as a Mendelian recessive

Hunter: Systemic mucopolysaccharidois (II); sex linked recessive

Hurler: Gargoylism; occurs sporadic or familial; autosomal recessive; manifestations become apparent during first year of life

Jadassohn-Lewandowski: Pachyonychia congenita; inherited by an autosomal dominant pattern with low penetrance

Klinefelter: Phenotypically males with positive female sex chromatin; karyotype shows 47 chromosomes, 44 autosomes and 3 sex-chromosomes; occurrence in 1 % of retarded males

Klippel-Feil: Congenital brevicollis; manifestations present at birth but often later; autosomal recessive inheritance, but possible autosomal dominance with poor penetrance and variable expression was also suggested

Klosepfer: Severe blistering of skin in sunlight; autosomal recessive with 100 % penetrance; manifestations present at 2months of age. Reduced life expectance (20 to 31 years of age)

Laurence-Moon-Bardet-Biedl: One dominant-autosomal and one recessive sex-linked gene. Male preponderance. Predominantly in Caucasians but also in Japanese and Egyptians. Onset in childhood

Leber: Optic atrophy-amaurosis-pituitary syndrome; male preponderance (sex linked recessive?), has been described in females, too.

Lenoble-Aubineau: Nystagmus-myoclonia syndrome; familial occurrence; chronic toxemia

Louis-Bar: Ataxia-telangiectasia syndrome; transmitted as an autosomal recessive trait

Lowe: Oculo-cerebro-renal syndrome; seems to be caused by a pathological gene. Since only observed in males transmittance as sex linked recessive trait has been suggested

Marchesani: Mode of transmission not established; hyperplastic form of dystrophia mesodermalis congenita, onset 9 months to 13 years of age

Marcus Gunn: Jaw-winking syndrome; familial occurrence rare. Ireegular dominant inheritance seems to exist in a few cases

Marfan: Dystrophic mesodermalis congenita; autosomal dominant, often with incomplete expression; recessive inheritance in few recorded cases; sporadic cases occur

Marinesco-Sjögren: Spinocerebellar ataxia-cataract-oligophrenia; apparently inherited as an autosomal recessive trait

271

Morgagni: Intracranial exostosis; dominant inheritance; mostly in females; onset about 45 years of age

Morquio-Bairlsford: Hereditary dystrophy of cartilage and bones; (MPS-IV); transmitted as a recessive mode

Naegeli: Melanophoric nevus syndrome; autosomal dominant inheritance; both sexes equally affected

Niemann-Pick: Essential lipoid histiocytosis; recessive mode of inheritance; onset of clinical signs during first months of life; predisposition among Jewish families

Noonan: Normal chromosomal analysis; familial disease with X-linked dominant inheritance or a multifactorial inheritance was suggested. Males and females equally affected (see Turner's syndrome)

Pelizaeus-Merzbacher: Aplasia axialis extracorticalis congenita; most often inherited as X-linked recessive, male members affected through normal-appearing carrier mothers

Refsum: Heredo-ataxia hemeralopica polyneuritiformis; recessive inheritance

Riegers: Dysgenesis mesostromalis; inherited by autosmal dominant mode

Riley-Day: Familial dysautonomia; inherited in autosomal recessive manner; occurs mainly in Jewish children

Romberg: Progressive hemifacial atrophy; autosomal dominant with little penetrance

Rothmund: Recessive heredofamilial disorder, ectodermal dysplasia; onset early childhood, often in siblings; females about twice more frequently affected than males

Rubinstein-Taybi: Possbily genetically determined; inheritance maybe polygenic or multifactorial

Sanfillipo-Good: Heparitinuria (MPS-III); autosomal recessive inheritance

Scheie: Mucopolysaccharidosis Type V; autosomal recessive inheritance

Sjögren-Larsson: Oligophrenia-ichthyosis-spastic diplegia; autosomal recessive mode of inheritance

Sturge-Weber: Encephalofacial angiomatosis; 47 chromosomes with trisomy for number 22 has been suggested as well as partial trisomy

Tapetal-like reflex syndrome: Sex-linked heterzygos

Tay-Sachs: Familial amaurotic idiocy (infantile type); Most often transmitted by an autosomal recessive gene or occasionally by dominant inheritance; mainly in Jewish children

Trisomy- 13–15: Extra chromosome in the D- group; fatal in first few months of life

Trisomy-18: Karyotype of 47 chromosomes with trisomy for chromosome number 18

Trisomy-22: 47 chromosomes and trisomy for chromosome number 22. (see tabulated page)

Turner: Genital dwarfism syndrome; females are generally involved (see Noonan's syndrome)

Unverrichts: Familial myoclonia syndrome; fatal disease, transmitted as an autosomal recessive trait

Hoeve, van der: Osteogenesis imperfecta; inherited as an autosomal dominant trait

Hippel-Lindau, von: Familial disease, dominantly transmitted, penetrance not always complete, power of expression variable; angiomata of the cerebellum and the walls of the fourth ventricle

Recklinghausen, von: Simple dominant; present at birth but usually not recognized until early childhood

Sallmann, von-Paton-Witkop: Hereditary benigne intraepithelial dyskeratosis; autosomal dominant trait with high penetrance

Waardenburg: Embryonic fixation syndrome; irregular dominant inheritance; penetrance of the different characteristica varies considerably in different pedigrees; persistance of embryonal development 8 to 10 weeks.

Waldenström: Macroglobulinemia; male preponderance 2:1; cromosomal abnormalities (number and form)

Werner: Simple recessive mode of inheritance; occurs mainly in second and third decade of life; aberration of hepatic metabolism of steroid compounds

Zinsser-Engman-Cole: Dyskeratosis congenita with pigmentation; suggestive of being recessively inherited with possible male linkage

GLOSSARY

Accommodation—The ability of the eye by means of changing the curvature and shape of the lens, to focus objects at various distances on the retina

Adiadochokinesia—Inability to perfom rapid alternating movements

Agenesia—Imperfect development

Agnosia—Total or partial loss of the perceptive faculty or of the ability to recognize or orientate objects or persons due to a disturbance in the cerebral associational areas, the sensory pathway and the receptor areas being intact. It is classified according to the sense affected, *e. g.,* visual agnosia, auditory agnosia.

Allocheiria—Reference of a sensation is made to the opposite side to which the stimulus is applied.

Alopecia—Baldness from disease

Anhidrosis—Abnormal deficiency of sweat

Anisocoria—Pupils of unequal diameter; may be physiological, as in antimetropia, or pathological as in Adie's syndrome, or in unilateral Argyll Robertson's pupil

Anorexia—Lack or loss of appetite for food

Anterior lenticonus—A rare congenital anomaly in which the anterior surface of the crystalline lens, usually in its axial region, has a conical bulging, as opposed to a spherical bulging

Aphtha—Small white spots on the mucous membrane of the mouth

Apraxia—Loss of previously acquired ability to perform coordinating movements

Areflexia—Absence of the reflexes

Athetosis—Continuous movements of fingers and toes

Autosome—Any chromosome other than a sex chromosome; autosomes normally occur in pairs in somatic cells and singly in gametes

Bitot's spot—White foamy conjunctival lesion at paralimbal region due to vitamin A deficiency

Blepharitis—Any inflammation of the eyelid without reference to any particular part of the eyelid, but commonly meaning the margin.

Blepharochalasis—Atrophy of the skin of the upper eyelids, usually bilateral and equal, following chronic or recurrent edematous swellings of the upper eyelids; characterized in its later stages by loose folds of wrinkled and venuled skin overhanging the upper eyelid margin

Blepharoptosis—Drooping of an upper eyelid

Blepharospasm—Tonic or clonic spasm of the orbicularis oculi muscle

Brachydactyly—Extremely short fingers and toes

Bradycardia—Abnormal slowness of the pulse

Bradycoria—Delayed and slow pupil reaction

Brevicollis—Shortness of the neck

Bulimia—Changes in dietary habits

Cataract—Opacity of the crystalline lens

Cephalalgia—Headaches

Cheilitis—Inflammation of a lip

Chemosis—Severe edema of the conjunctiva, least marked in the tarsal region

Chorioretinitis—Inflammation of the choroid and retina

Chromosomal aberration—Abnormality of chromosome number or structure

Concomitant—The condition in which the two eyes move as a unit, maintaining a constant or relatively constant angular relationship between the lines of sight for all directions of gaze, usually indicating absence of paresis or paralysis of the extraocular muscles

Confabulation—The relation of imaginary experience: a symptom seen in psychoses

Congenital—Present at birth, does not imply genetic

Convergence—The turning inward of the visual axes toward each other during near vision

Consanguinity—Descent from a common ancestor
Consensual reflex—Excited by reflex stimulation; especially the contraction of the contralateral pupil when the retina of only one eye is stimulated

Dermatoglyphics—Pattern of the ridged skin lines of fingers, palms, toes and soles
Diploid—Number of chromosomes (double the number of gametes. In man 46)
Diplopia—Double vision
Discoria (Dyscoria)—Abnormality in the shape of the pupil
Dominant—If a gene is expressed when heterozygous
Dysneuria—Impairment of nervous power
Dysopsia—Defective vision
Dysorexia—Impairment of appetite
Dysosmia—Impairment of the sense of smell
Dysostosis—Defective ossification
Dysphagia—Difficulties in swallowing
Dysphasia—Difficulty in uttering or understanding words
Dysphonia—Difficulty in speaking
Dysplasia—Abnormality of development
Dyspnea—Labored or difficult breathing
Dysraphia—Malformation due to defective or delayed closure of the embryonic neural tube

Ectopia lentis—Displacement, subluxation, or malposition of the crystalline lens
Embryotoxon—A ring opacity of the periphery of the cornea, situated in its deep layers, distinguished from an arcus senilis in that it appears to be continuous with the sclera, having no clear zone at the limbus
Emmetropia—An infinitely distant fixated object is sharply focused on the retina without accommodation
Enophthalmos—Recession of the eye ball into the orbit
Epicanthus— A fold of skin partially covering the inner canthus, the caruncle, and the plica semilunaris. It is normal in the fetus, in some infants, and in mongolians and other peoples characterized by low nasal bridges
Epiphora—Overflow of tears from obstruction of lacrimal drainage system
Exophthalmos—An abnormal protrusion or proptosis of the eyeball from the orbit
Expressivity—Extent to which a gene shows its effect

Fingerprint—(1) See dermatoglyphics; (2) term used for the method for combining electrophoresis and chromatography to separate components of proteins

Gamete—Mature germ cell with haploid chromosome number
Genotoype—Full set of genes in an individual
Gerontoxon'—Arcus senilis, a grayish-white ring opacity in the paralimbel area of the cornea due to lipid infiltration of the corneal stroma
Glaucoma—Increase of intraocular pressure above normal
Glossoptosis—Displacement of the tongue downward
Gynecomastia—Overdevelopment of mammary glands in the male

Haploid—One member of each chromosome pair, in man 23
Hemianopsia—Blindness in one half of the visual field of one or both eyes
Hemiparesis—Paresis affecting one side
Heterochromia iridis—Difference in color of the iris in the two eyes
Heterogeneity—If different genetic mechanisms can produce the same phenotype, genetic heterogeneity exists for that phenotype
Heterophoria—Deviation of the visual axis of one eye when the other eye is covered and fusion is prevented
Heterozygote—Two different alleles at a given locus on a pair of homologous chromosomes

Homozygote—A pair of identical alleles at a given locus on a pair of homologous chromosomes

Hypertelorism—Wide separtion of eyes

Hypopyon—An accumulation of pus in the anterior chamber of the eye associated with infectious diseases of the cornea, the iris, and the ciliary body.

Hyposphagma—Subconjunctival hemorrhage

Ichthyosis—Hypertrophy of the corneous layer of the skin, usually congenital, in which the skin becomes dry, hard, and scaly, and absence of secretion from the sweat or sebaceous glands. When affecting the eyelids, it may result in the loss of the eyelashes and in ectropion

Iridocyclitis—Inflammation of iris and ciliary body

Iridodialysis—Localized separation of the iris from its attachment to the ciliary body

Iridodonesis—Tremolus of the iris as present on movement of the eye in case of partial lens dislocation

Iridoschisis—Separation of the anterior from the posterior iris layers

Iseikonia—Size and shape of retinal images are equal in both eyes

Karyotype—Chromosome set of an individual

Keratitis—Inflammatory process of the cornea

Keratoconus—A developmental or dystrophic deformity of the cornea in which it becomes cone shaped, due to a thinning and stretching of the tissue in its central area

Leukoma—Dense, white opacity of the cornea

Leukoplakia—Focal epithelial hyperplasia involving mucous membranes, mainly mouth and occasionally the conjuntiva

Linkage—Genes with their loci on the same chromosome

Macrostomia—Excessive size of the mouth

Micromelia—Abnormal smallness of one or more extremities

Micrognathia—Undue smallness of jaws

Microtia—Abnormal smallness of the external ear

Miosis—(1) Reduction in pupil size. (2) The condition of having a very small pupil, *i. e.,* approximately 2 mm or less in diameter

Mosaic—Individual with at least two cell lines differing in genotype or karyotype, derived from a single zygote

Multifactorial (polygenic)—Inheritance by many genes at different loci

Mydriasis—(1) Increase in pupil size. (2) The condition of having an abnormally large pupil, *i. e.,* approximately 5mm or greater in diameter

Myoclonus—Chronic spasm of a muscle

Myotonia—Tonic spasm of a muscle

Nystagmus—A regularly repetitive, usually rapid, and characteristically involuntary movement or rotation of the eye, either oscillatory or with slow and fast phases in alternate directions

Ophthalmoplegia—Paralysis of one or more extra-ocular muscles

Oxycephaly—A condition in which the skull is conical in shape (tower skull), due to abnormal union of the cranial and the facial bones

Pachyonychia—Thickening of the nails

Papilledema—Edema of the optic disc (or nerve head) with elevation

Papillomacular bundle—A well-defined, oval-shaped bundle of ganglionic axons in the nerve fiber layer of the retina, extending from the region of the macula lutea to the optic disk, entering it from the temporal side. All other tempora fibers course around this bundle as they approach the disk

279

Pars planitis—Inflammation of the uveal tissue in the area of the pars plana

Phoria—Axis or meridian of one eye in relation to the other eye (presyllable designates the type of phoria, *i. e.,* esophoria, exophoria, heterophoria, hyperphoria, etc.)

Photophobia—An abnormal intolerance to light causing a painful sensation

Platybasia—A deformity in which the floor of the occipital bone is pushed up by the spine of the cervical vertebra

Poikiloderma—An atrophic condition of the skin

Poliosis—Grayness of the hair

Polydipsia—Excessive thirst

Polycoria—An anomaly consisting of more than one pupil in a single iris

Polyuria—Excess in amount of urine discharged

Prognathism—Projection of the jaws

Proptosis—An abnormal protrusion of the eyeball from the orbit

Ptosis—Drooping of the upper eyelid below its normal position

Pupillatonia—Failure of the pupil to react to light

Recessive—A trait which is expressed only in individuals homozygous for the gene

Retinopathy—Pathology of the retina of any etiology

Scotoma—An isolated area of absent vision or depressed sensitivity in the visual field, surrounded by an area of normal vision or of less depressed sensitivity

Scotopic Vision—Visual performance under low illuminance (dark adaptation)

Sex Chromatin—Chromatin mass in nucleus of interphase cells of females representing a single X chromosome

Sex Chromosomes—Responsible for sex determination; XX in females, XY in males

Sex-influenced—A trait not sex-linked in inheritance but expressed differently in males and females

Sex-limited—Trait expressed only in one sex or the other

Sex-linkage—(X-linked) Inheritance by genes on the sex chromosomes

Sibling—Brother or sister

Steatorrhea—Excess fat in the feces (usually due to pancrease disease)

Strabismus—The condition in which binocular fixation is not present under normal seeing condition, *i. e.,* the foveal line of sight of one eye fails to intersect the object of fixation

Symblepharon—A cicatrical attachment of the bulbar to the palpebral conjunctiva.

Syndactyly—Abnormal union of the fingers or toes

Synechiae—Adhesion of the iris to the cornea (anterior) or to the capsule of the crystalline lens (posterior)

Syringobulbia—Presence of cavities in the medulla oblongata

Syringomyelia—Presence of abnormal liquid-filled cavities in the spinal cord

Tinnitus—A noise in the ears, which may at times be heard by others than the patient

Translocation—Transfer of a piece of one chromosome to a non-homologous chromosome

Triploid—A cell having three times the normal haploid chromosome number

Triradius—In dermatoglyphics, a point from which the dermal lines go in three directions at angles of about 120°

Trisomy—Presence of one extra chromosome per cell

Uveitis—Inflammation of the uveal tract

Vitiligo—A disease of the skin characterized by patches of depigmentation of various sizes and shapes

Zygote—Fertilized ovum

Tables of Similar Syndromes

CRANIAL NERVE SYNDROMES

Syndrome	Nerves Involved	Lesion	Symptoms
Rochon-Duvigneaud	II, III, IV, V, VI	Sphenoidal fissure	Ophthalmoplegia, papilledema, decreased sensitivity V_1, visual loss
Foix	II, III, IV, V, VI	Lateral wall cavernous sinus	Ophthalmoplegia, optic atrophy, decreased sensitivity V_{1-2}
Jacod	II, III, IV, V, VI	Petrosphenoidal space	Ophthalmoplegia, optic atrophy, visual loss, trigeminal neuralgia
Rollet	II, III, IV, V, VI, sympathetic	Orbital apex	Ophthalmoplegia, ptosis, neuralgia V, optic atrophy, hyperesthesia or anesthesia forehead
Carotid arterycavernous sinus fistula	II, III, IV, V, VI	Cavernous sinus	Ophthalmoplegia, papilledema, loss of corneal sensitivity, chemosis, exophthalmos, headache, buzzing noise in head
Spheno cavernous	III, IV, VI	Cavernous sinus	Ophthalmoplegia, diplopia, paresis V_{2-3}
Cushing (3)	II	Suprasellarchiasmal	Hemianopsia, optic atrophy

CRANIAL NERVE SYNDROMES (cont'd.)

Syndrome	Nerves Involved	Lesion	Symptoms
Benedikt	III	Nucleus ruber	Oculomotor paralysis, hyperkinesis, tremor, ataxia, paresis of extremities
Nothnagel	III	Sup. cerebellar epduncle	Oculomotor paresis, cerebellar ataxia
Weber	III	Cerebral peduncle	Oculomotor paralysis, ptosis, fixed pupil, hemiplegia, hemifacial paralysis, polyuria
Raymond	VI	Pons (Level VI)	Paralysis VI, hemiplegia, anesthesia
Millard-Gubler	VI, VII	Pons (Level VI, VII)	Paralysis VI, hemifacial paralysis, hemiplegia
Claude	III, IV	Paramedian mesen-cephalic lesion	Ophthalmoplegia, ataxia, hemianesthesia
Gradenigro	V, VI	Apex of petrous bone	Paralysis VI, diplopia, decreased sensitivity V
Foville	(V), VI, VII	Pontine area	Abducence paralysis, peripheral facial palsy, hemiplegia (possible)
Cushing (2)	V, (VI), VII, VIII	Ponto cerebellar angle	Paraylsis VII, lateral rectus paresis (VI), decrease sensitivity V, papilledema, deafness, tinnitus, disturbed labyrinth function, nystagmus

ANGIOMATOSIS-RETINAE SYNDROMES

Syndromes	Findings	
	Ocular	Other
Bonnet-Dechaume-Blanc	Arteriovenous retinal angiomata, papilledema, reduced corneal sensitivity, anisocoria, strabismus	Angiomas mesencephalon and thalamus, facial angiomata, hydrocephalus, slow speech, hemiplegia, neurological symptoms
v. Hippel-Lindau	Retinal angiomatosis, vascular proliferation, retinal detachment, sec. glaucoma	Cerebral angiomatosis, epilepsy, psychic disturbances, dementia
Sturge-Weber	Chorioretinal angiomata, vascular proliferation, glioma, retinal detachment, conj. telangiectases, glaucoma	'Portwine' nevus, cerebral angiomata, hemiparesis, hemiatrophy, mental retardation, epilepsy

DEAFNESS-RETINOPATHY SYNDROMES

Syndromes	Inheritance	Findings	
		Ocular	Other
Alport	autosomal dominant, but some pedigrees show more complex mode	Fundus albi punctatus, lens changes	Progressive deafness (after 10 years of age). Vestibulary disturbances, hem. nephritis
Cockayne	autosomal recessive	Retinal pigmentary degeneration, optic atrophy	Deafness, dwarfism, mental retardation
Dialinas-Amalric	autosomal dominant	Retinal pigmentary degeneration, *No* nightblindness, normal ERG	Deafmutism
Hallgren	autosomal recessive	Retinitis pigmentosa, optic atrophy, lens changes, progressive blindness	(Congenital) deafness, ataxia, oligophrenia, skeletal anomalies
Laurence-Moon-Bardet-Biedl	one dominant autosomal gene and one recessive sex-linked gene was suggested	Retinitis pigmentosa, optic atrophy, progressive visual loss	Deafness(occasionally), obesity, mental retardation, skeletal anomalies
Usher	autosomal dominant	Retinitis pigmentosa (No ring scotomata)	Deaf-mutism

LIPID STORAGE DISEASES

Syndrome	Material	Inheritance	Findings	
			Ocular	Other
Fabry-Anderson	Ceremide-trihexoside	X-linked recessive	Conj. varicosis, corneal opacities	Angiokeratosis disturbed sweat secretion, pain in extremities
Gaucher	Glucocere-broside	Probably autosomal recessive, occasionally dominant. Preselection for Jews. Infantile form death in first 2 years	Brown-yellow conj. lesion, strabismus	Hepatospleno-megaly, Hypertonia, lymph-adenopathy
Niemann-Pick	Sphingomyelin and lecithin	Probably autosomal recessive Predisposition for Jews. Death in infancy	Retinopathy, reduced vision	Hepatospleno-megaly, mental retardation, seizures, skin pigmentation
Tay-Sachs	Ganglioside	Autosomal recessive dominant. Death in first 2 years of life. Predisposition for Jews	Macular red spot, optic atrophy	Mental retardation, seizures

OCULO-MUCO-CUTANEOUS SYNDROMES

Findings:	Behcet	Fuchs (2)	Reiter	Stevens-Johnson
Ocular:				
Conjunctivitis	++	+++	+/++	++
Conjunctival ulceration		++		++
Kerato conjunctivitis sicca	(+)			(+)
Keratitis	++	(+)	(+)	++
Corneal ulceration				+
Iritis	++		(+)	+
Uveitis	+			
Hypopion	+			+
Vitreous hemorrhages	(+)			
Retinal trombophlebitis	+			
Retinal hemorrhages	+			
Visual loss	+			+
Muscle palsies	(+)			
Nystagmus	(+)			
Mucous membranes:				
Oral aphthous lesions	+			
Oral ulcerations		+	(+)	++
Glossitis	+	+		
Rhinitis				+
Gastrointestinal ulcers				+
Genital ulcers	+	+	+	++
Balanitis	+			+
Vulvovaginitis	+			+
Urethritis	+		+	+
Cystitis			+	+
Nephritis				+
Cutaneous:				
Erythema multiforme	+	+	(+)	+++
bullosum	+			+
vesiculare		+		+
Joints:				
Arthritis	(+)		++	
Others:				
Headache		+		+
Fever	+	+	(+)	+
Lymphadenopathy			+	
Respiratory infection			+	+
CNS:			(+) — occasional findings	
Cerebellar signs	(+)		+, ++, +++, — degree	
Convulsions	(+)		of severity	
Paraplegia	(+)			

287

Syndrome	Inheritance	Excretion	Findings	
			Ocular	Other
MPS I Hurler	autosomal recessive	Chondroitin sulfate B and heparitin sulfate excretion	Ret. pigm. changes, corneal opacities, proptosis	Retarded development, skeletal deformities, hepatosplenomegaly, sinfantilism
MPS II Hunter	sex-linked recessive	Chondroitin B and heparitin sulfate excretion	Ret. pigm. changes, vis. field loss, corneal haze	Dwarfism, hepatosplenomegaly, deafness
MPS III Sanfillipo-Good	autosomal recessive	Heparitin sulfate excretion	Ret. pigm. changes, corneal opacities	Mental deficiency, seizures, mild gargoyl features
MPS IV Morquio-Brailsford	autosomal recessive	Keratosulfate	Corneal haze Horner's trias	Dwarfism, skeletal deformities, decreased muscle tone
MPS V Scheie	autosomal recessive	Chondroitin sulfate B excretion	Ret. pigmentosa possible, vis. field changes, corneal opacities	Aortic valvular disease, thickened joints

Syndromes Exhibiting Horner's Trial (Enophthalmos—Ptosis—Miosis)	
Babinsky-Nageotte	Pankoast
Cestan-Chenais	Raeder
Déjerine-Klumpke	V. Herrenschwand
Morquio-Brailsfora	Wallenberg

Reference Books

Adler, F.H.: Physiology of the Eye, 4th Ed., St. Louis, C.V. Mosby Co., 1965.

Ballantyne, A.J. and Michaelson, I.C.: The Fundus of the Eye, Edinburgh, E. & S. Livingstone Ltd., 1962.

Bender, M.B.: The Oculomotor System, New York, Harper & Row, 1964.

Cogan, D.G.: Neurogloy of the Ocular Muscles, 2nd Ed., Springfield, Charles C Thomas, 1956.

Cogan, D.G.: Neurology of the Visual System, 2nd. Ed., Springfield, Charles C Thomas, 1967.

Duke-Elder, Sir Stewart: Sytem of Ophthalmology, Vol. 1-X, St. Louis, C.V. Mosby Co.

Durham, R.H.: Medical Syndromes, New York, Paul B. Hoeber, Inc., 1960.

Ford, F.R.: Diseases of the Nervous System in Infancy, Childhood and Adolescence, 3rd. Ed., Springfield, Charles C Thomas, 1952.

Francois, J.: Heredity in Ophthalmology, St. Louis, C.V. Mosby Co., 1961.

Gardner, L.I.: Endocrine and Genetic Diseases of Childhood, Philadelphia, W.B. Saunders Co., 1969.

Gorlin R.J. and Pindborg, J.J.: Syndromes of the Head and Neck, New York, McGraw-Hill book Co. (Blakiston Division), 1964.

Hartmann, E. and Gilles, E.: Roentgenologic Diagnosis in Ophthalmology, Philadelphia, J.B. Lippincott Co., 1959.

Hogan, M. J. and Zimmerman, L.E.: Ophthalmic Pathology, 2nd. Ed., Philadelphia, W.B. Saunders Co., 1962.

Kestenbaum, A.: Clinical Methods of Neuro-Ophthalmologic Examination, 2nd. Ed., New York, Grune & Stratton, 1961.

Lombardi, G.: Radiology in Neuro-Ophthalmology, Baltimore, The Williams & Wilkins Co., 1957.

Mac Bryde, C.M.: Signs and Symptoms, 4th Ed., Philadelphia, W.B. Saunders, Co., 1961.

Mann, I: Developmental Abnormalities of the Eye, 2nd. Ed., Philadelphia, J.B. Lippincott Co., 1957.

McKusick, V.A. Heritable Disorders of Connective Tissue, St. Louis, C.V. Mosby Co., 1960.

McKusick, V.A.: Medical Genetics, St. Louis, C.V. Mosby Co., 1961.

Reese, A.B.: Tumors of the Eye, New York, 2nd. Ed., Paul B. Hoeber, Inc., 1963.

Schapero, M.; Cline, D. and Hofstetter, H.W.; Dictionary of Visual Science, 2nd. Ed., Philadelphia, Chiltion Book Co., 1968.

Smith, J.L.: Neuro-Ophthalmology, Vol. I. Springfield, Charles C Thomas Co., 1964; Vol. II-IV, St. Louis, C.V. Mosby Co., 1965/68.

Tassman, J.: The Eye Manifestations in Internal Disease, 3rd. Ed., St. Louis, C.V. Mosby Co., 1951.

Theodore, F.H. and Schlossman, A.: Ocular Allergy, Baltimore, The Williams & Wilkins Co., 1958.

Thiel, R.: Atlas of Diseases of the Eye. Amsterdam-London-New York, Elsevier Publ., Co. 1963.

Thompson, J.S. and Thompson, M.W.; Genetics in Medicine, Philadelphia, W.B. Saunders, Co., 1966.

Walsh, F.B.: Clinical Neuro-Ophthalmology, 2nd Ed., Baltimore, The Williams & Wilkins Co., 1957.

Woods, A.C.: Endogenous Inflammations of the Uveal Tract, Baltimore, The Williams & Wilkins Co., 1961.